Cracking the
Intercollegiate
General Surgery
FRCS Viva

A Revision Guide

Cracking the Intercollegiate General Surgery FRCS Viva

A Revision Guide

Edited by

Elizabeth Ball MBChB PhD FRCS
Consultant Oncoplastic Breast Surgeon
Ipswich Hospital NHS Trust, Ipswich, UK

Stewart Walsh MSc MCh FRCS
Associate Professor of Surgery and Consultant Vascular Surgeon
University Hospital Limerick, Limerick, Ireland

Tjun Tang MA(Hons) MD FRCS
Consultant Vascular Surgeon
Changi General Hospital, Singapore

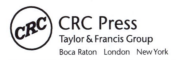

CRC Press
Taylor & Francis Group
Boca Raton London New York

CRC Press is an imprint of the
Taylor & Francis Group, an **informa** business

CRC Press
Taylor & Francis Group
6000 Broken Sound Parkway NW, Suite 300
Boca Raton, FL 33487-2742

© 2014 by Taylor & Francis Group, LLC
CRC Press is an imprint of Taylor & Francis Group, an Informa business

No claim to original U.S. Government works

Printed on acid-free paper
Version Date: 20130710

International Standard Book Number-13: 978-1-4441-8472-3 (Paperback)

Library of Congress Cataloging-in-Publication Data

Cracking the intercollegiate general surgery FRCS viva : a revision guide / editor, Elizabeth Ball, Stewart Walsh, and Tjun Tang.
    p. ; cm.
    Includes bibliographical references and index.
    ISBN 978-1-4441-8472-3 (softcover : alk. paper)
    I. Ball, Elizabeth, 1974- editor. II. Walsh, Stewart, editor. III. Tang, Tjun, editor.
    [DNLM: 1. General Surgery--Great Britain--Examination Questions. 2. General Surgery--Ireland--Examination Questions. 3. Certification--standards--Great Britain--Examination Questions. 4. Certification--standards--Ireland--Examination Questions. 5. Clinical Competence--standards--Great Britain--Examination Questions. 6. Clinical Competence--standards--Ireland--Examination Questions. 7. Education, Medical, Graduate--Great Britain--Examination Questions. 8. Education, Medical, Graduate--Ireland--Examination Questions. WO 18.2]

    RD37.2
    617.0076--dc23   2013024475

Visit the Taylor & Francis Web site at
http://www.taylorandfrancis.com

and the CRC Press Web site at
http://www.crcpress.com

*This book is dedicated to my nearest and dearest,
for their love, support and understanding.*

Elizabeth Ball

For Serena, who put up with it all from the beginning.

Stewart Walsh

*This book is gratefully dedicated to my wife and children: Nicole
the most supportive, loving and understanding person I know and
Eleanor and Leo, who give me the greatest joy in life. Thank you.*

Tjun Tang

Contents

Foreword

This is no question a high hurdle. But it's not something that cannot be done.

Lou Lamoriello

This observation was made about hockey but could equally be applied to the FRCS examination. 'The exit exam' sits in the mind of every surgeon throughout his or her final years of training. It is the last hurdle, the ultimate professional examination on the road to independent practice as a consultant surgeon. It is the surgical profession's final opportunity to ensure that the trainees reach the standards and calibre expected of consultant surgeons in the United Kingdom and Ireland. It was never meant to be straightforward.

For many exit FRCS candidates, it is often a number of years since they have been in an examination situation. Undergraduate and postgraduate medical education has changed radically over the last decade. Increasingly, FRCS candidates may have little or no experience of the 'viva voce' that forms a major component of the exit exam and which was the bread and butter of exams in my day. These examinations seek not only to evaluate the candidate's knowledge of various surgical topics but also to test the candidate's reasoning and decision-making skills through the use of multiple clinical scenarios. Patients are no longer passive recipients of our knowledge and wisdom and come prepared to their consultation armed with information gleaned from the Internet and prepared to interrogate the unwary practitioner. The 'viva voce' not only is an integral part of the examination, but also serves to prepare candidates for life as independent consultant surgeons.

The contributors to this book have all taken and passed the Intercollegiate FRCS in General Surgery in the last 5 years. They have not produced a textbook but instead have sought to provide a guide to approaching the viva for those yet to take the examination. By the time of the exit exam, candidates have many competing pressures compared to the MRCS earlier in training. Families, mortgages and 'getting that job' all add to the stress for candidates. Hopefully, by providing some advice on how to tackle the myriad of topics that may come up in the vivas, this book will go some way toward reducing the stress.

Dr Stansfield, an anatomist at the Royal College of Surgeons, sent my generation of surgeons off to their exams with the rejoinder, 'I don't wish you luck, I wish you justice'; reading this book will ensure justice is delivered.

The Lord Ribeiro Kt, CBE, FRCS

The Editors

Elizabeth Ball, MBChB, PhD, FRCS (Gen), graduated from the University of Wales College of Cardiff in 1998 and did her basic surgical training in South Wales. She spent 4 years researching the molecular genetics of human thyroid cancer and was awarded a PhD from Cardiff University in 2006. She then moved to East Anglia to complete 5 years of higher general surgical training before being awarded a prestigious National Oncoplastic Fellowship at the Royal Marsden Hospital, London, in 2011. During her fellowship, she began a postgraduate MS in oncoplastic surgery with the University of East Anglia. Miss Ball was appointed as a Consultant Oncoplastic Breast Surgeon at Ipswich Hospital, England, in 2012.

She has an active interest in teaching and the career development of junior surgical staff and has enrolled on the Trainer Development Programme with the University of Bedford. Miss Ball is a faculty member for the 'Training the Trainers' course on this programme. She has also served as a faculty member on the Basic Surgical Skills, ATLS and CCrISP courses all over the UK. She has written 12 peer-reviewed publications and several chapters in general surgical revision textbooks. Her research has been presented both nationally and internationally. She has peer-reviewed journals for the *European Journal of Surgery* and the *British Journal of Surgery*. She is a Fellow of the Royal Colleges of Surgeons of England and Edinburgh.

Stewart Walsh MSc, MCh, FRCS, is currently the Associate Professor of Surgery at the Graduate Entry Medical School, University of Limerick, and Consultant Vascular Surgeon at University Hospital Limerick. He qualified from University College Dublin in 1997. Following basic surgical training in north-west England, he completed a Master of Science degree at the University of Liverpool in 2002 and was appointed as a specialist registrar on the East of England surgical training rotation. From 2005 until 2007, he carried out research work at Addenbrooke's Hospital and the University of Cambridge, leading to a Master of Surgery Degree. Mr Walsh finished training as a vascular and endovascular surgeon in 2010, immediately prior to appointment as Associate Professor.

His research interest focuses on the perioperative care of major vascular surgery patients, utilising comparative-effectiveness methodology to evaluate current and potential interventions. He has over 120 peer-reviewed journal publications. Since 2011, he has been assistant editor at the *International Journal of Surgery*. In 2013, he was appointed as an editor with the Cochrane Peripheral Vascular Disease Group. He leads the surgery modules at the University of Limerick and has served as faculty member on the Basic Surgical Skills and CCrISP courses in the Eastern Deanery. He is a Fellow of the Royal College of Surgeons of Edinburgh.

Tjun Tang, MA (Hons), MD, FRCS (Gen), graduated from Queens' College in Cambridge and qualified from Addenbrooke's Hospital, Cambridge, in 2000 with a distinction in surgery. He trained on the higher surgical training program in East

Anglia and was awarded his Doctorate of Medicine (MD) by the University of Cambridge in 2009 for research into imaging carotid plaque inflammation. Just after his completion of surgical training in late 2012, he was awarded a prestigious British Society of Endovascular Therapy (BSET) fellowship and undertook further endovascular training at Leicester Royal Infirmary. Mr Tang is currently doing a senior fellowship at the Prince of Wales Hospital in Sydney, Australia, concentrating on subspecialising in complex lower limb revascularisation, prior to taking up a consultant post in vascular and endovascular surgery at Changi General Hospital in Singapore.

He has active research interests in carotid imaging and outcome modelling in vascular surgery and has published widely on these subjects. Mr Tang has over 100 peer-reviewed publications and has cowritten/edited five postgraduate revision textbooks in general surgery. He regularly reviews manuscripts for journals including *Circulation, Stroke* and the *British Journal of Surgery.* Furthermore, he is enthusiastic about training medical students and junior doctors alike. He has served as a clinical supervisor and Final MB examiner at the medical school in Cambridge and taught undergraduate anatomy for a number of years at Christ College in Cambridge. Mr Tang has also served as a faculty member on the Basic Surgical Skills and CCrISP courses in the Eastern Deanery. He is a Fellow of both the Royal College of Surgeons of England and Royal College of Physicians and Surgeons of Glasgow.

The Contributors

Jithesh Appukutty, MD, MRCA
Department of Anaesthetics
West Suffolk Hospital NHS Trust
Bury St Edmunds, Suffolk, England

Elizabeth Ball, MBChB, PhD, FRCS
Consultant Oncoplastic Breast Surgeon
Ipswich Hospital NHS Trust
Ipswich, Suffolk, England

Amy E E Burger, FRCS
Consultant Oncoplastic Surgeon
Queen Elizabeth Hospital King's Lym
    NHS Trust
King Lym, England

Edward Courtney, MBChB, FRCS
Consultant Colorectal and General
    Surgeon
Royal United Hospital Bath
Combe Park, Bath, England

**John Davidson, B Med Sci, BM, BS,
FRCA, FFICM**
Consultant Intensive Care Medicine and
    Anaesthesia
Freeman Hospital
Newcastle upon Tyne, England

Sue K Down, PhD, FRCS
Consultant Oncoplastic Breast Surgeon
James Paget University Hospital
Gorleston-on-Sea, Great Yarmouth
Norfolk, England
Honorary Senior Lecturer, University
    of East Anglia, England

**Naheed Farooq, FRCS, BSc(Hons),
PGCME**
Senior Upper GI fellow
Cambridge University Hospitals NHS
    Foundation Trust
Cambridge, England

Saurabh Jamdar, MD, FRCS
Consultant Hepatopancreatobiliary
    Surgeon
Manchester Royal Infirmary
Manchester, England

Nicole Keong, MPhil FRCS
Consultant Neurosurgeon
National Neurosciences Institute
Tan Tock Seng Hospital
Singapore

Ashish Lal, FRACS
Consultant General Surgeon
Mid Western Regional Hospital
Dooradoyle, Limerick, Ireland

**Jeffrey Lordan, BSc, MBBS, PhD,
FRCS**
Post-CCT Fellow in
    Hepatopancreatobiliary Surgery
Royal Marsden NHS Foundation Trust
London, England

Pankaj Mishra, MRCS, MS, MCh
Clinical Fellow in Paediatric Surgery
Norfolk and Norwich University
    Hospital NHS Trust
Norwich, England

Zia Moinuddin, MBBS, MRCS
Specialist Trainee (transplant and
    general surgery)
Department of Renal and Pancreas
    Transplantation
Manchester Royal Infirmary
Manchester, England

Dermot O'Riordan, MBBS, FRCS
Consultant General Surgeon and
    Medical Director
West Suffolk Hospital NHS Trust
Bury St Edmunds, Suffolk, England

Dimitri Pournaras, PhD, MRCS
Specialist Trainee General Surgery
West Suffolk Hospital NHS Trust
Bury St Edmunds, Suffolk, England

Manel Riera, MD, FRCS
Consultant Upper GI Surgeon
Shrewsbury and Telford Hospital NHS
    Trust
Shrewsbury, Shropshire, England

C J Shukla, PhD, FRCS
Consultant Urological Surgeon
Western General Hospital
Edinburgh, Scotland

**Vinodkumar Singh, FRCA, MRCP,
FFICM, MD**
Department of Anaesthetics
West Suffolk Hospital NHS Trust
Bury St Edmunds, Suffolk, England

Rajesh Sivaprakasam, MPhil, FRCS
Locum Consultant Transplant Surgeon
St George's Healthcare NHS Trust
London, England

Tjun Tang, MA (Hons), MD, FRCS
Consultant Vascular Surgeon and
    Endovascular Surgeon
Changi General Hospital
Singapore

Gillian Tierney, DM, FRCS
Consultant in General Surgery and
    Coloproctology
Department of Colorectal Surgery
Royal Derby Hospital
Derby, England

**Samson Tou, MS, FRCS,
M.MinInvSu**
Consultant Colorectal Surgeon
Department of Colorectal Surgery
Royal Derby Hospital
Derby, England

Andy Tsang, MD, FRCS
Consultant Upper GI Surgeon
Peterborough and Stamford Hospitals
    NHS Trust
Peterborough, Cambridgeshire, England

Thomas Tsang, FRCS
Consultant Paediatric Surgeon
Norfolk and Norwich University
    Hospital NHS Trust
Norwich, England

Janice Tsui, MD, FRCS
Senior Lecturer/Consultant Vascular
    Surgeon
UCL Division of Surgery and
    Interventional Science
Royal Free Vascular Unit
London, England

David van Dellen, MD, FRCS
Consultant Transplant and General
    Surgeon
Department of Renal and Pancreas
    Transplantation
Manchester Royal Infirmary
Manchester, England

Colin Walsh, PhD, MRCOG, MRCPI
Subspecialty Fellow
National Maternity Hospital
Dublin, Ireland

Stewart Walsh, MSc, MCh, FRCS
Associate Professor of Surgery and
    Consultant Vascular Surgeon
University Hospital Limerick
Dooradoyle, Limerick, Ireland

Michael Wu, BPharm, BMBS
Vascular Surgery Registrar
Box Hill Hospital
Melbourne, Australia

Introduction

Congratulations on passing the first part of the FRCS exam. This book will guide you through the second part.

STRUCTURE

The exam takes place over 2 days, and you will be allocated to start with either the clinicals or the vivas. If you start with the vivas, then the clinicals are held on the morning of the second day, and you finish at lunchtime. If you start with the clinicals, these are held on the afternoon of the second day, with the vivas on the third day.

The clinical section consists of two exams—one in general surgery and one in your chosen subspecialty. Both exams are 30 minutes long, with two examiners who swap around after 15 minutes. You should see six patients in each exam.

There are six vivas. You start with the academic vivas. You will have one general and one subspecialty paper to review in 1 hour and then a 10-minute viva on each paper. You can choose which paper you start with. The remaining vivas are paired into general and subspecialty (general is always first) and emergency surgery and critical care (you can choose which you do first). These four vivas cover three questions in 15 minutes (5 minutes per question).

The vivas are scored from 4 to 8. A score of 6 is a pass. Both examiners score you for each question. You need to average 6 or more for every question/patient to pass. It is an aggregate score, so you can fail one section but make up for it with a highly scoring question.

SURGICAL VIVAS

The first thing to do is to read the ISCP syllabus (https://www.iscp.ac.uk/surgical/syllabus.aspx). It is over 300 pages long, and any topic on the syllabus can be covered in the exam. You therefore need a very broad range of knowledge to pass, rather than depth of knowledge.

Ideally, you should be able to talk for 3–4 minutes on every topic. The examiners only have 5 minutes per question, and some of this will be taken up with them asking the question and you thinking.

The examiners have a list of points to cover for each topic, starting with a very basic level of knowledge for a pass, and then the questions become more difficult, to enable you to score a 7 or an 8.

You are likely to have most of the basic knowledge already just from training as a surgeon and being on call. The level of detail for the most part is MRCS level, but that does include quite detailed physiology for the critical care section.

The key to passing is to answer the questions as a consultant, not as a trainee. Examiners want to know what *YOU* would do if you saw the patient in clinic or on a post-take ward round, or the decision *YOU* would make in an MDT. The answer to every decision-based question should start with, 'I would...'—NOT 'you could/ the options are/my consultant would....' Do not refer every difficult scenario to a colleague. This is a general surgery exam, and you are meant to be able to cope with these things as a consultant. If you were by yourself in a small DGH, what would you actually do to control a difficult laparotomy? You may not have the surgical expertise (e.g., if you are a breast trainee), but you should know the principles of trauma surgery and how to get out of trouble safely.

For the subspecialty vivas, you will need a more detailed level of knowledge. This includes anatomy, physiology, embryology and pathology, as well as NICE guidelines, Cochrane reviews, other national guidelines and key papers and trials that have changed practice. You will pick up a lot from your own MDTs, and these meetings are a good time to practice interpreting radiological imaging and become familiar with the current chemotherapy trials.

The examiners are unlikely to give you any feedback during the questioning. This can be difficult, especially if you are used to getting nods and sounds of encouragement from colleagues when practicing. You must remember that you can aggregate marks. Therefore, if you have a bad question, take a breath, and start again. You have to be able to pick yourself up. Remember that, with no feedback from the examiners, you may not have done as badly as you think.

There is a definite halo effect, and a good first impression will go a long way. You want to sound and act like a colleague, not a terrified candidate (internal brown trousers, external calm). Smile, keep your head up and make eye contact. Take a few seconds to think and to compose your answer before you actually start speaking.

We have listed some of the books we found useful in the bibliography. It is not essential to buy the entire Core Companion series. They can be a little out of date by the time they are published. We would recommend reading the *Core Topics in General and Emergency Surgery* book and your own subspecialty book as a starting point. However, you will need quite detailed physiology and critical care knowledge, over and above the ATLS and CCrISP manuals. *Schein's Common Sense Emergency Abdominal Surgery* book is also a must-read to help you through the emergency viva.

ACADEMIC VIVA

This should be one part of the exam when it is relatively easy to score highly, as you have the papers in front of you. You need to practice reading and reviewing a paper in 25 minutes, giving yourself an extra 5 minutes per paper to make notes.

The general paper is often from the previous 6 months' worth of the *British Journal of Surgery*. We strongly encourage you to start practicing early, and with a bit of luck, you may have already seen one of the papers you are given. You should also read the last 6 months' worth of the key journals in your subspeciality.

During the reading time, other candidates will enter and leave the room. You are spaced quite close to the person next to you. Some candidates will be talking to themselves, so you need to get used to working in a noisy room with distractions. You are given pencils and markers and the papers. You can take your own pencils, pens and highlighters in with you. It is also worth taking a watch so that you can more easily keep track of time.

A good starting point is to flick through the paper to see how many tables and graphs you need to analyse. The examiners will have had the papers for a couple of weeks, so they will be a lot more familiar with the data than you are. Then, read the abstract and the conclusions. Often, the author critiques his or her own paper in the discussion and also explains missing patients or data. This can save time flicking back and forth through the methods and results sections looking for excluded patients and the reasons for this. You will naturally develop your own method for reading a paper with practice.

You then need to practice making notes on the paper. Some candidates use red and green pens to highlight good and bad points; others find this distracting and just use a pencil to star the relevant points. Finally, practice giving a 5- to 10-minute summary of the paper. The list of points to cover is included in the academic section of the book. Some examiners will let you talk for 5–8 minutes without interrupting, whilst others will keep butting in every 30 seconds or so. This can be very distracting because you never get into a rhythm, and you need to practice with colleagues so that you can cope with both examining styles.

The end point to get across is whether the paper would change your own practice. You are not critiquing a paper for a journal club; you are critiquing it as a surgeon reviewing the evidence. You may be asked if you would publish it. And remember that your examiner may have written the paper you are about to critique.

CLINICALS

These stations often scare candidates the most, but you should simply treat them as minivivas. With only 5 minutes to see, examine and talk to a patient, there is not a lot of time to do a full formal examination. Most of the time you will be asked to look at a scar/examine a lump/take a history, and then the examiners will show you scans or start a discussion about the patient's surgical history and proposed treatment.

You should be able to interpret basic CT scans of the abdomen and pelvis, angiograms, ERCPs, mammograms—the images that you would request during a normal clinic and when on-call.

Remember that you may be taken to see patients from other subspecialties in your general exam (that includes breast and transplant patients). It is therefore worth trying to get to a couple of clinics and MDTs outside your own subspecialty in the weeks before the exam to refresh yourself. There are often lots of skin lesions, neck lumps and patients with rare diseases who turn up at every clinical exam. We have listed useful books to read in the bibliography at the back of the book.

HOW TO PASS THE EXAM

Passing this exam is all about technique. People who fail usually do not do so because of lack of knowledge. The exam is a bit like a game, and you need to learn how to play it. As we mentioned earlier, you have to sound like a consultant giving an opinion. It is all very well to quote 10 papers' worth of evidence, but if you cannot make a decision, then you are not ready to become a consultant.

You must also be safe in your answers. When several options are available to treat a patient in your viva, start with the most widely practiced option that has the greatest evidence base. You can then talk about new techniques and the pros and cons, but you do not want to come across as a maverick. It is also unwise to get into an argument with your examiner.

There are several courses available, and if you can afford it, they can be invaluable. It is very helpful to be put under pressure in a viva situation before the exam and to make the mistakes on the course, instead of on the day. It is also useful to hear how other candidates answer questions and to see how much you improve over the duration of the course.

This is a selection of available viva revision courses.

Edinburgh, Scotland – FRCS Viva Preparation Course
http://www.rcsed.ac.uk/education/courses-and-events/general-surgery.aspx

Les Alps, France – Alpine FRCS Course
http://www.surgicalcourses.org.uk/courses/alpine-frcs

Liverpool, England – Intensive FRCS Part III Course
http://www.liv.ac.uk/cancerstudies/courses/FRCS_Course/

Llantrisant, Wales – Practice Course for Clinical and Viva Examination in FRCS (Gen Surg)
http://www.doctorsacademy.org/academycms/default.asp?contentID=868

London, England – Whipps Cross Higher Surgery Course
http://www.wxmec.org.uk/courses/HSC.html

Manchester, England – The Christie FRCS Exit Exam Course in General Surgery
http://www.doctorsacademy.org/AcademyCMS/default.asp?contentID=987

FINAL PREPARATION

If you can afford it, stay in a nice hotel rather than the cheapest one available. We know that the exam is already expensive before you add on the cost of courses, books and travel. But a decent hotel can make a huge difference to your preparation. Ask the receptionist when you book the hotel to find you a room in a quiet part of the hotel. Tell him or her that you are sitting an important exam. You do not want a room by a lift overlooking the back streets where the nightclubs empty at 1 a.m.

On the day, you may find taking music and headphones helps to distract you from hearing other candidates talking whilst you are waiting. However, sometimes it can be helpful to know what questions have been asked of other candidates. Try not to spend your last hour beforehand flicking through books and pages of notes. Everyone does it, but it rarely helps you in the exam.

Good luck!

Elizabeth Ball
Stewart Walsh
Tjun Tang

Abbreviations

AAA: abdominal aortic aneurysm
AAST: American Association of Surgery for Trauma
ABCs: airway, breathing and circulation
ABS: Association of Breast Surgery
ACE: acetylcholinesterase
ACPGB: Association of Coloproctology of Great Britain
ACS: abdominal compartment syndrome
ACTH: adrenocorticotropic hormone
ADH: antidiuretic hormone
ADH: atypical ductal hyperplasia (in breast section)
ADRCs: adipose-derived regenerative stem cells
AF: atrial fibrillation
AFP: alphafetoprotein
AI: aromatase inhibitor
AIDS: acquired immune deficiency syndrome
ALI: acute lung injury
ALT: anterolateral thigh
AMPLE: allergies, medication, past medical history, last meal, events surrounding trauma
AMR: antibody-mediated rejection
ANC: axillary node clearance
APACHE: acute physiology and chronic health evaluation
APC: adenomatous polyposis coli
APER: abdominoperineal excision of rectum
APTT: activated partial thromboplastin time
ARDS: acute respiratory distress syndrome
ASA: American Society of Anesthetists
ASGBI: Association of Surgeons of Great Britain and Ireland
AT: anaerobic threshold
ATLS: advanced trauma life support
ATN: acute tubular necrosis
ATP: adenosine triphosphate
AUC: area under the curve
AV: arteriovenous
AXR: abdominal x-ray
BADS: British Association of Day Surgery
BCC: basal cell carcinoma
BCS: breast conserving surgery
BCSH: British Committee for Standards in Haematology
BE: Barrett's oesophagus (UGI section)
BE: base excess

BK: below knee
BM: Boehringer Mannheim (blood glucose test)
BMI: body mass index
BMT: best medical treatment
BP: blood pressure
BPD with DS: biliopancreatic diversion with duodenal switch
BPH: benign prostatic hypertrophy
BSA: body surface area
BSD: brain-stem dead
BXO: balanitis xerotica obliterans
Ca: calcium
CAD: coronary artery disease
cAMP: cyclic adenosine monophosphate
CBD: common bile duct
CCRISP: care of the critically ill surgical patient
CDT: catheter-directed thrombolysis
CEA: carcinoembryonic antigen
CEA: carotid endarterectomy (vascular section)
CFA: common femoral artery
CHOP: cyclophosphamide, doxorubicin, vincristine and prednisolone
CISH: chromogenic in situ hybridisation
CKD: chronic kidney disease
Cl: chloride
CMF: cyclophosphamide, methotrexate and fluorouracil
CMI: chronic mesenteric ischaemia
CMV: cytomegalovirus
CNI: calcineurin inhibitor
CNS: central nervous system
CO: carbon monoxide
COPD: chronic obstructive pulmonary disease
COX 2: cyclo-oxygenase 2
CPAP: continuous positive airway pressure
CPD: continuing professional development
CPEX: cardiopulmonary exercise testing
CPP: cerebral perfusion pressure
CPR: cardiopulmonary resuscitation
CRM: circumferential margin
CRP: c-reactive protein
CRT: capillary refill time
CSF: cerebrospinal fluid
CT: computerised tomography scan
CTA: computerised tomographic angiography
CTD: chronic transplant dysfunction
CVA: cerebrovascular accident
CVC: central venous catheter

CVP: central venous pressure
CVS: cardiovascular system
CXR: chest x-ray
D+V: diarrhoea and vomiting
D2: second part of duodenum
DBD: donation after brain-stem death
DCD: donation after cardiac death
DCIS: ductal carcinoma in situ
DCL: damage-control laparotomy
DDAVP: desmopressin acetate
DEXA: dual-energy x-ray absorptiometry
DGH: glutamate dehydrogenase
DIC: disseminated intravascular coagulopathy
DIEP: deep inferior epigastric perforator
DM: diabetes mellitus
DNA: deoxyribonucleic acid
DO$_2$: oxygen delivery
DOH: Department of Health
DPG: diphosphoglycerate
DRI: donor risk index
DRIL: distal revascularisation and interval ligation
DSA: digital subtraction angiography
DVT: deep vein thrombosis
EBV: Epstein–Barr virus
ECF: extracellular fluid
ECG: electrocardiogram
ECMO: extracorporeal membrane oxygenation
eGFR: estimated glomerular filtration rate
EIA: enzyme immunoassay
ER: oestrogen receptor
ERCP: endoscopic retrograde cholangiopancreatography
ESBL: extended-spectrum beta-lactamases
ESR: erythrocyte sedimentation rate
ESRF: end stage renal failure
ET: endotracheal
EUA: examination under anaesthesia
EUS: endoscopic ultrasound scan
EVAR: endovascular aneurysm repair
FAP: familial adenomatous polyposis
FAST: focussed assessment of sonography in trauma
FBC: full blood count
FDG-PET: fludeoxyglucose positron emission tomography
FDP: fibrin degradation products
FeNa: fractional excretion of sodium
FEV1: forced expiratory volume in 1 second

FFP: fresh frozen plasma
FiO$_2$: concentration of inspired oxygen
FISH: fluorescent in situ hybridisation
FNA: fine needle aspiration
FOB: faecal occult blood
FRC: functional residual capacity
FRCS: Fellow of the Royal College of Surgeons
FSH: follicle-stimulating hormone
FU: follow-up
FY1: foundation year 1 doctor
FY2: foundation year 2 doctor
G+S: group and save
GA: general anaesthetic
GCS: Glasgow coma scale
GCSF: granulocyte colony-stimulating factor
GFR: glomerular filtration rate
GI(T): gastrointestinal (tract)
GIST: gastrointestinal stromal tumours
Glc: glucose
GM: gynaecomastia
GN: Gram negative
GN: glomerulonephropathy (in transplant section)
GOJ: gastro-oesophageal junction
GOO: gastric outlet obstruction
GORD: gastro-oesophageal reflux disease
GP: general practitioner
GTN: glyceryl trinitrate
GU: genitourinary
Hb: haemoglobin
HBV: hepatitis B virus
HCC: hepatocellular carcinoma
HCG: human choriogonadotrophin
HCO$_3$: bicarbonate
HCV: hepatitis C virus
HDU: high-dependency unit
HER2: herceptin 2 receptor
HIAA: hydroxyindoleacetic acid
HIT: heparin-induced thrombocytopaenia
HIV: human immunodeficiency virus
HLA: human leukocyte antigen
HNA: human neutophil antigen
HNPCC: hereditary nonpolyposis colorectal cancer
HPB: hepatopancreaticobiliary
HPV: human papilloma virus
HR: heart rate
HRS: hepatorenal syndrome

HRT: hormone replacement therapy
IAH: intra-abdominal hypertension
IAP: intra-abdominal pressure
IBD: inflammatory bowel disease
ICAP: intercostal artery perforator
ICD: implantable cardioverter defibrillator
ICP: intracranial pressure
IFTA: interstitial fibrosis and tubular atrophy
IgG: immunoglobulin G
IMA: inferior mesenteric artery
IMCA: independent mental capacity advocate
INR: international normalised ratio
IOC: intraoperative cholangiography
IPMN: intraductal papillary mucinous neoplasm
ISCP: Intercollegiate Surgical Curriculum Project
ITC: isolated tumour cells
ITGCN: intratesticular germ cell neoplasia
ITP: idiopathic thrombocytopenic purpura
ITU/ICU: intensive treatment/care unit
IV: intravenous
IVC: inferior vena cava
IVF: in vitro fertilisation
K: potassium
KCl: potassium chloride
LA: local anaesthetic
LAGB: laparoscopic adjustable gastric band
LDH: lactate dehydrogenase
LFTs: liver function tests
LH: luteinising hormone
LHRH: luteinising hormone receptor hormone
LIF: left iliac fossa
LIFT: ligation of the intersphincteric fistula tract
LLQ: left lower quadrant
LMA: laryngeal mask airway
LRTI: lower respiratory tract infection
LRYGB: laparoscopic Roux-en-Y gastric bypass
LSG: laparoscopic sleeve gastrectomy
LSV: long saphenous vein
LVEF: left ventricular ejection fraction
MAP: mean arterial pressure
MBL: massive blood loss
MC+S: microscopy, culture and sensitivity
MCN: mucinous cystic neoplasm
MDT: multidisciplinary team/meeting
MEN: multiple endocrine neoplasia
Met-Hb: methaemoglobin

Mg: magnesium
MI: myocardial infarction
MIP: minimally invasive parathyroidectomy
MMF: mycophenolate mofetil
MNG: multinodular goitre
MRA: magnetic resonance angiography
MRCP: magnetic resonance cholangiopancreatography
MRI: magnetic resonance imaging
MRSA: methicillin-resistant *Staphyloccus aureus*
MS: multiple sclerosis
MSU: midstream urine
MTOR: mammalian target of rapamycin
MUGA: multigated acquisition
Na: sodium
NAC: nipple–areolar complex
NaCl: sodium chloride
NASH: nonalcoholic steatohepatitis
NBM: nil by mouth
NBO: nil by oral route
NF: neurofibromatosis
NGT: nasogastric tube
NHS: National Health Service
NHSBSP: NHS Breast Screening Programme
NICE: National Institute for Clinical Excellence
NIDDM: non-insulin-dependent diabetes mellitus
NJ: nasojejunal
NODAT: new-onset diabetes after transplantation
NOMI: nonocclusive mesenteric ischaemia
NSAID: nonsteroidal anti-inflammatory drugs
NSGCT: nonseminomatous germ cell tumours
OCP: oral contraceptive pill
OGD: oesophagogastroduodenoscopy
OPSI: overwhelming postsplenectomy infection
OR: odds ratio
OSNA: one-step nucleic acid amplification
PAWP: pulmonary artery wedge pressure
PBC: primary biliary cirrhosis
PCA: patient-controlled analgesia
PCC: prothrombin complex concentrate
PCR: polymerase chain reaction
PE: pulmonary embolism
PEEP: positive end-expiratory pressure
PEG: percutaneous endoscopic gastrostomy
PEI: percutaneous ethanol injection
PMHx: past medical history
PN: parenteral nutrition

PNS: parasympathetic nervous system
PO: per oral
PO$_4$: phosphate
PONV: postoperative nausea and vomiting
POSSUM: physiological and operative severity score for the enumeration of mortality and morbidity
PPIs: proton pump inhibitors
PPPD: pylorus preserving pancreatico-duodenectomy
PPV: positive predictive value
PR: per rectum
PR: progesterone receptor (breast section)
PRBC: packed red blood cells
PSA: prostate-specific antigen
PT: prothrombin time
PTC: percutaneous transhepatic cholangiogram
PTFE: polytetrafluoroethylene
PTH: parathyroid hormone
PTLD: post-transplant lymphoproliferative disorder
PTS: post-thrombotic syndrome
PVS: persistent vegetative state
QA: quality assurance
QARC: quality assurance reference centre
QoL: quality of life
QPTH: quick parathyroid hormone assay
RBCs: red blood cells
RCT: randomised controlled trial
RFA: radiofrequency ablation
Rh: rhesus
RIF: right iliac fossa
RLN: recurrent laryngeal nerve
RLQ: right lower quadrant
RNA: ribonucleic acid
ROC: receiver operating characteristic
RT: radiotherapy
RUQ: right upper quadrant
SAFARI: subintimal arterial flossing with antegrade–retrograde intervention
S/C: subcutaneous
SCC: squamous cell carcinoma
SCF: supraclavicular fossa
SCM: sternocleidomastoid
SFA: superficial femoral artery
SGAP: superior gluteal artery perforator
SHA: Strategic Health Authority
SIADH: syndrome of inappropriate antidiuretic hormone secretion
SIRI: serious incident requiring investigation
SIRS: systemic inflammatory response syndrome

SISH: silver in situ hybridisation
SLE: systemic lupus erythematosus
SLN(B): sentinel lymph node (biopsy)
SMA: superior mesenteric artery
SNS: sacral nerve stimulation (colorectal section)
SNS: sympathetic nervous system (critical care viva)
SOB: short of breath
SPECT: single-photon emission computed tomography
SSI: surgical site infection
SSV: short saphenous vein
ST (5,6,7): speciality trainee doctor (year 5, 6, 7)
STARR: stapled transanal rectal resection
STC: slow transit constipation
SVC: superior vena cava
SVR: systemic vascular resistance
TAPP: transabdominal preperitoneal mesh repair
TB: tuberculosis
Tc: technetium
TEMS: transanal endoscopic microsurgery
TEO: transanal endoscopic operation
TEP: total extra peritoneal mesh repair
TFT: thyroid function tests
Tg: thyroglobulin
TIA: transient ischaemic attack
TIC: touch imprint cytology
TIPS: transjugular intrahepatic portosystemic shunt
TM: therapeutic mammoplasty
TME: total mesorectal excision
TNF: tumour necrosis factor
TPN: total parenteral nutrition
TRALI: transfusion-related lung injury
TRAM: transverse rectus abdominis myocutaneous
TSH: thyroid-stimulating hormone
TT: thrombin time
TTG: antitissue transglutaminase
TUG: transverse upper gracilis
U+E: urea and electrolytes
UC: ulcerative colitis
UGI: upper gastrointestinal
UIQ: upper inner quadrant
US(S): ultrasound scan
UTI: urinary tract infection
VAB: vacuum-assisted biopsy
VAP: ventilator-associated pneumonia
VEGF-A: vascular endothelial growth factor A
VMA: vanillylmandelic acid

VRD: von Recklinghausen's disease
vWF: von Willebrand factor
WCC: white cell count
WHO: World Health Organisation
WLE: wide local excision

1 Academic Viva

Elizabeth Ball, Tjun Tang and Stewart Walsh

CONTENTS

ACADEMIC VIVA—HOW TO REVIEW A PAPER

Abstract
- Does the abstract reflect accurately the content of the paper?

Introduction
- Has the background to the study been given appropriately?
- Is the aim of the study clearly stated?
- What was the hypothesis?

Methodology
- Was there selection bias by the authors?
- What patients were excluded from the study?
- Were the patients included in the study representative of the patients encountered in general surgical practice?
- Are the methods appropriate?

- If it is a randomised study, was a power calculation used?
- What information is required to undertake a power calculation?
- Was the end point valid?
- Was the difference sought in the study of clinical relevance?

Results

- Are the results well set out?
- Was statistical analysis appropriate or needed?
- Are all patients accounted for?
- What is type I or type II error?
- What is sensitivity/specificity?
- Can you explain the Forest plots/ROC curves?
- Have the results been presented in a biased way?
- Is follow-up adequate?
- Are significant complications excluded from the analysis?

Discussion

- Are the results discussed fairly and compared to what is known in the literature?
- What are the novel observations?
- Are you aware whether the topic is covered in existing guidelines or published papers?
- Are the conclusions supported by the data presented?
- What are the healthcare issues?

Final summary

- You can give this at the beginning or the end, depending on the examining style.
- Summarise it in five or six sentences.
- Pick out the good and bad points.
- Form an opinion—is it good/average/bad?
- Decide whether it will change your practice
- How would you have designed the study differently?
- If you were the editor, would you publish it?

BASIC STATISTIC DEFINITIONS

Mode
Most common value in a data set
Median
Middle value in a data set
Mean
Sum of all values/number of values
Standard deviation (SD)
Describes degree of data spread about the mean
Square root of the variance (only with parametric data)
1 SD = 68% observations; 2 SD = 95% observations
Standard error (SE)
Standard deviation of the sample mean

Confidence interval (CI)
Measure uncertainty in measurements.

Width of the CI = precision of estimate.

95% CI = range in which 95% of population lies.

CI that includes 0 is not significant.

The larger the sample is, the smaller the variability, and the more likely the results are true.

When quoted alongside a ratio (e.g., relative risk, odds ratio), an interval including 1 is not significant.

When comparing two groups, if the CI of each group does not overlap, this is a significant result.

Prevalence
Proportion of population with disease at given time point

Incidence
Rate of occurrence of new cases over a period of time

Odds
Number of times an event is likely to occur/number of times it is likely not to occur

Odds of having a girl = 1/1 = 1

Odds ratio (OR)
Odds of having the disorder in the experimental group relative to the odds in favour of having the disorder in the control group

OR = 1: no effect

OR > 1: higher chance of disease in exposed group

Risk
Probability of something happening

Number of times that an event is likely to occur/total number of events possible

Risk of having a girl = 1/2 = 50%

Absolute risk
Incidence rate of outcome in the group

Relative risk (RR)
Experimental absolute risk/control absolute risk:

RR = 1—no risk difference

RR > 1—greater risk with the exposed factor

RR < 1—factor is protective

Number needed to treat
Number of subjects that must be treated for one extra person to experience a benefit

Hazard
Instantaneous probability of an end point event

Degree of increased and decreased risk of a clinical outcome due to a factor

Hazard ratio
Comparison of hazard between two groups:

>1: Factor increases the chance of the outcome.

<1: Factor decreases the chance of the outcome.

Null hypothesis

Any difference between the study groups is chance.

P value

Probability of results given a true null hypothesis

<0.05: Result due to chance is less than 1 in 20

Threshold for statistical significance

Type I error (alpha)

False positive

Null hypothesis is rejected when it is true

Due to bias, confounding variables

Type II error (beta)

False negative

Null hypothesis accepted when it is false

Due to a sample size that is too small

Intention-to-treat analysis

All the patients are included in the analysis, regardless of whether they completed the study. If not accounted for, it leads to attrition bias.

Dropouts increase the chance of a type I or II error.

Power

Ability to detect a true difference in outcome between each arm

Probability that a type II error will not occur

The larger the sample size, the greater the power

Power of 0.8 = 80% probability of finding a significant difference, if one existed, having excluded the role of chance

Power = 1 − Type II error (beta—arbitrarily set at 0.2)

Sensitivity

True-positive rate:

Proportion of subjects with the disorder who will have a positive result

SnNout: highly sensitive test—negative result will rule out the disorder

Specificity

True-negative rate:

Proportion of subjects without the disorder who will have a negative result

SpPin: highly specific test—positive result will rule in the disorder

Clinical end point

Measurement of direct outcome (e.g., mortality, disability)

Surrogate end point

Outcome used as substitute for clinically meaningful end point

Believed to be predictive but cannot guarantee relationship

Composite end point

Combines several measurements into algorithm—overcomes underpowering:

Primary end point—health parameter measured in all subjects to detect a response to treatment

Secondary end point—other parameters measured in all subjects to help describe effects of treatment

Validity
Extent to which a test measures what it is supposed to measure
Reliability
How consistent a test is in repeated measurements

BIAS

Selection bias
- Recruitment of unrepresentative sample population
- Sampling bias—introduced by researchers
- Response bias—introduced by study population

Observation bias
- Result of failure to classify or measure the exposure or outcomes correctly

Attrition bias
- Number of dropouts differs significantly in the different arms.
- Those left at the end may not be representative of the original study sample.

Confounding factors
- Confounder is associated with exposure but not a consequence of exposure.
- It is also associated with outcome, independent of exposure.
- For example, coffee (exposure), ischaemic heart disease (outcome), smoking (confounder).
- Not due to bias (cannot be created).
- Must be identified so you can take measures to eliminate.
- Control confounding factors with matching and randomisation, and at time of analysis by stratification, standardisation and statistical adjustment (multivariate analysis).

COHORT STUDIES

What is a cohort study?

- This is an observational study in which a group of people without a certain condition are followed over time to establish the incidence of the condition of interest.
- It allows for the identification and evaluation of potential risk factors for development of the condition of interest.
- In the hierarchy of evidence, cohort studies lie beneath randomised controlled trials because they are more vulnerable to bias.
- They are also more likely to be influenced by confounders.
- The cohort is a group of people who share a certain characteristic.
- Cohort studies may be prospective or retrospective.
- The key difference with other study designs is that the exposure status is always assessed before the outcome status.

If randomised trials are superior, what purpose do cohort studies serve?

- Cohort studies are extremely useful as a means of proving a causative link between a putative risk factor and disease.
- The key feature is that the cohort is identified before the development of the disease in question and then followed over time.
- They provide strong circumstantial evidence of causality.
- Prospective cohort studies have the advantage of reducing recall error as data are all collected as the study progresses.

What are the advantages of cohort studies?

- They can clearly demonstrate an appropriate temporal relationship between exposure and disease development.
- They allow direct estimation of incidence rates in both exposed and unexposed groups.
- Multiple outcomes can be assessed in the same study (e.g., the Million Women Study).
- They provide insight into the latent period or incubation period for communicable and noncommunicable diseases.
- They can be used to study exposures that are relatively uncommon.

What are the disadvantages?

- They often need a large sample size to ensure enough cases are captured to allow meaningful analysis, particularly for rarer conditions.
- Long follow-up periods are necessary.
- Frequent re-evaluations of exposure are required.
- Outcomes must be determined as they develop.
- Portions of the cohort may be lost to follow-up, which may then introduce bias.
- Outcomes may be misdiagnosed or misallocated, particularly if diagnostic criteria or technology changes in the course of the study.
- Outcome assessment is vulnerable to diagnostic suspicion bias (i.e., if the investigator strongly believes that the exposure causes the disease, he or she may be more inclined to reach diagnoses in the exposed population).

CONSORT AND PRISMA

What is the CONSORT statement?

- CONSORT (consolidated standards of reporting trials) is a set of recommendations for papers reporting the results of randomised clinical trials.
- The first version was published in 1996, the latest in 2010.
- The document is regularly updated as new evidence regarding clinical trial design and conduct emerges.

- It provides a framework to evaluate the quality of randomised clinical trials.

What guidance does the statement provide?

- The 2010 version provides a 25-item checklist and a template participant flow diagram.
- The checklist provides guidance for each section of the paper: title, abstract, introduction, methods, results, discussion and other information.
- The current checklist can be downloaded at www.consort-statement.org.

What is the PRISMA statement?

- The PRISMA (preferred reporting items for systematic reviews and meta-analysis) statement is a set of evidence-based guidelines intended to improve the quality of reports of systematic reviews.
- It was originally called the QUOROM statement, but was renamed in the 2009 update.
- In addition to providing a guide for researchers undertaking systematic reviews, it can be used a framework to critique reports of such reviews.
- Like CONSORT, PRISMA provides an itemised checklist providing guidance for each section of the paper together with a template flow diagram to describe the identification and inclusion/exclusion of trials/studies in the review.
- The current checklist can be downloaded at www.prisma-statement.org.

IMPACT FACTOR

You should know the impact factor of the key journals in your subspeciality.

How can you evaluate the impact of academic work?

- Directly—numbers of citations, impact factor of journals, patents obtained
- Indirectly—invitations for expert advice, participation in expert bodies and citations in support of major specialty guidelines

What is an impact factor (IF)?

- It is an objective measure of a particular journal's relative importance in its field; in general, the higher the impact factor is, the more significant is the journal.
- Impact factors are calculated each year, based on a 3-year period and published in the *Journal of Citation Reports.*
- It is the average number of times published papers are cited up to 2 years after publication.
- The 2012 IF for a journal would be calculated as follows:
  - A = the number of times articles published in 2010–2011 were cited in indexed journals during 2012

- B = the number of articles, reviews, proceedings or notes published in 2010–2011
- 2012 impact factor = A/B
- 2012 impact factors:
  - *British Journal of Surgery:* 4.61
  - *British Medical Journal:* 14.09
  - *The Lancet:* 38.28
  - *The New England Journal of Medicine:* 53.30

How valid is the impact factor as an index of importance?

- It is discipline dependent as some disciplines tend to cite faster than others; thus, it is unreliable when comparing journals across disciplines.
- It is calculated using an arithmetic mean, which is statistically inappropriate, as citations are not normally distributed, instead tending to be left-skewed.
- Journal rankings based on impact factor only moderately correlate with journal rankings based on expert survey.
- Impact factor can be influenced by deliberate editorial policies (e.g., publishing the most significant papers early in the year to maximise time to accrue citations).

LEVELS OF EVIDENCE

What are levels of evidence?

- They provide an index of the strength of evidence for a particular recommendation in evidence-based medicine.
- Differing levels are defined for evidence of interventions and evidence of diagnostic ability.
- The Oxford taxonomy is commonly used for studies of interventions.

Can you outline the Oxford system for studies of interventions?

- 1a Systematic reviews (with homogeneity) of randomised clinical trials
- 1b High-quality individual randomised controlled trials with narrow confidence intervals
- 1c All or none randomised controlled trials
- 2a Systematic reviews (with homogeneity) of cohort studies
- 2b Individual cohort study or low-quality randomised controlled trials
- 2c Outcomes research and ecology studies
- 3a Systematic reviews (with homogeneity) of case-control studies
- 3b Individual case-control study
- 4 Case series, poor quality cohort or poor-quality case control studies
- 5 Expert opinion

Do you know of any alternatives?

- The National Institute for Health and Care Excellence (NICE) and the Scottish Intercollegiate Guidelines Network (SIGN) recommend an alternative classification.
- The advantage of this system is that it provides guidance as to which levels of evidence should not be used to form the basis of a recommendation.
- Levels are ranked from 1 to 4 with various sublevels.

Can you explain the SIGN system?

- 1++ High-quality meta-analyses, systematic reviews of randomised controlled trials (RCTs) or RCTs with a very low risk of bias
- 1+ Well-conducted meta-analyses, systematic reviews of RCTs or RCTs with a low risk of bias
- 1– Meta-analyses, systematic reviews of RCTs or RCTs with a high risk of bias (should not be used as a basis for a recommendation)
- 2++ High-quality systematic reviews of case-control or cohort studies; high-quality case-control or cohort studies with a very low risk of confounding, bias or chance and a high likelihood that the relationship is causal
- 2+ Well-conducted case-control or cohort studies with a low risk of confounding, bias or chance and a moderate probability that the relationship is causal
- 2– Case-control or cohort studies with a high risk of confounding bias or chance and a significant risk that the relationship is not causal (should not be used as the basis for a recommendation)
- 3 Nonanalytic studies (e.g., case series, case reports)
- 4 Expert opinion, formal consensus

META-ANALYSIS[1]

What is a meta-analysis?

- The Cochrane collaboration defines meta-analysis as the use of statistical methods to combine results of individual studies.
- Meta-analysis allows investigators to determine a more precise estimate of treatment effect.
- Meta-analysis is applied to studies of interventions, most often randomised controlled trials.

What is a systematic review?

- This is a secondary research study in which a literature review is conducted according to a strict protocol in order to identify all studies relevant to the question under consideration.

- They often include attempts to identify and obtain data from unpublished studies relevant to the question at hand.
- Rigorous inclusion and exclusion criteria are applied in order to ensure that no selection bias occurs with respect to study eligibility.
- They should be conducted in accordance with the current PRISMA guidelines.

Do systematic reviews and meta-analyses provide a high level of evidence?

- Systematic review and meta-analysis of high-quality, homogenous, randomised controlled trials currently constitute the pinnacle of the hierarchy of evidence, ranked as level 1a evidence in the Oxford taxonomy.

What elements comprise a good systematic review/meta-analysis?

- It should have a well-constructed, relevant, clinical question, ideally expressed in PICO terms: population, intervention, controls and outcomes.
- Objective inclusion and exclusion criteria should be defined at the outset.
- The key outcomes should also be explicitly defined in the review protocol.
- The review should use a structured search strategy in order to identify all relevant studies, ideally both published and unpublished.
- Where necessary, efforts should be made to obtain missing but relevant data from published papers, to avoid propagating publication bias.
- Data should be extracted by two or more observers independently using a prepared extraction pro forma.
- An assessment of the validity of the eligible studies must be included.
- Outcome measures should be standardised and defined in advance.

Do you know any commonly used pooled outcome measures in meta-analyses?

- Continuous variables (e.g., length of stay) are usually pooled in the form of a weighted mean difference.
- Categorical variables (e.g., death) are often combined in the form of a pooled odds ratio for intervention studies and a risk ratio or relative risk for epidemiological studies.

What are the advantages of meta-analyses compared to traditional literature reviews?

- Meta-analysis controls for between-study variation.
- The result can be generalised to the study population.
- It allows an evaluation of whether bias exists in the literature.
- It has greater statistical power to detect an effect than a single study would.
- It provides a more reliable synthesis of the available literature, allowing clinicians to cope with information overload.
- By combining results from several studies, it is less likely to be influenced by local factors peculiar to single institutions.

Are there any disadvantages to meta-analyses?

- Pooling results from several small studies may not reliably predict the results of a single large study. Some meta-analyses have later been contradicted by large, well-conducted RCTs.
- If the source studies are poorly designed, the meta-analysis will produce unreliable results.
- They are vulnerable to publication- and agenda-driven bias.

What is publication bias and how is it tested for?

- Studies with positive results are more likely to be published than those with negative results.
- Consequently, meta-analyses restricted to published studies only may produce an exaggerated effect-size estimate as the unpublished studies with negative results are missing.
- Publication or other bias is detected using a funnel plot.
- A funnel plot exploits the observation that in small studies, effect-size estimates should vary quite a lot while, in larger studies, the variability should be much less.
- Consequently, a plot of effect-size estimate against sample size would be expected to form an inverted funnel.
- An asymmetric funnel suggests an absence of studies, usually small, negative studies.
- This is usually due to publication bias, though it could also arise from selection or agenda-driven bias on the part of the meta-analysts.

Why do a meta-analysis? Why not simply add up the results of all the individual studies?

- This is known as the pooling participants approach and is not considered a valid approach.
- Mixing participants from different studies and calculating a simple effect-size estimate negates the effects of randomisation.
- It also gives equal weighting to all results, rather than taking account of more precise results from larger studies.
- A meta-analysis avoids these pitfalls by calculating an effect-size estimate for each individual study and then assigning a weight to each study based upon the sample size to generate an overall summary effect-size estimate.

What is a Forest plot?

- It is a graphical demonstration of the results of the meta-analysis.
- It has a vertical line of no effect.
- The area of the box is proportional to the weight of the study in meta-analysis.
- Larger sample sizes and studies with tighter CIs are given more weight.

- Horizontal line = 95% CI; if CI crosses the vertical line of no effect, either the sample size is too small or the result is not statistically significant.
- Diamond = point estimate of pooled result.
- Horizontal width of diamond is pooled 95% CI.

PARAMETRIC AND NONPARAMETRIC STATISTICAL TESTS

What are parametric tests?

- They are based on assumptions about the shape of the distribution and form of distribution of the characteristic being tested in the population.
- Parametric tests require the population characteristics to have a normal (i.e., Gaussian) distribution.
- An example of a simple parametric test would be the Student t-test.

What are nonparametric tests?

- These tests do not rely on assumptions about the distribution of the characteristic in the underlying population.
- There is less scope for erroneous or improper use of nonparametric tests compared to the parametric equivalents.
- An example of a simple nonparametric test is the Mann–Whitney U-test.
- Nonparametric tests can be used to compare inherently subjective data (e.g., pain scores).
- Nonparametric tests are widely used to study data that take on a ranked order (e.g., patient preferences regarding four different types of postoperative analgesia).

Why not always just use a nonparametric test, if it makes no assumptions about the underlying data?

- Nonparametric tests have two drawbacks compared to their parametric equivalents.
- Firstly, they are less statistically powerful, which means that there is a smaller probability that the test will tell us that two variables are related when they are, in fact, related to each other.
  - Consequently, nonparametric tests require a slightly larger sample size to achieve the same power as their parametric equivalents.
- The other main drawback is that results of nonparametric tests are less easy to interpret.
- They also tend to rely on ranking the values in the data set rather than using the actual data.

What tests should be used for categorical, non-normal and normal data?
See Table 1.1.

TABLE 1.1

Statistical Tests Used to Analyse a Given Data Set

	Categorical	Non-normal Compare median	Normal Compare mean
One sample	Chi^2	Wilcoxon's signed rank test	One-sample t-test
Two groups, unpaired	Chi^2 (unpaired)	Mann–Whitney	t-Test
Two groups, paired	McNemar's test	Wilcoxon's matched pairs	t-Test
More than two groups, unpaired	Chi^2	Kruskall–Wallis ANOVA	ANOVA
More than two groups, paired	McNemar's test	Friedman's test	ANOVA

POWER

What do you understand by the term 'power' in medical studies?

- It is the measure of the ability of the study findings to conclude that an observed effect really occurred, rather than simply being the result of inaccurate observations or experimental error.
- It is related to the sample size. Generally, the larger the sample size is, the greater the study's power to detect increasingly small differences.
- Large studies may detect small differences that reach statistical significance but are of dubious clinical significance.

Explain the difference between clinical and statistical significance.

- Statistical significance indicates that the study findings are not likely to have occurred by chance alone.
- This differs from clinical significance, which is the clinical importance or meaning of the findings.
- Large studies may find tiny differences between patient groups that reach statistical significance but are unlikely to have any great clinical significance.
- Conversely, small studies may identify large clinical differences between patient groups that fail to reach statistical significance, but would be of great clinical importance if true, warranting further, larger studies with adequate power.

How do you undertake a power calculation for a randomised controlled trial?

- This should involve assistance from an experienced clinical trials statistician.
- Realistic data regarding the proportion of patients with the outcome of interest in the control group will be required as a baseline.

- An assumption then has to be made about the expected effect size of the intervention under investigation.
- Generally, the larger the effect-size estimate is, the smaller the number of patients required in each arm of the trial.
- However, large effect sizes may be unrealistic.
- This, in turn, may result in the incorrect conclusion that the intervention has no effect.
- Numbers needed in each arm of the trial are determined using precalculated tables for the common statistical tests.

What do you understand by the term *stratification*?

- Stratification is a method of ensuring an equal distribution of key confounding factors between the arms of a randomised trial.
- It avoids relying on chance to produce an even distribution of these key confounders.
- Stratification is particularly useful in small trials, which are particularly vulnerable to an uneven distribution of key confounders occurring by chance.
- For example, in a pilot trial of vitamin C for prevention of contrast-induced nephropathy, participants were stratified according to baseline eGFR < 60 or > 60 (i.e., baseline renal impairment). Separate randomisation schedules were prepared for each of these two groups to ensure that they were evenly distributed between the arms of the trial.

RANDOMISED CONTROLLED TRIALS

What is a randomised controlled trial?

- This type of study design permits comparison of two or more possible interventions.
- Participants enrolled in the study are randomly allocated to one or the other treatment arm.
- Apart from the intervention being tested, all other care received by the participants should be intrinsic to the treatments being studied.
- Properly conducted and reported randomised controlled trials provide level 1b evidence of treatment efficacy.

What are the advantages and disadvantages of randomised trials?

- A key advantage is that randomisation should minimise the risk of introducing bias, especially allocation bias, into the study by balancing both known and unknown prognostic factors between the arms of the trial.
- Properly conducted trials have high internal validity (i.e., a causal relationship between two variables is demonstrated).

- A causal relationship can be inferred provided that the supposed cause precedes effect in time, the cause and effect are related and there is no other potential explanation for the observed cause–effect relationship.
- The results of randomised controlled trials can be combined in systematic reviews to provide level 1a evidence of a treatment's efficacy, thus guiding healthcare policy.
- While internal validity is often very good, external validity is often limited.
- External validity is the extent to which the trial findings can be applied outside the setting of the actual trial (i.e., the generalisability of the trial findings).
- The external validity may be affected by the physical location of the trial, exclusion criteria that render the trial population different or more selected than the general population, the use of outcome measures infrequently used in clinical practice and inadequate adverse event reporting.
- Time and cost are two other frequent limitations. The time taken to conduct a good-quality trial often renders the results of limited interest as medical technology has progressed in the time taken to perform the trial. Large-scale trials are expensive to run.
- It is often difficult to continue trials for the time necessary to obtain long-term follow-up data.
- Trials often tend to focus on one narrow area of the patient's condition and thus may not be reflective of a complex medical situation.

What are different phases of randomised trials?

- Phase 1: test new drug/intervention in HEALTHY people
  - Assess safety, dose range, side effects
  - No financial incentives
- Phase 2: test on people with RELEVANT ILLNESS
  - Assess effectiveness and safety profile
  - A phase 2A trial aims to establish dosing requirements whilst a phase 2B study aims to establish efficacy.
- Phase 3: large groups of people in CLINICAL SETTINGS
  - Assess effectiveness, dose range, duration of treatment, monitor side effects, as large multicentre RCTs
  - Compare with current gold standard treatment—marketing authorisation
- Phase 4 trials: POSTMARKETING surveillance studies, after drug has been proven to work, granted a licence and marketed
  - Assess benefits and side effects in different populations; data on long-term usage
  - Can identify new safety concerns and refute them
  - Aim to prove that drug works

What types of randomised trials are you aware of?

- Parallel-group trials—participants are randomly assigned to a group and all members of that group then receive or do not receive an intervention.

- Crossover trials—participant receives the intervention and then does not receive the intervention in a random sequence over time.
- Factorial trials—participants are randomly assigned to groups with differing combinations of the intervention elements.
- Cluster trial—pre-existing groups of participants are randomised en masse to receive one intervention or another (e.g., entire wards are randomised to use a new or old type of hand-wash).

What methods are available to randomise patients taking part in trials?

- Simple randomisation:
  - Toss coin, roll dice at time of entry to study or use computer-generated numbers
- Block:
  - Ensure equal number of patients in each arm
  - Patients put into blocks that, when filled, are divided equally between different arms
- Stratified:
  - Subgroups of confounding factors formed and each subgroup block randomised
- Adaptive:
  - Probability of being allocated to a certain arm adjusted to maintain similarity between the arms

What is allocation concealment?

- This ensures that the trial assignment of the next recruited participant remains unknown before successful recruitment of the patient.
- Successful allocation concealment is considered critical to minimising selection bias in the trial.
- Various methods are available including sequentially numbered opaque sealed envelopes, sealed containers, pharmacy randomisation or central randomisation.
- Ideally, randomisation should be undertaken by a third party not involved in the recruitment or care of the patient. This helps to preserve allocation concealment.

How does allocation concealment differ from blinding?

- Allocation concealment is the method used to prevent clinicians working out the trial allocation of the next participant, thus influencing their decision as to whether or not to recruit the next eligible patient.
- Blinding refers to the intervention under investigation. In a blinded study, combinations of the clinicians, patients and outcome assessors are unaware of whether the patient has received one intervention or another.

- Allocation concealment should always be used but blinding is often not feasible or possible.

REGRESSION ANALYSIS

What is meant by regression analysis?

- A statistical technique which aims to model the relationship between multiple variables.
- In medicine, it is most often used to identify and control for the effect of possible confounding variables in an experiment.
- It is frequently applied in case series aiming to compare nonrandomised cohorts.
- Occasionally, it is used in randomised trials if random chance has created an imbalance in key confounders, though this is unlikely in large, properly designed trials.
- Regression analysis may also be used for prediction and is essential in the development of risk prediction models in surgery such as POSSUM and VBHOM.

What types of regression analysis do you know?

- Linear regression—the dependent variable (the outcome) is continuous.
  - For example, a cohort of vascular surgery patients receives aspirin or clopidogrel or dipyridamole preoperatively and we wish to determine whether any of the three increases blood loss measured in millilitres.
  - Linear regression using the amount of blood loss as the dependent variable will evaluate the possible effect of each of the three antiplatelets on blood loss.
- Logistic regression—the dependent variable is categorical (i.e., a yes or no variable).
  - If the data held on blood loss in our vascular surgery cohort were simply recorded as >1 l or <1 l, logistic regression would be used to evaluate the influence of the different antiplatelets.
- Cox regression—the influence of multiple variables on survival is evaluated.
  - Cox regression is generally only used under the expert guidance of a statistician as it relies upon multiple complex assumptions.

What are the limitations of regression?

- It is based upon assumptions about which variables should be entered at the start. Incorrect assumptions will lead to flawed models and the selection criteria for including/deleting variables, especially in stepwise models, are controversial.
- In surgical series, the models are often applied to small cohorts. The models then lack sufficient power to tease out the relationship between competing

variables, which are erroneously determined to be 'independent' of each other.
- As a rule of thumb, in order to construct an adequately powered model, there should be at least 10 patients with the outcome of interest for each of the candidate variables entered into the model. For example, if you read a report of a regression analysis of factors influencing complications following colorectal surgery, 10 variables were entered into the model but there were only 50 patients with a complication. The model is likely to be underpowered.

ROC CURVES

What are ROC curves?

- They are receiver operating characteristic curves.
- An ROC curve is a graphical plot which illustrates the performance of a test as its threshold of discrimination varies. The test must have a threshold value above which a positive result is returned, and vice versa.
- The curve is generated by plotting the fraction of true positives out of all the positives against the fraction of false positives out of the negatives at various thresholds.
- It is a trade-off between sensitivity and specificity.

How do you interpret ROC curves?

- The ROC curve is drawn based on the true positive rate and false positive rate.
- The best possible prediction method would have a sensitivity of 100% (i.e., no false negatives) and 100% specificity (i.e., no false positives).
- This would be plotted on the curve as co-ordinates 0,1, which would lie in the upper left corner of the ROC space.
- The better the test is, the closer it will lie to the upper left corner of the ROC space.
- A test that is performing no better than random chance will yield a point along a diagonal line running from the bottom left to the top right of the ROC space. This is called the line of nonsignificance.

What does the area under the curve (AUC) mean?

- The area under the ROC curve is a summary statistic that is used to summarise the performance of the test at various thresholds.
- A perfect test would have an AUC of 1.0 but, in reality, this is never attained.
- A poorly performing test would have an AUC of 0.5 or less.
- The AUC is sometimes also referred to as the c-statistic.
- In medicine, a test with a c-statistic of 0.8 or greater is considered to have good discrimination.

- Values of 0.6 to 0.8 are considered to indicate moderate discrimination and anything below 0.6 is poorly discriminating.

SCREENING TESTS

What is screening?

- Screening is a population-based strategy which aims to identify disease before it is clinically obvious, thus allowing earlier and hopefully more effective treatment.
- The overall aim is to reduce disease-related mortality.
- Screening tests differ from other tests in that they are generally performed in apparently healthy people.

What criteria need to be fulfilled to justify a screening test?

- A test must be available with reasonable sensitivity.
- A test must be available with reasonable specificity.
- The disease must be a significant public health problem (i.e., sufficiently common to justify screening).
- The test must be acceptable to the population at large.
- The test must carry minimal risks.
- The test should be economically viable.
- An effective treatment must be available for the target disease of the screening exercise. It is probably not ethical to screen for incurable disease.
- There should be a latent period between the establishment of the disease process and clinical presentation.
- Sufficient facilities and resources must exist to allow treatment of those individuals who screen positive for the disease under consideration.

What types of screening do you know?

- There are two types of screening:
- Universal screening screens an entire population defined by a certain characteristic (e.g., all men between 65 and 67 years of age for abdominal aortic aneurysm).
- Case selection is more focussed screening in which only members of the population with certain risk factors are selected for screening (e.g., all men between 65 and 67 years of age with a smoking history for abdominal aortic aneurysm).

What are the disadvantages of screening?

- There is a risk of false positives (i.e., the screening test suggests the person has the disease when he or she actually does not). This may lead to unnecessary anxiety or treatment.

- Conversely, there is a risk of false negatives (i.e., the test fails to detect the disease in a person with the condition, resulting in misplaced reassurance and possibly delayed treatment.
- Screening exposes large numbers of people to tests who ultimately do not require any form of treatment.
- If the disease detected is at an advanced, incurable stage, the screening simply prolongs stress and anxiety without affecting the ultimate prognosis.

STATISTICAL ERROR

What are the types of statistical error?

- There are type 1 and type 2 errors.
- Statistical testing depends upon a null hypothesis which the test aims to accept or reject (e.g., blue-eyed men are no more likely than brown-eyed men to have abdominal aortic aneurysms).
- Type 1 and 2 errors can occur if the null hypothesis is erroneously accepted or rejected.

What is meant by a type 1 error?

- When the null hypothesis is actually true but is accidentally rejected, this results in an erroneous conclusion. In the example of the blue-eyed and brown-eyed men, a type 1 error would involve a conclusion that eye colour did influence AAA risk when, in fact, no such relationship exists.
- In simple terms, a type 1 error occurs when we fail to recognise a falsehood.
- The rate of type 1 errors usually equals the significance level of the test.
- At the 5% significance level, the investigator accepts that 1 in 20 tests will result in an erroneous rejection of the null hypothesis.

What is meant by a type 2 error?

- A type 2 error occurs when the null hypothesis is false but is not rejected. In the example of eye colour and AAA risk, a type 2 error would occur if there was, in fact, a connection between blue eyes and AAA risk but the null hypothesis (that no such relationship exists) was not rejected.
- In simple terms, type 2 errors occur when we fail to recognise the truth.
- The rate of type 2 errors relates to the power of the test.
- A statistical test can either reject a null hypothesis (i.e., prove it to be false) or fail to reject a null hypothesis (i.e., not prove it to be false). However, a statistical test can never prove the null hypothesis to be true.

What is a type 3 error?

- A type 3 error is said to occur when the null hypothesis is correctly rejected, but the effect is attributed to the wrong cause.

- For example, the null hypothesis regarding eye colour and AAA is correctly rejected but the investigators incorrectly attribute the difference to eye colour when, in fact, another difference (e.g., smoking) exists between the groups.

How can you avoid type 1 errors?

- Reducing the amount of acceptable error reduces the chances of a type 1 error.
- Type 1 errors tend to be viewed as more serious than type 2 and thus more important to avoid.
- In practice, reducing the chance of a type 1 error means reducing the level at which significance is assumed from 5% to 1% or lower.
- Reducing the risk of a type 1 error does involve a converse increase in the risk of a type 2 error.

SUBGROUP ANALYSES[2]

What is a subgroup analysis?

- Subgroup analysis is the term applied to searching for a pattern within a subset of subjects in a study. It may be encountered in every study design but tends to be seen most frequently in large randomised trials.
- Large studies aim to assess general, representative patient populations, but clinical decision making often relies on individual patient characteristics, thus providing an impetus for analysis of particular subgroups with particular characteristics of interest.
- The broad aim is to determine whether the treatment effect observed in the whole trial population differs in magnitude in selected subsets of interest.
- Ethically, such analysis can be justified as identifying patient subsets who are unlikely to benefit and may suffer harm as a result of an intervention that, in their case, is likely to be futile.
- The term is used equivocally, sometimes referring to analysis of effect-size estimates within subgroups (subgroup analysis) or between subgroups (interaction analysis).

How would you assess the quality of a subgroup analysis?

- Use DARA: design, analysis, reporting, applicability.
- Design: Is there a rational indication for the subgroup analysis? Was it pre-defined or suggested post hoc? Was the subgroup small? Did the original power calculation take account of subgroup analysis? Was randomisation stratified for subgroup variables? Were subgroup definitions based on pre-randomisation patient characteristics?
- Analysis: Were interaction tests used? Were the tests adjusted to account for multiple comparisons? Were the subgroups checked for an even distribution of prognostic factors?

- Reporting: Did the authors report all the subgroup analyses or just a few? Does the overall discussion remain largely focussed on the overall treatment effect or is there undue emphasis on particular subgroups? Are the subgroup analyses reported as relative risk reductions?
- Applicability: Is the observed subgroup effect clinically relevant? Is it observed consistently across other similar studies?

What are the problems with subgroup analyses?

- Sometimes they are performed and designed post hoc, when the main trial has not yielded the expected or desired result. This may lead to distortions in the trial manuscript, as authors emphasise the subgroup analyses and gloss over the main results.
- They are often underpowered and can be vulnerable to type 2 errors, resulting in erroneous conclusions about treatment efficacy.
- If the subgroup analysis was not planned from the outset, and possibly randomisation stratified accordingly, there may be an imbalance of key prognostic factors between the subgroups, resulting in faulty conclusions about treatment effects.

SURVIVAL ANALYSIS

What is survival analysis?

- Survival analysis is a branch of statistics which considers comparisons of time to event data.
- It can be applied to any event but is frequently encountered in the analysis of time to death or recurrence in cancer patients.
- The analysis depends on well-defined events occurring at specific times.
- Generally, survival analysis can only be applied to events which only occur once.

What is censoring?

- Censoring is a technique used in survival analysis to account for missing data.
- If the occurrence of the event of interest is not known for a particular participant in the analysis, his or her data are censored at the date of last contact.

What is a Kaplan–Meier curve?[3]

- A Kaplan–Meier curve is a form of survival analysis widely used in medical research.
- It shows the event rates over a study period rather than at a specific time point.

- It can be used to measure the fraction of patients living a certain time following treatment.
- A key advantage is that the technique can take account of patients who are censored due to losses to follow-up.
- By convention, censored patients are indicated by a tick on the plot at the time point at which they were censored.

How do you compare two Kaplan–Meier curves?

- The curves are often compared using the log-rank test.
- This is a nonparametric test which is used when the data are skewed (often the case in survival data) and when some data are censored.
- If there are no censored data (unlikely in medical research), the Wilcoxon rank sum test can be used as an alternative.
- The test involves computing the expected and observed events in each group at each observed event time.
- The log-rank test gives equal weight to each event regardless of when it happened; the Peto test applies a greater weighting to earlier events.

What information should be presented with Kaplan–Meier curves to allow adequate interpretation?

- Definition of patients (T-stage, treatment groups, etc.) and study groups with dates of enrolment.
- The actual number of patients in each group at the start of the analysis together with revised numbers at reasonable time intervals along the curves. These numbers should be presented with 95% confidence intervals.
- Definitions of events and censoring.
- Median follow-up time and method of calculation.
- Numbers of missing data and losses to follow-up in each group, together with information on how these issues were handled.
- Results of a test statistic (e.g., log rank test if appropriate).

How far should the plot extend?

- Theoretically, the plot can extend as far as the last point of contact with the last patient, but this results in wide confidence intervals and consequently much uncertainty at the far right of the plot due to small numbers.
- Conventionally, the plot should be curtailed when <20% of patients remain under follow-up.

REFERENCES

1. Panesar, Sukhmeet S., Mohit Bhandari, Ara Darzi and Thanos Athanasiou. 2009. Meta-analysis: A practical decision making tool for surgeons. *International Journal of Surgery (London, England)* 7 (4): 291–296.

2. Dijkman, Bernadette, Bauke Kooistra and Mohit Bhandari, Evidence-Based Surgery Working Group. 2009. How to work with a subgroup analysis. *Canadian Journal of Surgery* 52 (6): 515–522.
3. Bollschweiler, Elfriede. 2003. Benefits and limitations of Kaplan–Meier calculations of survival chance in cancer surgery. *Langenbeck's Archives of Surgery/Deutsche Gesellschaft Für Chirurgie* 388 (4): 239–244.

2 Critical Care

Jithesh Appukutty, Elizabeth Ball, John Davidson, Vinodkumar Singh, Nicole Keong, Tjun Tang and Stewart Walsh

CONTENTS

ABDOMINAL COMPARTMENT SYNDROME

You have been asked to review a 71-year-old male patient in ITU who is 48 hr postoperative following a laparotomy for a diverticular perforation. The nurses are concerned that his intra-abdominal pressure reading is 21 mmHg. What would you do?

- The patient could be developing abdominal compartment syndrome.
- I would speak to the staff involved in his care and ask about their concerns.
- After checking the ABCs, I would review the patient by looking at the past medical history and medications, the operative note, current medication (including nephrotoxic drugs), nursing and medical notes, and the observation and fluid balance charts.
- I would examine the patient, looking for signs of peritonism, an increase in abdominal girth, basal creptitations, and evidence of a DVT or PE.
- I would check his pulse, blood pressure, CVP, respiratory rate and ventilation pressure, urine output, nasogastric aspirate, and the most recent bloods and blood gases.
- I would check the IAP reading and look at the trend over the last 24 hr.
- If the patient is oliguric, I would exclude other causes of acute kidney injury (ACS is not necessarily due to postop distension):
  - Prerenal—shock (haemorrhagic, septic, third-space losses, pump failure), acute MI, ACS
  - Intrarenal—acute tubular necrosis due to hypotension, nephrotoxins
  - Postrenal—catheter problems (kink, clogged), bilateral ureteral occlusion/injury (rare)
- If ACS is confirmed, I would inform the patient's consultant and intensivist and resuscitate the patient whilst investigating the cause.

What is abdominal compartment syndrome?

- ACS is defined as the presence of BOTH:
  - An IAP > 20 mmHg recorded by a minimum of three standardised measurements conducted 1–6 hr apart
  - Single or multiple organ system failure which was not previously present
- The underlying cause is capillary permeability due to SIRS, leading to leakage of fluid out of the capillary beds into the interstitial space (including gut wall, mesentery and retroperitoneal tissue).
- There are three categories:
  - Primary—due to peritoneal injury/disease or following abdominal surgery
  - Secondary—injuries outside the abdomen causing fluid accumulation (pancreatitis, ruptured AAA, sepsis, burns)
- Chronic—cirrhosis, ascites

How is IAP measured?

- IAP should be measured at end-expiration with the patient in a supine position after ensuring that abdominal muscle contractions are absent and the transducer is zeroed at the level of the midaxillary line.
- To measure IAP, I would use a bladder catheter and inject 25 ml of sterile saline into the aspiration port. I would cross-clamp the urinary drainage bag just distal to the culture aspiration port, ensuring the tubing proximal to the clamp is filled with urine. I would then Y-connect a pressure transducer to the drainage bag via the culture aspiration port of the tubing, using a 16-gauge needle, and determine the IAP from the transducer using the top of the symphysis pubis bone as the zero reference point with the patient in the supine position.
- It is expressed in mmHg (normal value is 5–7 mmHg or <10 cm water). An IAP > 15 mmHg can cause significant end-organ dysfunction, failure and patient death.
- Failure to intervene when IAP rises above 25 mmHg is associated with a poor outcome.
- Intra-abdominal hypertension (IAH) is graded as follows:
  - Grade I   IAP of 12–15 mmHg
  - Grade II   IAP of 16–20 mmHg
  - Grade III   IAP of 21–25 mmHg
  - Grade IV   IAP > 25 mmHg

What are the pathophysiologic changes of ACS?

- Visceral—decreased visceral perfusion and splanchnic blood flow, GI mucosal ischaemia (leads to stress ulcers and colitis)
- Renal—decreased renal blood flow and GFR (renal impairment occurs at 15 mmHg, oliguria at 20 mmHg, anuria at 30 mmHg)
- Pulmonary—diaphragmatic splinting, decreased ventilation and compliance, decreased tidal volumes, increased $PaCO_2$ and respiratory acidosis
- Cardiovascular—decreased cardiac output, BP and stroke volume, increased pulse, CVP, SVR and PAWP, DVT due to venous stasis
- Cerebral—elevated ICP and reduced cerebral perfusion pressure

When would you operate to treat ACS?

- Treatment of ACS is based upon four general principles:
  - Serial monitoring of IAP
  - Optimisation of systemic perfusion and organ function
  - Appropriate medical procedures to reduce IAP and end-organ consequences
  - Prompt surgical decompression for refractory IAH
- I would use a trial of medical treatment, particularly for secondary causes of ACS, using sedation, analgesia, neuromuscular blockade and body positioning to improve abdominal wall compliance.

- I would consider endoscopic decompression or neostigmine for pseudo-obstruction, and percutaneous drainage of abdominal fluid
- If the IAP persists at >20 mmHg, or the patient was oliguric, I would perform a laparostomy.

There are two options available—say which one YOU would use:

- Bogota bag: a presterilised 3 l fluid irrigation bag; suture or staple it to the skin (option of placing vacuum drains on top).
  - Sandwich technique: cover viscera with fenestrated polyethylene sheet, moist surgical towels, vacuum drains and an iodoform-impregnated adhesive drape. Connect to wall suction.
- I would cover the patient with broad spectrum IV antibiotics whilst the abdomen is open.
- The sudden release may lead to an ischemia-reperfusion injury, causing acidosis, vasodilatation, cardiac dysfunction, arrhythmias and cardiac arrest. I would liase with the anaesthetist, so that the patient was adequately resuscitated prior to opening the abdomen.

ACUTE KIDNEY INJURY

You have been asked to review a 72-year-old male who is day 5 postop following a left hemicolectomy. His HR is 90 bpm but his BP is normal, and he is apyrexial. His urine output has deteriorated in the last 6 hr, and in the past 3 hr it has been <10 ml/hr. How will you manage this patient?

- This patient is oliguric. The commonest cause in postop patients is hypovolaemia.
- I will take a history—is he thirsty, does he have any pain, is he short of breath?
- I will examine the patient:
  - Assess hydration status, signs of heart failure, sepsis and peritonism/anastomotic leak
- Review the observation, fluid and drug charts, and then look at the medical notes (co-morbidities, operative note details, previous renal failure)
- Check a full blood count and urea, creatinine and electrolytes and request urinalysis.

The patient is not obviously septic. He has had 500 ml of IV saline today and is not really eating and drinking yet. You think he might have an acute kidney injury. How do you define acute kidney injury?

- A sudden rise in serum creatinine of 50 mmol/l, or >50% from baseline
- Oliguria with urine output < 400 ml/day
- Need for renal replacement therapy

What are the RIFLE criteria?

- Classification of the severity of renal failure
- Risk, Injury, Failure, Loss, End-stage disease
- Based on the increase in serum creatinine/decrease in GFR, and the degree of oliguria (volume of urine passed and length of time the patient has been oliguric)

What are common causes of acute kidney injury?

- Prerenal:
  - Reversible if the underlying cause is corrected
  - Due to reduced renal perfusion
    - Loss of blood (e.g., UGI haemorrhage)
    - Loss of fluid (e.g., hypovolaemia, D+V, third space losses, pancreatitis, burns, septic shock)
    - Pump failure—cardiogenic shock, septic shock
    - Drugs—NSAIDs, ACE inhibitors
- Renal
  - Intrinsic renal failure
    - Glomerular disease—glomerulonephritis, SLE, DIC
    - Interstitial nephritis—drug-induced (NSAIDs, antibiotics), sarcoidosis, pyelonephritis, lymphoma
    - Acute tubular necrosis—ischaemic (prolonged renal hypoperfusion, vasculitis), nephrotoxic (contrast media, aminoglycosides)
- Postrenal:
  - Obstruction of outflow of both kidneys, or a single functioning kidney
  - Renal stones, blocked catheter, transected ureter, extrinsic obstruction from pelvic tumour, BPH and urethral strictures

You thought the patient was dehydrated, and gave a 500 ml fluid challenge. He has some atelectasis since he came back to the ward. His hydration status has improved, but he remains oliguric. Now what will you do?

- Firstly, check that there are no obvious causes (drugs, sepsis, blocked catheter, MI) that can be treated.
- Liaise with ITU for ongoing support whilst establishing and treating the cause.
- The patient may need central line monitoring to ensure that he is adequately filled (CVP > 8).
- If still oliguric, despite being well filled, he will need either an inotrope (dobutamine) or vasopressor (noradrenaline) to optimise cardiac output and improve renal perfusion.

One of your juniors prescribes another 1 l of fluid. The patient is taken to HDU and a central line records a CVP of 18 mmHg. He is now SOB, his respiratory rate has increased and he remains oliguric. How would this change your management?

- The dyspnoea and elevated CVP reading suggest that the patient is fluid overloaded, which will further decrease renal perfusion.
- His acute kidney injury has probably been triggered by sepsis.
- As the patient is day 5 postop, the likely cause is an anastomotic leak. Other causes would include a chest infection, wound infection and a catheter or cannula site infection.
- I would like a CT scan to confirm the diagnosis, but the contrast could worsen his renal failure.
- He now is likely to require renal replacement therapy.

How can you determine if he is still in reversible prerenal failure or has developed intrinsic renal damage?

- In prerenal failure, kidney function is preserved; therefore, urea excretion and sodium conservation are possible.
- Urinary sodium and osmolality and urine microscopy will confirm the diagnosis:
- Prerenal failure
  - Urinary sodium < 20 mmol/l
  - Urinary osmolality > 500
  - Urine: plasma urea ratio > 20
  - Microscopy—normal
  - Fractional excretion of sodium (FeNa) < 1% (FeNa = urine Na x plasma Cr/urine Cr x plasma Na) is a sensitive indicator.
- Renal failure
  - Urinary sodium > 40 mmol/l
  - Urinary osmolality < 350
  - Urine: plasma urea ratio < 10
  - Microscopy—tubular casts
  - FeNa > 2%

What is the pathophysiology of acute tubular necrosis (ATN)?

- The kidneys receive 20% of the cardiac output.
- The renal medulla is relatively hypoxic under normal physiologic conditions and therefore is very susceptible to ischaemic injury.
- A drop in renal perfusion leads to decreased sodium reabsorption.
- This causes arteriolar constriction and a drop in GFR.
- The ischaemic cells swell, causing cytokine activation, resulting in ATN.
- The anuric phase of ATN classically lasts 7–21 days.
- Once renal perfusion and oxygen supply are restored, viable cells still adherent to the tubular basement membrane can spread to cover denuded areas.
- They reproduce normal tubular architecture and function.
- A polyuric phase follows when glomerular filtration has normalised, but tubular function remains deranged.
- The kidneys may eventually regain full normal function.

Before requesting the CT scan, you check the latest blood tests. The patient's potassium is 7.3. How will you treat this?

- Ask for an urgent ECG whilst prescribing the necessary drugs; there may be tall T waves, absent P wave, broad QRS complex.
- Stabilise cardiac myocytes with 10 ml 10% calcium chloride intravenously over 10 min.
- Sodium bicarbonate can be given as the alkalosis causes a shift of K^+ into cells.
- Increase cellular uptake of potassium—IV insulin dextrose infusion or nebulised salbutamol.
- Increase potassium excretion in stool with calcium resonium.
- Stop K-sparing diuretics and ACE inhibitors.
- Renal replacement therapy may be needed.
- Haemodialysis is more effective than haemofiltration and can have an immediate effect on potassium excretion.

What are the indications for renal replacement therapy?

- Symptomatic uraemia, uraemic encephalopathy/pericarditis
- Metabolic acidosis (pH < 7.1)
- Severe hyperkalaemia, unresponsive to medical therapy
- Pulmonary oedema not responding to medical treatment
- Poisoning (dialyzable toxin)
- High urea and creatinine—relative indications

What are the different types of renal replacement therapy?

- In critical care units, haemofiltration and haemodialysis are used for renal replacement. For patients requiring long-term renal replacement therapy, peritoneal dialysis is also an option.
- Haemofiltration:
  - Blood is pumped through a semipermeable membrane.
  - The hydrostatic pressure on the blood side of the filter drives plasma water across the filter (ultrafiltration).
  - Small molecules (Na, urea, HCO_3, creatinine) are dragged across the membrane with the water by convection.
  - The filtered fluid (ultrafiltrate) is discarded and replaced with fluid buffered with HCO_3 and lactate.
- Haemodialysis:
  - Blood is pumped through a dialyser.
  - In the dialyser, blood is separated from a crystalloid solution (dialysate) by a semipermeable membrane.
  - Solutes move across the membrane along their concentration gradient from one compartment to the other by diffusion.

- – Bicarbonate moves from dialysate to blood.
- – Urea and potassium move from blood to dialysate.
- To maintain concentration gradients, the dialysate flows counter to the flow of blood.
- When removal of water is required, the pressure on the blood side of the membrane has to be increased, forcing water molecules to pass into the dialysate.

ACUTE RESPIRATORY DISTRESS SYNDROME

What is the definition of ARDS?

- Acute respiratory failure with noncardiogenic pulmonary oedema leading to decreased lung compliance and hypoxaemia refractory to oxygen therapy
- Characterised by:
  - Diffuse pulmonary infiltrates on CXR
  - A normal pulmonary artery wedge pressure (PAWP < 18 mmHg)
    - – Excludes pulmonary oedema secondary to elevated left atrial pressure
  - PaO_2/FiO_2 ratio < 26.6 kPa

What are the clinical features of ARDS?

- There must be a known precipitating cause and the onset of symptoms is acute.
  - Dyspnoea
  - Tachypnoea
  - Hypoxia refractory to oxygen therapy
  - New bilateral diffuse infiltrates on chest radiograph:
    - – May lag behind clinical picture by 12–24 hr
  - No clinical evidence of a raised left atrial pressure
- The severity of the hypoxic insult can be quantified into acute lung injury (ALI) or ARDS depending on the fraction of inspired oxygen that the patient is breathing:
  - In ALI the PaO_2/FiO_2 ratio is <40 kPa (300 mmHg).
  - In ARDS the PaO_2/FiO_2 ratio is <26.6 kPa (200 mmHg).
- The following are associated clinical findings (but are not included as diagnostic criteria):
  - Need for mechanical ventilation
  - Low lung compliance
  - High airway pressures during positive pressure ventilation

What are the causes of ARDS?
The causes are divided into direct and indirect causes:

- Direct/pulmonary causes:
  - Infection

- Contusion from blunt trauma
- Aspiration of gastric contents
- Near drowning
- Smoke inhalation
- Indirect or nonpulmonary causes:
  - Sepsis
  - Major trauma
  - Severe hypotension and prolonged haemorrhage
  - Fat/amniotic fluid/thrombotic embolism
  - Burns
  - Pancreatitis
  - Massive blood transfusion
  - DIC
  - Cardiopulmonary bypass

What pathological processes cause ARDS?

- Respiratory component of systemic inflammatory response syndrome (SIRS)
- Acute inflammatory response—immediate exudative phase
  - Activated neutrophils and macrophages secrete cytokine mediators of acute inflammation (IL-6, TNF-α, proteases, prostaglandins and free radicals)
- Complement system and clotting cascades are also activated:
- Increases capillary permeability by local endothelial injury
  - Decrease of type II pneumocytes and reduced pulmonary surfactant
  - Reduces lung compliance by increasing the pressure required to open the alveoli
- A proliferative phase 5–10 days later:
  - Hyperplasia of type II pneumocytes and fibroblasts
  - Causes progressive interstitial fibrosis and a restrictive picture
  - May persist after the patient has recovered
- Pathological changes result in:
  - Decreased lung compliance
  - Increased atelectasis and reduced FRC
  - Increased shunt and V/Q mismatch
  - Increased pulmonary vascular resistance and pulmonary hypertension

What are the treatment options for ARDS?

- Most patients will need to be managed in ITU.
- Identify and treat the cause (if known).
- Provide nutritional support.
- Supply mechanical ventilation to aid oxygenation, decrease the work of breathing and improve clearance of CO_2.
- Avoid ventilator-induced lung injury:

- Limit mean airway pressures (<30 cmH$_2$O) and tidal volume (6–8 ml/kg ideal body weight).
- Use PEEP to aid alveolar recruitment.
- Strict fluid management—ensure that patient does not develop cardiogenic pulmonary oedema as a result of fluid overload:
  - Prone ventilation—usually for 4–8 hr at a time; redistributes secretions
  - Minimises basal atelectasis with regular turning
  - Improves V/Q mismatch, thereby improving oxygenation
- Inhaled prostacyclins, ECMO (extracorporeal membrane oxygenator), high-frequency oscillatory ventilation, nitric oxide and steroids may also help.

What is the prognosis?

- Outcome usually poor
- 50%–60% mortality rate overall
- 90% mortality rate if associated with sepsis
- Death of most patients due to sepsis and multiorgan failure, not hypoxaemia
- Considerable morbidity with progressive interstitial fibrosis and pulmonary hypertension

What is the role of decreased surfactant and inhaled nitric oxide in ARDS?

- Surfactant:
  - No RCTs show a mortality benefit.
  - Some case series demonstrate successful use in the neonates.
- Nitric oxide acts as a potent local pulmonary vasodilator:
  - Improves perfusion to better ventilated areas of lung and reduces shunt.
  - No class I evidence to show any mortality benefit.
  - Some evidence of morbidity benefit; seldom used in the UK.

AIRWAY ASSESSMENT

A 25-year-old driver of a car has been involved in a head-on collision. There was no airbag in the vehicle. He is hypoxic in A+E, with obvious bruising to his face and torso. How would you assess him?

- I would first assess his airway whilst maintaining cervical spine control and delivering high-flow oxygen through a nonrebreathing mask.
- I would look for the use of accessory muscles of respiration, obvious airway injury, foreign bodies, evidence of aspiration and cyanosis.
- I would listen for sounds of upper airway obstruction (stridor, grunting and gurgling), hoarse voice or absent breath sounds.
- I would feel for crepitus, equal chest wall movement and the tracheal position.
- I would then assess the circulation with capillary refill, pulse and blood pressure, assess the GCS and check for papillary size following which I would complete the primary survey with full exposure.

What are the causes of airway obstruction?

- Soft tissues (e.g., tongue) blocking oropharynx
- Vomit/blood/foreign body
- Laryngospasm
- Facial trauma/neck trauma
- Airway oedema secondary to burns/smoke inhalation

After your initial ABC assessment, his saturation is 86% on high-flow oxygen, and there is bruising and dried blood over his mouth and nose. His pulse is 100, and his respiratory rate is 25. His GCS is 10. What will you do?

- Suction the airway and perform a chin lift whilst maintaining cervical spine control.
- If this improves the oxygenation, I would insert an oral airway to keep the upper airway patent.

This initially improves things, and the saturation rises to 92%. A chest x-ray shows bilateral rib fractures, and he clinically has a midfacial and mandibular fracture. His GCS is now 7. The anaesthetist is busy with another patient. What will you do?

- This patient now needs a definitive airway (cuffed endotracheal tube). In view of his facial trauma, a surgical airway would be my first choice here.
- I would perform a surgical cricothyroidotomy. I would incise through the skin and the cricothyroid membrane, dilate the opening with a curved haemostat and insert a small (5–7 mm) ET tube, then reapply the surgical collar.

Do you know any other types of surgical airways?

- A needle cricothyroidotomy:
  - Converts an emergency intubation to an urgent intubation
  - Does not protect the airway, and there is only minimal exhalation, so CO_2 levels accumulate
  - Can only be used for 30–40 min

Can you describe how you would assess a patient for a difficult intubation?

- I would use the LEMON technique as described in the ATLS manual:
  - Look for external injuries, beard, protruding incisors, neck
  - Evaluate 3,3,2 (interincisor, hyomental and thyromandibular distance in finger breaths)
  - Mallampati classification
  - Obstruction: epiglottitis, peritonsillar abscess, trauma
  - Neck mobility: none if wearing a hard cervical collar

BLEEDING DISORDERS

What is a bleeding disorder and how do you screen for it?

- A congenital or acquired disorder that predisposes the patient to bleeding
- Diagnosed with the following blood tests:
  - FBC and blood film
  - APTT—intrinsic and common (X to fibrin) pathways
  - PT—extrinsic (VII) and common pathways; expressed as INR
  - TT—deficiencies of fibrinogen or thrombin inhibition
  - Coagulation factor tests—VIII, IX etc.
  - FDP levels—useful in DIC

What are the common congenital bleeding disorders?

- Haemophilia A:
  - X-linked recessive disorder with deficiency/abnormality of factor VIII
  - Bleeding into soft tissues, muscles and joints
  - Mild, moderate and severe disease
  - Treat with Desmopressin or factor VIII concentrate pre-op
- Haemophilia B:
  - X-linked recessive disorder with defect/deficiency in factor IX
  - Identical clinical picture to haemophilia A
  - Treat with prothrombin complex concentrate or factor XI
- Von Willebrand's disease:
  - vWF (von Willebrand factor) aids platelet adhesion at sites of vascular injury and is a plasma carrier protein for factor VIII
  - Autosomal dominant and recessive inheritance, with reduction or loss of vWF
  - Mucosal bleeding, petechiae, epistaxis
  - Treat with cryoprecipitate, factor VIII or desmopressin

What are the common acquired bleeding disorders?

- Thrombocytopaenia:
  - Decreased platelet production (marrow failure/infiltration and alcoholism)
  - Decreased platelet survival (drugs, ITP)
  - Increased consumption (DIC, infection)
- Platelet dysfunction:
  - NSAIDs, heparin, alcohol, antiplatelet drugs (e.g., clopidogrel, aspirin)
- Vitamin K deficiency (leads to deficiency of activated factors II, VII, IX, X):
  - Poor diet, malabsorption, lack of bile salts
- Liver failure:
  - Decreased synthesis of coagulation factors (except VIII) and coagulation inhibitors (protein C, S and antithrombin III)
  - Impaired absorption and metabolism of vitamin K

- Renal failure:
  - Decrease in platelet aggregation and adhesion

What is a thrombophilia?

- Abnormality of blood coagulation that increases the risk of thrombosis
- Can be congenital (overactivity of coagulation factors or deficiency of anti-coagulant proteins) or acquired (disease or generic risk factors)

When would you suspect a thrombophilia?

- History of recurrent thromboembolism
- History of idiopathic thromboembolism
- DVT < 40 years of age
- Family history of thrombosis
- Thrombosis in unusual sites (mesenteric vein, renal vein, hepatic and cerebral thrombosis)
- About 50% of patients presenting with their first idiopathic venous thrombosis have an underlying thrombophilia.

What are the congenital thrombophilias?

- Overactivity of coagulation factors:
  - Factor V Leiden (resistant to inactivation by protein C/S)—most common
  - Prothrombin G20210A (triples risk of thrombosis)
- Anticoagulant deficiency:
  - Protein C deficiency—impaired neutralisation of Va
  - Protein S deficiency—impaired neutralisation of Va
  - Antithrombin deficiency—impaired neutralisation of Xa and thrombin

What are the causes of acquired thrombophilia?

- Antiphospholipid syndrome—antibodies against lupus anticoagulant
- Myeloproliferative disorders
- Sickle cell disease—sluggish blood flow
- DIC
- Risk factors—advanced age, immobility, inflammation, pregnancy, OCP, obesity, HRT, cancer
  - Procoagulants released in cancer and pregnancy

How do you treat thrombophilia?

- Consider primary anticoagulation or prophylaxis in patients at risk
- Primary prophylaxis—prolonged hospitalisation postoperatively, immobilisation and in patients with active cancer.

- Long-term prophylaxis—complex assessment of all risk factors; liaise with haematology colleagues
  - Benefits of anticoagulation must outweigh the risk of bleeding, especially in elderly patients.

BRAIN-STEM DEATH

A 25-year-old male motorcyclist is admitted under your care to the intensive care unit. He arrived in the emergency department following a road traffic accident with a Glasgow coma scale of 3. A CT scan of his head demonstrated diffuse cerebral oedema. The intensivists assess him after 36 hr and find that he has suffered brain-stem death.

What is brain-stem death?

- Irreversible loss of the capacity for consciousness, combined with irreversible loss of the capacity to breathe
- Equates with the death of the individual

Why is brain-stem function important to life?

- The brain stem contains nuclei controlling the body's major homeostatic mechanisms, including:
  - Respiratory centres
  - Cardiovascular centres (autonomic—particularly vagus nerve nuclei)
  - Arousal centres (reticular activating system)
  - Cranial nerve nuclei III–XII
- Loss of these nuclei is incompatible with life.

How is brain-stem death diagnosed?

- I would demonstrate that all brain-stem reflexes are absent.
- The pupils are fixed and do not respond to light:
  - Mediated by cranial nerves II and III
- There is no corneal reflex:
  - Sensory Va, motor VII cranial nerves
- The vestibulo-ocular reflexes are absent:
  - No eye movements seen during or following the slow injection of at least 50 ml of ice cold water over 1 min into each external auditory meatus in turn
  - Clear access to the tympanic membrane established by direct inspection and the head should be at 30° to the horizontal plane
- There are no motor responses within the cranial nerve distribution:
  - Cranial nerves VII and Vc
    - Can be elicited by adequate stimulation of any somatic area
  - No limb response to supraorbital pressure
- There is no gag reflex or reflex response to bronchial stimulation with a suction catheter placed down the trachea:
  - Sensory IX, motor X cranial nerves

- No respiratory movements occur when the patient is disconnected from the mechanical ventilator for 5 min following preoxygenation with 100% oxygen for 10 min, a systolic pressure >90 mmHg and a $PaCO_2$ of 6 kPa. The apnoea testing has to be abandoned if there are cardiac arrhythmias, hypotension; but the tests can be repeated after stabilisation of the patient.
  - $PaCO_2$ must exceed threshold for respiratory stimulation (>6.5 kPa) (i.e., the $PaCO_2$ should reach 6.5 kPa). This should be ensured by measurement of the blood gases. The pH should be kept below 7.4
  - Hypoxia during disconnection should be prevented by delivering oxygen at 6 l/min through a catheter in the trachea.

What medical criteria need to be satisfied in order for a diagnosis of brain-stem death to be valid?

- No sedation: barbiturates and benzodiazepines can accumulate and need to be stopped for some time before brain-stem testing can begin.
- No muscle relaxants: this must be confirmed by the use of a standard neuromuscular stimulator on one of the limbs.
- Patient must be normothermic.
- Patient must have normal electrolyte levels and be normoglycaemic.
- Decerebrate or decorticate posturing is incompatible with brain-stem death, although true spinal-mediated reflexes may be compatible with the diagnosis.
- Brain-stem death testing cannot be performed in children <2 months of age and with anencephaly.
- In anencephalic children, the organs can be procured only after two non-transplant clinicians confirm apnoea.

Who can diagnose brain-stem death?

- Two medical practitioners who have been registered for more than 5 years can diagnose brain-stem death.
- Both must be competent in this field and neither can be a member of the transplant team.
- At least one of the doctors should be a consultant.
- Two sets of tests should always be performed by the two doctors acting together.
- The timing between these two sets of tests will vary according to the pathology in question and the individual situation but brain-stem death can be diagnosed only after two full sets of criteria have been met.
- The legal time of death is at the end of the first set of tests.
- Confirmatory tests such as electroencephalography, cerebral angiography and transcranial Doppler are not required in the UK but are used in other countries.

Your patient's family agree to consider organ donation and ask about the process involved. What is the pathway to organ explantation and retrieval?

- Pathway to transplantation:
  - Transplant coordinator involved
  - Relatives consulted
  - Brain-stem death diagnosed
  - Coroner informed (if necessary)
  - Blood tests (including virology and serology) and other screening tests
  - Donor screened for malignancy (including glioblastoma)
  - Surgical and anaesthetic interventions to assess viability of organs
  - Organ retrieval by dedicated transplant team (heart/lung last)

When should these cases be referred to the coroner?

- Brain-stem death is not clearly the result of natural causes.
- In England, the coroner and, in Scotland, the procurator fiscal must be consulted.
- The transplant coordinator is usually responsible for identifying who is in lawful possession of the body and for obtaining the necessary authorisation for organ removal.

What is the position if the patient carries a donor card?

- A donor card signed by the patient is binding by law and overrides any concerns voiced by the relatives.
- In practice, organs are rarely retrieved against the relatives' wishes.

What is a persistent vegetative state (PVS)? Does it constitute brain-stem death?

- PVS is where there is no evidence of higher brain function but brain-stem reflexes are intact.
- There is much controversy about its definition and prognosis.
- There are reports of PVS being at least partially reversible.
- Some functional brain studies have shown that some PVS patients have higher brain activity as a result of somatic stimuli despite no outward clinical evidence of this.
- It is not equivalent to brain-stem death.

BURNS[1]

A 25-year-old man is rescued from a house fire and taken to A+E. How would you assess him?

- Resuscitate according to ATLS principles: airway control, stop the burning process, gain IV access and start IV crystalloid infusion.
- Airway: assess for inhalation injury (face/neck burns, hair singeing, stridor, carbon deposits in oropharynx, carbonaceous sputum, hoarseness, CO > 10%):

- Give high-flow oxygen and take ABG/CoHb levels.
- If inhalation injury is present, intubate to protect airway and transfer to burns centre.
    - There is a risk of airway compromise due to oedema and obstruction.
- Stop burning process: remove clothing (do not peel adherent clothing), cover with warm, dry linens to prevent hypothermia, analgesia.
- IV access: arms are preferable to legs; needles can go through burned skin (high incidence of phlebitis when saphenous vein is used for cut down).
- Catheterise to monitor urine output.

How much fluid would you give?

- First assess burn size and depth:
    - Wallace's rule of 9s, patient's palmar surface = 1% body surface area, Lund and Brouder chart
- Depth:
    - First degree (sunburn)—erythema, pain, no blisters, no IV fluids
    - Second degree (partial thickness)—red/mottled, swelling, blisters
    - Third degree (full thickness)—dark/leathery, waxy/white skin, may be painful or painless, do not blanch
- Infuse fluids to produce 0.5–1 ml/kg/hr urine (1–2 ml/kg in children).
    - Parkland formula: 4 ml/kg/% BSA in first 24 hr (Hartmann's solution)
        - 50% in first 8 hr, 50% in second 16 hr
        - Additional maintenance fluids as required

What are the principles of burns management?

- There are seven principles (National Burn Care Review):
    - Rescue
    - Resuscitate
    - Retrieve
    - Resurface
    - Rehabilitate
    - Reconstruct
    - Review

The patient has circumferential burns on his upper arms. What would you do?

- Perform an escharotomy to prevent compartment syndrome.
- Make multiple checkerboard incisions down to fat.

When would you transfer patient to a burns centre?

- Second/third degree burns > 10% in <10 years, >50 years of age
- Second/third degree burns > 20% BSA

- Burns to hands, feet, face, genitalia, joints
- Inhalation injury
- Significant electrical/chemical injury

What is the pathophysiology of a burns injury?

- Local effects:
  - Inflammatory mediators—vasodilatation, vessel permeability
  - Leads to fluid loss from the circulation into the interstitial space and hypovolaemia
- Systemic effects:
  - Hypermetabolic—increased catecholamines and glucagon leading to reduced insulin sensitivity and protein catabolism
  - Poor temperature regulation
  - Immunosuppression and increased susceptibility to infection.
  - Bacterial translocation due to reduced splanchnic blood flow
  - ARDS—increased mucus production, reduced compliance
  - Anaemia—coagulopathy in muscle and soft tissue, haemolysis
  - Renal failure—hypovolaemia, ATN, rhabdomyolysis

CARDIOVASCULAR EFFECTS OF AORTIC CROSS-CLAMPING

What are the cardiovascular effects of aortic cross-clamping?

- Increase in after-load leading to:
  - Hypertension
  - Myocardial ischaemia
  - Arrhythmias
  - Left ventricular failure
- Techniques to reduce after-load include:
  - Use of increased volatile anaesthetic
  - Vasodilators (e.g., GTN/sodium nitroprusside)
  - Epidural anaesthesia to provide sympathetic blockade
- May be insignificant effects if significant aorto-occlusive disease due to collateral circulation

What are the cardiovascular effects of releasing the aortic cross-clamp?

- Effects secondary to decreased after-load
- Release of vasodilatory metabolites from legs/lower part of body
- Decreased myocardial contractility due to acidosis (increased lactate and $PaCO_2$)
- Hypotension and arrhythmias

How can you prevent these effects from happening?

- Ensure that the patient is adequately filled.
- Stop vasodilators prior to releasing the clamp.
- Slowly releasing cross-clamp over several minutes, with partial clamping by surgeon to maintain systemic vascular resistance, can prevent harm.

DISSEMINATED INTRAVASCULAR COAGULATION

What is DIC?

- Pathological activation of the coagulation and fibrinolytic pathways:
  - Release of cytokines and tissue factors by damaged tissues
- Leads to widespread microvascular thrombosis and fibrin occlusion of small and large vessels
- Results in shock and end-organ failure:
  - Low cardiac output, tachycardia and hypotension
- Patient develops a bleeding tendency due to consumption of clotting factors and platelets:
  - Petechial rash and bleeding from mucosal surfaces

What are the causes of DIC?

- Any disorder that causes activation of coagulation
- Severe sepsis:
  - Gram negative/anaerobes
  - Viruses—CMV, HIV, hepatitis
- Organ destruction (e.g., severe pancreatitis)
- Trauma/tissue injury
- Transfusion reactions
- Obstetric emergencies:
  - Amniotic fluid embolism, placental abruption and pre-eclampsia
- Severe hepatic failure
- Malignancy—neoplastic cells express tissue factor

Why do patients with DIC develop anaemia?

- Red blood cells get fragmented by the fibrin deposits.
- A microangiopathic haemolytic anaemia is caused.

What are the blood results in DIC?

- Raised D-dimer—fibrin degradation product, which indicates activation of the fibrinolytic pathway

- Platelet count $< 15 \times 10^9/l$—consumption with activation of the clotting cascade
- Decreased fibrinogen
- Prolonged PT, TT and APTT
- Reduction in the individual clotting factors
- Red blood cell fragments on a blood film
- Prolonged clotting, low platelets and elevated D-Dimer/FDP is enough to diagnose DIC

How do you treat DIC?

- Treat the underlying disorder.
- Platelets and FFP to replenish consumed factors:
  - Only if the patient is bleeding or there is a risk of bleeding
  - $<50 \times 10^9/l$ in presence of bleeding, and if $<10 \times 10^9/l$ without bleeding
  - Cryoprecipitate and fibrinogen possibly needed in high-risk patients
- Packed red cells may also be required if the haemolytic anaemia is severe.
- Early haematology advice and support is recommended.

EPIDURAL ANALGESIA

A 57-year-old woman is on your elective list for an open right hemicolectomy. The anaesthetic junior doctor has suggested to her that she have an epidural for postoperative analgesia. She is not sure whether she wants to have one and asks to discuss it with you. What is the epidural space?

- A fat-filled space in the spinal canal, just outside the dura

What are the indications for an epidural catheter?

- Adjunct to GA to reduce opioid requirements:
  - Thoracoabdominal, pelvic and leg surgery
- Sole technique for surgery (e.g., caesarean section)
- Analgesia (e.g., childbirth)
- Postoperative analgesia
- Flail chest—to improve ventilation pattern

What drugs are infused through an epidural, and what are their side effects?

- Local anaesthetic agents
- Opioids (e.g., fentanyl)—reduce LA requirement
- Clonidine, ketamine and magnesium (but rarely used)
- Side effects include:
  - Nausea and vomiting

- Pruritus
- Sedation
- Reduced sensation of needing to urinate (therefore need catheter)
- Delayed respiratory compromise (intercostal motor blockade)
- Respiratory centre depression
- Hypotension

How does an epidural work?

- Local anaesthetic blocks sensory afferent nerve roots and reduces transmission of pain:
  - It also causes a degree of SNS and motor blockade.
  - SNS block causes vasodilatation and hypotension (SNS chain runs from T1 to L2).
    - Reducing infusion rate may improve blood pressure:
  - A high T1-5 block affects SNS cardiac fibres, causing bradycardia, reduced stroke volume and further hypotension.
- Opioids modulate pain pathways by diffusing through dura into CSF to reach spinal cord opioid receptors.

What are the benefits of an epidural?

- Better analgesia—decreased oral opioid requirements
- Reduced respiratory problems postop
- Better GIT function (due to SNS blockade)
- Reduced DVT/PE risk—better blood flow and vasodilatation and a reduction in thrombogenic factors
- Decreased surgical stress response

What are the contraindications for siting an epidural?

- The contraindications may be divided into absolute and relative:
- Absolute:
  - Sepsis at planned site
  - Coagulopathy
  - Raised ICP
  - Patient refusal
- Relative
  - Anticoagulation
  - Systemic sepsis
  - Previous spinal surgery
  - Planned ITU sedation
  - Aortic stenosis (cannot tolerate resulting hypotension)

For patients on anticoagulant therapy, when can you insert and remove an epidural catheter?

- 4 hr after unfractionated heparin:
  - APTT checked prior to insertion/removal
- 12 hr after prophylactic low molecular weight heparin, and 24 hr after a treatment dose
- Platelets > 100
- INR < 1.5
- Aspirin is not a contraindication to insertion or removal

What are the complications of epidural catheters?

- Failure to achieve block or partial block:
  - Higher in obesity, multiparity, previous failure of epidural
  - For partial blocks—catheter withdrawn 1–2 cm, reposition patient and try increasing volume of infusion
- Dural puncture—total spinal block—get headache (1:100)
- Infection:
  - Can cause abscess with devastating CNS sequelae
    - MRI and removal of catheter
- Haematoma—urgent spinal decompression to prevent permanent CNS damage

What is the mechanism of hypotension in epidural and spinal anaesthesia and what is the treatment?

- The mechanism is blockade of the sympathetic outflow to the vasculature causing vasodilatation.
- The treatment is reduction of the epidural rate, if possible, colloids to increase blood volume and, rarely, vasoconstrictors.

FLUIDS

What are the average daily fluid and electrolyte requirements?

- Approximately 40 ml/kg/day of fluid
- Sodium: 1–2 mmol/kg/day
- Potassium: 0.5–1 mmol/kg/day

What are volumes and electrolyte concentrations of fluids secreted at different levels of the GI tract?

- Saliva: 1.5 l/day
- Gastric secretions: 2.5 l/day
- Bile/pancreatic secretions: 1 l/day
- Small intestine: 3 l/day

See Table 2.1.

TABLE 2.1
Concentrations of Electrolytes in Gastrointestinal Secretions (mmol/l)

	Plasma	Saliva	Gastric	Pancreas	Bile	Small intestine
Na^+	140	10	60	140	145	140
K^+	4	26	10	5	5	5
Cl^-	110	10	130	75	100	125–135
HCO_3^-	30	30	0	115	35	8–30

What electrolytes are contained in 1 l of Hartmann's solution?

- Sodium: 131 mmol
- Potassium: 5 mmol
- Chloride: 111 mmol
- Calcium: 2 mmol
- Bicarbonate: 29 mmol

What are the volumes of the fluid compartments of the body?

- Intracellular—28 l
- Extracellular—14 l:
  - Plasma—3 l
  - Interstitium—10 l
  - Transcellular—1 l

A patient has a high duodenal fistula following failed repair of a perforated duodenal ulcer. What are the daily fluid and electrolyte losses? Why do they occur?

- Patients can lose up to 4 l/day (saliva + gastric fluid).
- High concentration of excreted H^+ and chloride ions (hypochloraemia) leads to metabolic alkalosis.
- Develop hypokalaemia secondary to fistula losses.

What is your approach to fluid management for this patient?

- Ensure adequate hydration.
- Patient will need 6–8 l/day to replace fistula losses and cover maintenance fluid requirements.
- Replace electrolytes (mainly K and Cl), ideally via enteral route as World Health Organisation solution or double strength Dioralyte.
- Consider a proton pump inhibitor to decrease volume of gastric secretions and reduce chloride content of secretions.
- Consider loperamide to slow GI transit and delay gastric emptying.
- Strict daily input–output charting is essential.

See Table 2.2.

TABLE 2.2

Concentrations of Electrolytes in Oral Rehydration Solutions

	WHO solution	Dioralyte (single strength)
Na^+ (mmol/l)	75	60
K^+ (mmol/l)	20	20
Cl^- (mmol/l)	65	60
Glucose (mmol/l)	75	90
Citrate (mmol/l)	10	10

HAEMOSTASIS

What are the basic components of blood haemostasis?

- Balance between the coagulation, complement and fibrinolytic pathways, with complex interactions between plasma proteins, platelets, blood flow and viscosity, and the endothelium
- Essential requirements are:
  - Normal vascular endothelial function and tissue integrity
  - Normal platelet number and function
  - Normal amounts of the coagulation factors and their normal function
  - Presence of cofactors (e.g., vitamin K and calcium)

Describe coagulation.

- A haemostatic plug is formed at the site of a damaged vessel to control bleeding.
- The von Willebrand factor binds to the subendothelium—platelet activation, adhesion and generation of a platelet plug.
- There is a coagulation cascade—formation of strong fibrin mesh through the primary platelet plug. There is a sequence of enzymes and cofactors that generate thrombin, which cleaves fibrinogen to produce fibrin.
- Extrinsic pathway: VII is present in plasma, binds tissue factor in the presence of calcium. This catalyses the activation of factor VII, which then activates IX and X.
- Intrinsic pathway: kallikrein activates XII, in presence of kininogen, on damaged endothelium, which activates XI and IX.
- Both pathways activate IXa, which binds to cofactor VIIIa in the presence of calcium that activates factor X. Xa complexes with factor Va, phospholipid and calcium to form prothrombin complex, which converts prothrombin to thrombin.
- Thrombin cleaves fibrinogen releasing fibrin, activates XIII (responsible for cross-linking the fibrin polymer, rendering it resistant to fibrinolysis), and activates factors V and VIII, generating factors Va and VIIIa, which are cofactors for factors Xa and IXa.

What is the function of vitamin K?

- It carboxylates factors II, VII, IX and X, allowing them to bind to calcium and therefore the platelet surface.

What are the natural anticoagulant mechanisms?

- Antithrombin inhibits thrombin, factor Xa and other activated clotting factors.
- Protein C pathway degrades and inactivates factors Va and VIIIa, thereby blocking thrombin generation.
- Tissue factor pathway inhibitor inactivates Xa and VIIa.
- Plasmin causes fibrinolysis by degrading fibrin into fibrin degradation products. It also inactivates Va and VIIIa and disrupts platelet function. Plasminogen activators tPA and uPA activate plasminogen to produce plasmin.

What are the causes of coagulopathy in a surgical patient?

- Hypothermia causes platelet dysfunction.
- Massive blood transfusion: packed RBCs do not contain platelets, and stored blood rapidly loses the function of V and VII.
- Aspirin reduces platelet function by interfering with thromboxane A2 synthesis.
- Heparin directly interferes with clotting and can also lead to thrombocytopenia (HIT).
- Sepsis can lead to DIC.
- Postoperative acute renal or liver failure can occur.

How would you recognise coagulopathy in the surgical patient?

- Persisting small vessel bleeding intraoperatively, despite achieving adequate haemostasis
- Postoperative excess blood loss from the drains
- Purpuric rash—suggestive of platelet depletion
- Bleeding from unusual sites (e.g., cannulation sites), haematuria from uncomplicated catheterisation

How would you confirm a coagulopathy?

- The platelet count
- Bleeding time (3–8 min)—tests platelet function
- Prothrombin time (9–15 s)—testing extrinsic and common pathways and the degree of warfarinisation
- Activated partial thromboplastin time (30–40 s)—testing intrinsic and common pathways and heparin therapy
- Thrombin time (14–16 s)—testing final common pathway

- Individual factor assay
- Fibrin-degradation products when testing for DIC
- Thromboelastogram—providing the whole blood haemostasis testing for platelet and coagulation cascade disorders

HAEMOSTATIC AGENTS

A patient on warfarin presents with fresh rectal bleeding and an INR of 8. How will you correct his INR?

- If the patient is haemodynamically stable, and has only had a small rectal bleed, I would manage the patient with 1–3 mg IV vitamin K.
  - IV dosing works more quickly than oral vitamin K, and the INR should return to normal within 6–8 hr.
  - Large doses of vitamin K can make re-warfarinisation difficult.
- If the patient was unstable and had lost a lot of blood, I would contact the haematology consultant on call. The patient needs prothrombin complex concentrate (PCC; Beriplex/Octaplex) at 25–50 μ/kg.
  - Warfarin reduces levels of factors II, VII, IX and X, and PCC rapidly corrects this within 10 min.
  - The factors have a finite half-life, so 5 mg IV vitamin K is given at the same time.
  - FFP is no longer given; it has a dilute concentration of clotting factors, it is difficult to infuse in large volumes (15–30 ml/kg) rapidly and produces suboptimal anticoagulation reversal.

You are doing a trauma laparotomy on a patient who has been stabbed in the abdomen and has several lacerations to the large bowel mesentery with mesenteric and retroperitoneal haematomas. All the vessels have been tied or cauterised but the patient is still oozing. What else can be done to control the bleeding?

- Firstly, I would liaise with the anaesthetist.
  - Is the patient physiologically stable (normothermic, well transfused, not acidotic), or are we approaching a damage-control situation?
  - I would check the full blood count with coagulation parameters.
  - If necessary, I would instigate the massive transfusion protocol.
- To control intraoperative bleeding, there are three further options:
  - Argon beam coagulation
    - May help liver capsule bleeding but not available in every hospital
  - Topical agents to oozing sites
  - Haemostatic drugs

What topical haemostatic agents could you use?

- Fibrin sealants/glues (e.g., Crosseal):
  - Contain human fibrinogen and thrombin

- Form a stable fibrin clot; work best in a dry field
- Gelatin sealants (e.g., Floseal):
  - Gelatin matrix with calcium chloride and thrombin
  - Allow high concentrations of thrombin to react with patient's fibrinogen to form a stable clot. As blood flows through the matrix, the granules swell and cause a tamponade effect.
  - They need blood at the surgical field to work.
- Oxidised regenerated methylcellulose (e.g., Surgicel):
  - After topical application, they absorb blood, forming a gel over the bleeding vessel. Moisture triggers the release of cellulosic acid which lowers the topical pH and aids vasoconstriction.
  - The main action is providing a matrix for platelet adhesion.

What haemostatic drugs are available to control intraoperative bleeding?

- Desmopressin acetate (DDAVP) is a synthetic vasopressin analogue:
  - It stimulates release of factor VIII and von Willebrand factor into the plasma.
  - Generally, it is used in haemophiliacs prior to surgery.
  - It may help in patients on aspirin as it shortens the bleeding time in these patients.
- There are antifibrinolytic agents (aprotinin, tranexamic acid):
  - Aprotinin inhibits circulating plasmin, thrombin and activated protein C.
  - Tranexamic acid inhibits the conversion of plasminogen to plasmin and impairs fibrin dissolution. It is recommended for trauma patients with or at risk of significant bleeding, where it significantly reduces all-cause mortality. Loading dose of 1 g infused over 10 min within 8 hr of injury followed by maintenance infusion of 1 g over 8 hr (CRASH-2 RCT protocol).
- Recombinant activated factor VIIa:
  - It enhances the coagulation pathway by forming tissue factor–VIIa complexes at site of endothelial damage.
  - It is used in patients with haemophilia.
  - Its use in trauma is not supported by the literature; there is also a significant risk of arterial thrombosis.
  - Liaise with the haematologists before using factor VIIa.
  - Confirm that the platelets and clotting are within normal range.

HEPATORENAL SYNDROME

Your registrar admits a 37-year-old known alcoholic with vague abdominal discomfort, distension and jaundice. Her serum creatinine is elevated and your registrar is concerned that she has hepatorenal syndrome. What is hepatorenal syndrome (HRS)?

- HRS is the development of renal failure in patients with advanced chronic liver disease, portal hypertension and ascites
- At least 40% of patients with cirrhosis and ascites will develop HRS during the natural history of their disease.
- It is usually fatal unless a liver transplant is performed.
- There are two types:
  - Type 1—rapid, progressive decline in renal function, commonly due to spontaneous bacterial peritonitis; median survival < 2 weeks; majority of patients die within 10 weeks of onset
  - Type 2—moderate, stable reduction in renal function, associated with development of ascites that does not improve with diuretics; median survival of 3–6 months

What precipitates it?

- Infection (e.g., spontaneous bacterial peritonitis)
- Acute alcoholic hepatitis
- Bleeding in the gastrointestinal tract
- Overuse of diuretic medications
  - These cause a rapid deterioration in liver function.

How do you diagnose HRS?

- The diagnosis of HRS is one of exclusion.
- There is reduced GFR (creatinine > 150) in the absence of other causes of renal failure in patients with chronic liver disease.

What is the pathogenesis of HRS?

- Underfill theory
- Portal hypertension causing splanchnic vasodilatation (nitric oxide, prostaglandins)
- Causes reduced arterial blood volume and renal vasoconstriction via activation of renin–angiotensin–aldosterone axis
- Renal vasoconstriction insufficient to counteract splanchnic mediators
- Results in persistent underfilling and worsening renal vasoconstriction, and acute renal failure

How do you treat HRS?

- The only curative treatment is liver transplantation, but most patients die before a donor is found.
- Medical treatments:
  - Splanchnic vasoconstrictors (terlipressin)
  - Somatostatin analogues (octreotide)
  - Noradrenaline

- Surgical treatments:
  - Transjugular intrahepatic portosystemic shunt (TIPS)

HYPONATRAEMIA

What is hyponatraemia?

- Serum sodium < 135 mmol/l and low plasma osmolality < 280 mOsm/kg:
  - If serum osmolality is normal (280–300), this is pseudohyponatraemia (occurs in hyperglycaemia and hyperlipidaemia).
- Onset can be acute or chronic.
- Three main types:
  - Hypovolaemic—total body water decreases, total body sodium decreased to greater extent, ECF volume decreases.
  - Euvolaemic—total body water increases; total sodium remains normal. ECF volume is decreased
  - Hypervolaemic—total body sodium is increased; total body water increases to a greater extent. ECF volume increases markedly.

Your FY1 tells you that a postoperative elderly patient has a Na of 127 mmol/l. What do you do?

- Take a history—vomiting/diarrhoea/high stoma losses, drug history (e.g., diuretics), past medical history (adrenal disease, diabetes, etc.)—and review old blood tests for chronicity.
- Perform an examination—assess volume status (pulse, BP, JVP, urine output, mucous membranes, CRT, peripheral oedema), evidence of confusion/lethargy/seizures.
- Arrange blood and urine tests—FBC, U+Es, LFTs, glucose, serum and urine osmolality and urinary sodium.

What are the symptoms of hyponatraemia, and who is at risk?

- There is gradation from lethargy and anorexia to seizures and coma.
- Symptoms are often initially vague and nonspecific.
- They depend on degree of hyponatraemia and whether acute or chronic.
- Acute cases can present with coning due to cerebral oedema.
- Patients at risk include alcoholics, malnourished patients, elderly patients taking thiazide diuretics, burns patients, hypovolaemic patients.
- Symptoms depend on:
  - Rapidity of onset
  - Severity of low Na

What are the causes of hyponatraemia?

- Hypovolaemic:
  - Urinary sodium < 20 mEq/l—GI losses, third space losses, diuretics (late)
  - Urinary sodium > 20 mEq/l—renal loss, diuretics (early)

- Euvolaemic:
  - SIADH (urine osmolality > 200 mOsm/kg, urinary sodium > 20 mEq/l)
  - Hypothyroidism
  - Adrenal insufficiency
  - Iatrogenic administration of hypotonic fluids
  - Drugs (e.g., tramadol, selective serotonin reuptake inhibitors)
- Hypervolaemic:
  - Urinary sodium < 20 mEq/l—liver disease, heart failure
  - Urinary sodium > 20 mEq/l—renal failure

How is the serum sodium level regulated?

- Increase in serum osmolarity (>280–300 mOsm/kg) stimulates hypothalamic osmoreceptors, which cause thirst and an increase in ADH.
- ADH increases free water reabsorption from the urine (low volume, high osmolarity), returning serum osmolarity to normal.
- Aldosterone is released in response to hypovolemia through the renin–angiotensin–aldosterone axis. This causes absorption of sodium at the distal renal tubule, which encourages water retention.
- Hypovolemic states increase sodium absorption in the proximal tubule.
- Hypervolaemic states suppress tubular sodium reabsorption, resulting in natriuresis.

How do you treat hyponatraemia?

- Hypovolaemic—restore volume with isotonic saline:
  - Inhibits ADH secretion and corrects low Na
- Euvolaemic—restrict water and treat underlying disorder.
- Hypervolaemic—water restriction and diuretics
- In acute symptomatic cases:
  - Correct with hypertonic saline (1.8% or 3%) and 20 mg IV Frusemide.
  - Raise serum Na by 1–2 mmol/hr.
  - Do not raise by >10–12 mmol/24 hr.
- Treatment can cause central pontine myelinolysis if sodium is corrected too quickly. Risk is higher in alcoholic and malnourished patients.
  - Focal demyelination in the pons and extrapontine areas is associated with serious neurologic sequelae (irreversible).

INOTROPES AND MONITORING

What is an inotrope, and how would you classify it?

- An inotrope is a drug which increases myocardial contractility.
- There are three main types:
  - Catecholamines
  - Phosphodiesterase inhibitors

- Cardiac glycosides
- Others: calcium, aminophylline, levosimendan, glucagon
- Catecholamines are naturally occurring or synthetic:
  - They increase cAMP and intracellular Ca^{2+}.
  - Affinity for different subclasses of adrenergic receptor explains the range of clinical effects.
  - Stimulation of α receptors mediates vasoconstriction.
  - Stimulation of β_1 receptors improves myocardial contractility.
  - Stimulation of β_2 receptors increases heart rate.

See Table 2.3.

- Phosphodiesterase inhibitors inhibit breakdown of cAMP in myocytes:
  - They cause positive inotropism, ± vasodilatation (inodilators)
  - They include enoximone, milrinone and amrinone.
- Cardiac glycosides inhibit Na^+/K^+ ATPase in cell membranes.
  - The increase intracellular sodium concentrations, thus displacing bound intracellular calcium ions.
  - They decrease calcium outflow, raising calcium concentration.
  - An example is digoxin.

Would you use the same inotropes in cardiogenic and septic shock?

- No
- Cardiogenic shock involves low cardiac output, high filling pressures and high systemic vascular resistance (SVR):
  - Inodilators (phosphodiesterase inhibitors or dobutamine) improve contractility while also decreasing SVR.
  - Adrenaline is also appropriate as its predominant effect is on contractility.
  - Specific vasodilators such as GTN may decrease after-load and myocardial work.
- Septic shock is characterised by a low SVR and high cardiac output:
  - Vasoconstrictors such as noradrenaline increase SVR.
  - Dobutamine or adrenaline is sometimes used to improve contractility and oxygen delivery.

TABLE 2.3
Inotropes and Their Target Receptors

	α_1	α_2	β_1	β_2
Adrenaline	+++	+++	++++	+++
Noradrenaline	+++	+++	++	+
Isoprenaline			+++	++
Dobutamine	+	+	++++	++
Dopamine	++	+	++++	++

How does a transducer for arterial/central venous pressure work?

- Components of an invasive monitoring system include:
  - Intravascular catheter
  - Continuous column of fluid
  - Transducer—usually a strain gauge connected to a distensible diaphragm
  - Amplifier
  - Display
- Pressure wave is transmitted via the column of fluid to the diaphragm.
- Distension of the diaphragm affects an electrical signal through the strain gauge.
- This signal is amplified and converted to a graphical output on the display.

How can cardiac output be measured noninvasively?

- There are three techniques, and all rely on assumption or estimation:
- Analysis of an arterial pressure waveform (can be calibrated or uncalibrated)
  - Allows calculation of cardiovascular parameters (e.g., stroke volume, cardiac output, systemic vascular resistance).
  - Lidco, PiCCO monitors rely on analysis of the arterial waveform measured in a peripheral or central artery.
  - Uncalibrated monitors rely on inbuilt nomograms.
- Oesophageal Doppler monitor
  - Estimation of aortic valve area based on height/weight.
  - Probe estimates velocity of blood in descending thoracic aorta.
  - NICE recommended this in high-risk surgical patients to guide perioperative fluid and vasopressor management.
- Thoracic impedance techniques (now superseded by bioreactance).
  - Flow of current through thorax is affected by blood volume in thoracic aorta.

LEVELS OF CARE

How are the different levels of care available in hospital defined?

- Level 0:
  - Normal ward care
  - Less than 4 hourly observations
- Level 1:
  - At least 4 hourly observations
  - Requiring outreach support
  - Additional monitoring or interventions including:
    - Continuous oxygen
    - Epidural/PCA
    - Tracheostomy or chest drain in situ

- Level 2:
  - Receiving single organ support (excluding advanced respiratory support—i.e., mechanical ventilation)
  - Patients needing extended postoperative care
  - Patients stepping down from level 3
- Level 3
  - Advanced respiratory support
  - Support of two or more organ systems

Why is it important to know the level of care?

- The level of care needed is used to work out the safe levels of staffing for an intensive care unit.
- A single nurse may only care for one level 3 patient at a time.
- It may be possible for two level 2 patients to be cared for by the same nurse.
- The funding received by an intensive care unit could depend on the number of level 2 or level 3 patients.

Following a road traffic accident, a 20-year-old male with rib fractures has an intercostal drain for a haemothorax. He needed a laparotomy to control bleeding from a ruptured spleen. He is currently being monitored with an arterial line and is requiring an infusion of noradrenaline to maintain his blood pressure. What is an appropriate level of care for him postoperatively?

- Currently receiving two organ support measures (basic respiratory and cardiovascular)
- Qualifies as level 3—therefore HDU/ITU care
- High chance of deteriorating respiratory function after laparotomy (pulmonary contusions, rib fractures and the haemothorax)
- May require postoperative mechanical ventilation or noninvasive ventilation to maintain adequate oxygenation

How do you decide on the appropriate level of care for a patient postoperatively?

- Depends on patient and local factors
  - Local factors—some general wards cannot look after epidural infusions or central lines, so patients remain on the Critical Care Unit until the lines are removed
  - Patient factors—surgical, anaesthetic, patient related
  - Surgical factors:
    - Higher frequency of observations than can be provided on a general ward (e.g., free flap observations)
    - Drains (e.g., intercostal drains)
    - Need for continuous infusions (e.g., heparin, inotropes)
    - High risk of bleeding

- Prolonged or major surgery (e.g., AAA repair, Whipple's procedure)
- Anaesthetic factors:
  - Prolonged anaesthesia
  - Type of analgesia (epidural catheter)
  - Need for vasoactive drugs
- Patient factors
- Identified as high risk preoperatively due to comorbidities (e.g., high P-POSSUM score)

How would you assess a patient's fitness for major surgery?

- Take a history (e.g., exertional dyspnoea, ankle swelling, orthopnoea, history of atrial fibrillation, previous myocardial infarction or coronary intervention, previous stroke, diabetes, medication use).
- Examine the patient for signs of respiratory and cardiac disease (e.g., ankle oedema, lung crepitations on auscultation, etc.).
- CPEX testing has recently been introduced for these patients:
  - It is able to quantify surgical risk more accurately.
  - The patient rides an exercise bike whilst O_2 consumption and CO_2 production are measured.
  - A report with measure of anaerobic threshold (AT) is generated.
  - AT < 11 ml/kg/min = high-risk patient
  - The patient should be looked after on ICU postoperatively.

What is the most commonly used disease severity scoring system in the UK?

- The most commonly used is the APACHE score—the acute physiology and chronic health evaluation II system (APACHE II).
- It combines 12 physiological parameters with age and a chronic health score.
- Physiological parameters include temperature, blood pressure, heart rate, respiratory rate, oxygen therapy required, arterial pH, serum sodium, potassium, creatinine, packed cell volume, white cell count and neurological score.
- Data are entered on admission to intensive care and then reassessed after 24 hr.
- The resulting score provides an index of disease severity and risk of death.
- Predicted risk of death with an APACHE score > 40 is 100%.

LOCAL ANAESTHETICS

How do local anaesthetics work?

- They reversibly block neuronal transmission and stabilise electrically excitable membranes by two mechanisms:

- Sodium channel blockade—un-ionised lipid-soluble drug passes through the phospholipid membrane, becomes ionised and binds to the intracellular surface of fast sodium channels to prevent further depolarisation.
- Membrane expansion—un-ionised drug dissolves into the phospholipid membrane, expanding and disrupting the Na^+ channel/lipoprotein matrix and causing inactivation of the Na channel.

What are the different classes of local anaesthetics?

- Esters:
  - Cocaine, procaine, amethocaine
- Amides:
  - Lidocaine—short acting (2 hr for skin infiltration)
  - Prilocaine—highest therapeutic index, safest agent for intravenous blockade
  - Bupivacaine—longer acting than lidocaine (4 hr)
  - Levobupivicaine—now used extensively for local infiltration to minimise wound pain postoperatively; less vasodilatation and less motor block compared with bupivicaine; has a better cardiovascular toxicity profile compared to bupivacaine.
  - Ropivicaine—produces a better motor block compared to bupivicaine

What are the maximum doses of lidocaine and bupivacaine?

- Lidocaine: 3 mg/kg
- Lidocaine with adrenaline: 5–7 mg/kg
- Bupivicaine: 2 mg/kg
- Bupivicaine with adrenaline: 3 mg/kg

Why do we add adrenaline to local anaesthetics and when is it used?

- Adrenaline is a vasoconstricting agent.
- When mixed with local anaesthetics, it reduces the local anaesthetic absorption, prolongs block duration and reduces toxicity.
- Local vasoconstriction is also useful to the surgeon—blanching of the skin allows the surgeon to see exactly where the anaesthetic has infiltrated and it provides a more bloodless surgical field.
- It must not be used near end-arteries (e.g., digital blocks and penile surgery), as there is a risk of gangrene.

How much anaesthetic is in a 1% solution?

- In 1 ml of a 1% solution there are 10 mg of local anaesthetic.
- Likewise, 1 ml of 2% solution contains 20 mg.

How are local anaesthetics administered?

- Local infiltration
- Field blocks and nerve blocks (e.g., femoral nerve block for neck of femur fracture analgesia)
- Spinal anaesthesia—one-off, medium to short acting
- Epidural anaesthesia—longer acting, indwelling catheter
- Intravenous (e.g., Bier's block for manipulation of a Colles' fracture)

What are the complications of local anaesthetics?

- All related to their membrane-stabilising effects
- CNS—fitting, coma
- CVS—hypotension, cardiac arrhythmias, cardiac arrest

Why are local anaesthetics not as effective in areas of infection?

- Infection promotes an acidic environment in the tissues.
- Local anaesthetics penetrate the cell membrane in an un-ionised form.
- In an acidic environment, the molecules become ionised and cannot therefore penetrate the membrane and exert their effect.

MASSIVE BLOOD TRANSFUSION

A 56-year-old man is brought into A+E with a PR bleed. On examination, you find him pale and confused, with a pulse of 140 bpm, a BP of 70/30 and a large amount of fresh and clotted blood between his legs. How would you manage him?

- I would resuscitate him using an ABC protocol for assessment.
- I would ensure adequate ventilation and oxygenation. Insert at least two large bore cannulae for venous access, take routine bloods, including FBC, coagulation and cross-match, and commence monitoring.
- I would treat profound hypotension initially with warm crystalloid (1 l given as an IV bolus).
- Hypothermia, which increases the risk of end-organ failure and coagulopathy, should be avoided.
- If he is not responding to fluids, I would arrange a blood transfusion.
- Once stabilised, he needs an emergency upper GI endoscopy as a torrential bleed from a duodenal ulcer is the most likely source of blood loss.

His Hb comes back as 6 g/dl. What blood would you give him?

- Group-specific blood is usually available in 5–10 min and fully cross-matched blood in 30 min.
- I would initially give four units via fluid warmer, aiming for Hb > 8 g/dl.

- Blood loss of >40% blood volume is immediately life threatening. In this situation, I would give Group O Rh D negative if blood group were unknown.
- In cases of extreme blood loss or shortages in O RhD negative, blood group O RhD positive units may be given to all males and females beyond reproductive age (>60 years).

How would you define a massive blood transfusion?

- Massive transfusion is arbitrarily defined as replacement of a patient's entire circulating blood volume within a 24 hr period or half the blood volume in 3 hr or by a rate of loss of 150 ml/min.

Does your hospital have a protocol for massive blood loss?

- Yes and it is based on the British Committee for Standards in Haematology (BCSH) guidelines on the management of massive blood loss (2006).
- Goals are:
  - Maintenance of blood volume to ensure adequate tissue perfusion and oxygenation
  - Control of bleeding by surgical intervention and use of blood and blood component therapies or other pharmacological interventions to stem bleeding
- I would initiate it by contacting the blood transfusion service, senior members of clinical team (haematologist, theatres, anaesthetics and radiologists), senior ward nurses and portering services immediately for collaboration.

What else needs to be considered during a massive blood transfusion?

- There is a risk of coagulopathy after four units of blood replacement and continuing bleeding, and the patient would need platelets and FFP.
- I would prevent this by transfusing the massive blood loss (MBL) pack (PRBC: five units; FFP: four units).
- I would request a secondary MBL pack (PRBC five units, FFP four units, one pool platelets, two pools cryoprecipitate).
- FBC and coagulation samples sent after every five units of blood given.
- Hypothermia needs to be corrected.
- Hypocalcaemia needs to be corrected (keep ionised calcium > 1.13 mmol/l).
- I would contact haematologist/appropriate clinical team to stop bleeding.

What is the point of massive blood loss packs?

- To minimise the length of time needed to arrange blood products and treat patients in an efficient and timely manner, and to prevent development of coagulopathy

When do you consider giving platelets, FFP and cryoprecipitate in this scenario?

- Platelets should be kept >75 × 10⁹/l and should be administered in the presence of ongoing blood loss, or if interventional procedures are anticipated:
  - Anticipate platelet count is <50 × 10⁹/l after 2 × blood volume replacement.
  - Allow a safety margin to ensure platelet count > 50 × 10⁹/l.
  - Aim for platelet count > 100 × 10⁹/l if there is multiple or central nervous system trauma or if platelet function is abnormal.
  - Platelets are stored in a central facility, so their requirement should be anticipated well in advance.
- Fresh frozen plasma (FFP) (12–15 ml/kg) should be administered if prothrombin time is 1.5 times higher than normal.
  - PT and APTT values around 1.5 times mean values are associated with clinically significant coagulopathy and need to be corrected.
  - It should be anticipated if more than one circulating volume is transfused when fibrinogen levels fall initially with the critical level of 1 g/l.
  - A therapeutic dosage of FFP for a 70 kg adult would be three to four units.
- Cryoprecipitate is rarely needed except in DIC.
  - The need for cryoprecipitate after 1.5 times blood volume replacement needs to be anticipated.
  - Maintain fibrinogen > 1 g/l.
  - If it is not corrected by FFP, give cryoprecipitate (two pooled packs). Allow 30 min thawing time.

What are the potential complications of a massive blood transfusion?

- There can be volume overload leading to acute pulmonary oedema.
- Thrombocytopenia—following storage, there is a reduction of functioning platelets, causing a dilutional thrombocytopenia.
- Coagulation factor deficiency leads to a coagulopathy.
- Hypothermia is usually from shock due to loss of thermal regulation.
  - Rapid transfusion of blood at 4°C and a cold environment add to this, so the patient should always be kept warm and a blood warmer should be used when the infusion rate is above 50 ml/kg/hr.
- Tissue oxygenation is ineffective due to reduced levels of 2,3 DPG.
- Hypocalcaemia is due to chelation by the citrate in the additive solution. It may compound the coagulation defect:
  - Red cell units, FFP and platelets contain citrate anticoagulant, which lowers plasma calcium levels; this is problematic in patients with impaired liver function, hypothermic patients and neonates.
- Hyperkalaemia due to progressive potassium leakage from the stored red cells is possible.
- Metabolic acidosis—lactic acid and citrate present may contribute to metabolic acidosis.

- Transfusion-related lung injury (TRALI) can occur within 6 hr of transfusion.
    - 1/5,000 transfusions—six times more common following platelet or FFP transfusion
    - Immune mediated—human leukocyte (HLA) and human neutophil antigen (HNA) thought to be the cause
    - Blood from multiparous women is more likely to cause these reactions due to sensitisation from foetal blood allowing antibody formation
- Immunomodulation
- Infections—HIV, Hep B and C, CMV, prion diseases

What is cell salvage?

- This is the process of collecting blood from the surgical field and then filtering and washing it before it can be transfused back to the patient.
- Red blood cells are retained while plasma and platelets are discarded with the washing solution.
- It can decrease the allogenic transfusion requirements.
- Cell salvage is appropriate if significant blood loss is expected or if a patient is anaemic preoperatively. It may be acceptable to some Jehovah's Witnesses.
- Cell salvage has been used in surgery for some types of malignancy (urology) without an increased risk of recurrence.
- It can also be used safely in bowel surgery and obstetrics as long as fluid contaminated with bowel contents or amniotic fluid is not suctioned into the apparatus.
- Cell salvage machines have been used to wash bank blood prior to its use in cases of massive transfusion (e.g., liver transplant surgery). The potassium concentration in packed red cells available from a blood bank increases with increasing age of the unit of blood due to cell death. It can reach 20 mmol/l. By washing the blood prior to transfusion, the risks of hyperkalaemia can be reduced.

NOSOCOMIAL INFECTIONS

Why are nosocomial infections important?

- They are associated with increased morbidity, mortality, length of stay and costs
- They are more common in ICU patients than in those on the general wards.
- ICU patients have a higher incidence of respiratory, wound and bloodstream infections.

Describe the risk factors for nosocomial infection.

- Patient factors:
    - Illness severity
    - Underlying comorbidity (e.g., diabetes)

- • Poor nutritional state
- • Immunocompromised patients
- • Surgical wounds
- • Invasive devices
- • Mechanical ventilation
- • Prolonged antibiotic therapy or several courses
- • Environmental factors:
  - • Poor hand hygiene
  - • Inadequate space at bedside
  - • Inadequate staffing ratios
- • Organism factors:
  - • Antibiotic resistance
  - • Pathogenicity

What is a care bundle and how is one used to reduce the incidence of ventilator-associated pneumonia (VAP)?

- • A care bundle is a group of interventions that, when all applied together, reduce morbidity.
- • Mechanically ventilated patients recurrently aspirate small amounts of oro-pharyngeal secretions; the cuffs on tracheal tubes and tracheostomies cannot completely prevent this.
- • Organisms present in the digestive tract can colonise the trachea and bronchi and can cause clinically significant infection.
- • The ventilator care bundle aims to decrease the likelihood of VAP and limit the duration of mechanical ventilation. It includes:
  - • Maintaining the bed at 30°–45° head–up
  - • Oral decontamination with chlorhexidine and regular mouth care
  - • Maintaining tracheal cuff pressures of 20–30 cmH$_2$O
  - • Daily sedation hold
  - • DVT and stress ulcer prophylaxis
  - • Subglottic aspiration

How is the diagnosis of ventilator-associated pneumonia made?

- • The diagnosis of VAP is usually made with:
  - • Clinical signs of infection (e.g., pyrexia, raised WBC and CRP)
  - • New purulent sputum
  - • New infiltrates on CXR
  - • Positive cultures from blood or sputum
- • Pulmonary secretions are often colonised with bacteria. Not all positive cultures should be treated, as this could select resistant bacteria. The results can be used to guide antimicrobial choice in the event of progression to VAP.
- • Close liaison with the microbiology team is essential in identification and treatment of VAP.

What bacteria are typically responsible for VAP and how would you treat them?

- These are Gram-negative organisms including *Pseudomonas aeruginosa, Enterobacter* sp., *Klebsiella* and *E. coli.*
- Antimicrobial choice will depend on local patterns of resistance and should be guided by microbiology advice targeted to specific organisms.
- Some bacteria produce beta-lactamases, inducing resistance to several classes of antibiotic including fluoroquinolones, aminoglycosides and those containing β-lactam. These ESBL are often seen with *Klebsiella, Enterobacter* sp. and *E. coli* infections.

Describe the risk factors for central venous catheter (CVC) infection and methods that can be used to minimise these.

- Five to forty percent of central venous catheters are colonised with bacteria; this may occur without causing any morbidity.
- Catheter-related bloodstream infection is potentially difficult to diagnose and relies on growing the same bacteria from peripheral blood and the CVC in a patient with clinical signs of infection and no other apparent source.
- Risk factors include:
  - Site of insertion (femoral > internal jugular > subclavian)
  - Poor technique during insertion
  - Multilumen catheters
  - Poor hand hygiene or aseptic technique used when accessing catheters
  - Frequent dressing changes
  - Long duration of catheter
- Risks can be reduced by:
  - Using meticulous aseptic technique and 2% alcoholic chlorhexidine
  - Avoiding the femoral route if possible
  - Antiseptic (often silver-impregnated) or antimicrobial-impregnated catheters possibly to reduce the rate of colonisation and bloodstream infections
  - Review of catheters on a daily basis and removal if they are no longer required

What are the risk factors for developing a *Candida* infection on ICU?

- *Candida* species are common commensals on the skin, mouth, gut and genitals. They are mostly nonpathogenic but several risk factors have been identified:
  - Abdominal surgery
  - Central venous catheter
  - Parenteral nutrition
  - Multiple courses of antibiotics
  - Acute renal failure
  - Chronic hepatic failure

- Prolonged ICU stay
- *Candida* isolated from other sites

How is a clinically significant infection with *Candida* identified and how should it be treated?

- All isolates from blood should be considered important.
- Patients at risk with *Candida* isolated from two sites and clinical signs of infection should be presumed to have a clinically significant infection.
- Antifungal treatment should be based on the resistance profile of the organism, isolated and guided by local microbiological advice.
- Removal of existing intravascular catheters may reduce the duration of candidaemia.
- Fundoscopy should be performed as up to 15% of patients may have endophthalmitis associated with the candidaemia.
- Treatment should be continued for at least 14 days following the last negative blood culture

NUTRITION

Why is nutrition important to maintain in surgical patients?

- Malnutrition has several deleterious consequences:
    - Impairs wound healing
    - Prolongs requirements for mechanical ventilatory support
    - Increases infective complications

What are the pros and cons of enteral and parenteral (PN) feeding?

- Enteral feeding—pros:
    - Fewer infective complications than PN
    - Maintains normal integrity of gut mucosa
    - Attenuates physiological stress response to injury and surgery
    - Lower cost
- Enteral feeding—cons:
    - Difficulty meeting requirements due to poor absorption/ileus
    - Diarrhoea
    - Increased risk of ventilator-associated pneumonia and sinusitis
- Parenteral feeding—pros:
    - Easier to provide full energy requirements
    - Does not depend on gut integrity and function
- Parenteral feeding—cons:
    - Risk of access-related infections
    - Liver dysfunction
    - Trace element deficiency

What are the indications for parenteral nutrition?

- These are divided into absolute and relative.
- The only absolute indication is an enterocutaneous fistula where complete bowel rest is required to allow the fistula to close.
- Relative indications include:
    - Moderate or severe malnutrition
    - Severe inflammatory bowel disease
    - Abdominal sepsis
    - Acute pancreatitis
    - Trauma and burns
    - Prolonged ileus

What routes are available for total parenteral nutrition (TPN)?

- TPN may be administered centrally or peripherally.
- Central TPN is usually administered via a line in the internal jugular or subclavian vein.
- The advantage is that concentrated solution can be used.
- Up to 10% of TPN central lines develop complications (line sepsis, thrombosis, pneumothorax during placement, line breakage).
- Peripheral TPN is administered via a peripheral vein using a more dilute solution.
- The peripheral site needs to be changed every 48 hr and there is a high rate of thrombophlebitis

What is refeeding syndrome? Who is at greatest risk?

- This occurs when nutrition is recommenced after a period of starvation.
- Metabolic disturbances include hypophosphataemia, hypokalaemia and hypomagnesaemia.
- Insulin levels rise in response to glycaemia, causing cellular uptake of these ions (K, PO_4, Mg).
- Hypophosphataemia can deplete ATP and 2,3 DPG, causing cellular dysfunction that can cause respiratory and cardiac failure. Seizures have also been reported, as have renal and hepatic failures.
- Any patient with poor nutrient intake for 5 days is at risk of refeeding syndrome. Specific groups include:
    - Chronic alcoholics
    - Drug abusers
    - Chronically malnourished (e.g., the elderly)
    - Patients with anorexia nervosa
    - Patients who are nil by mouth for prolonged periods

What is the approach to feeding in a patient at risk of refeeding syndrome?

- Liaise with a dietician.
- Check baseline K/PO_4/Mg and replace as necessary.
- Start thiamine/multivitamins.
- Initiate feeding at low rate (e.g., 25%–50% target and check electrolytes every 6–12 hr).
- Achieving full feed may take 72 hr.
- Those patients at the highest risk (BMI < 14 and not fed for 15 days) should be monitored for cardiac arrhythmias on the critical care unit whilst feed is established.

What are the typical requirements for components of TPN?

- Fluid: 30 ml/kg/day
- Calories: 25–30 kcal/kg/day
- Protein: 1–2 g/kg/day
- Sodium: 1–2 mmol/kg/day
- Potassium: 1 mmol/kg/day
- Calcium: 0.1–0.3 mmol/kg/day
- Magnesium: 0.1–0.3 mmol/kg/day
- Energy should be approximately 30% lipid and 70% carbohydrate.

How should glycaemic control be managed on intensive care?

- Hyperglycaemia is common in critically ill patients due to insulin resistance as part of the stress response.
- Hyperglycaemia is associated with increased morbidity and mortality.
- Early studies from surgical intensive care units showed a mortality benefit with 'tight' glycaemic control (target range of 4.4–6.1 mmol/l).
- More recent studies in mixed intensive care populations have found that a more relaxed approach (target glucose < 10 mmol/l) is associated with a lower mortality and lower incidence of hypoglycaemia than the traditional 'tight' control.
- Hyperglycaemia on intensive care should therefore be treated to maintain a target blood glucose of <10 mmol/l.

ORGAN DONATION

What strategies are used to maximise organ donation?

- Early identification and optimal care of donors
- Careful assessment and procurement of organs
- Use of organs from marginal donors

What types of donors are used for solid organ donation?

- Solid organs for abdominal organ transplantation are donated by live and deceased donors.

- Despite increased numbers of live donors, the deceased donors continue to be the main course of allografts for transplantation.
- Deceased donors are divided into donation after brain-stem death (DBD) and after cardiac death (DCD).
- The non-heart-beating donors are grouped by Maastricht as follows:
  - I: Brought in dead—uncontrolled
  - II: Unsuccessful resuscitation—uncontrolled
  - III: Awaiting cardiac arrest—controlled
  - IV: Cardiac arrest after brain-stem death—controlled
  - V: Cardiac arrest in a hospital inpatient—uncontrolled

What are the selection criteria for cadaveric organ donation?

- All potential donors need to be considered for organ donation.
- Intensive care units must be encouraged to liaise with the specialist nurse for organ donation to facilitate discussion with the transplant centres.
- Contraindications vary based on the donated organ; they are AIDS (not HIV infection), Creutzfeldt–Jacob disease, malignancy within the last 5 years and grade IV CNS malignancy.
- Organs can be considered from donors in the following clinical states with appropriate caution and advice from the relevant clinical teams:
  - Active infection—need to gain information on the treatment received and appropriate advice from microbiologists. In cases with severe systemic fungal sepsis, a biopsy can be considered prior to transplantation.
  - Expanded criteria or marginal donors—age > 60 years, age 50–60 years with hypertension/creatinine > 133 μmol/l per cerebrovascular incident as the cause of death
  - CNS tumours—astrocytoma (grade IV), glioblastoma multiformae, intracranial sarcomas, malignant meninigiomas and lymphomas

What is a donor risk index?

- A donor risk index (DRI) is an objective evaluation with the premise that every donor has a definable risk which can be measured for each donor/recipient pair.
- There are DRIs for liver, pancreas and kidney allografts, which will assist the transplant team to quantify the potential outcome following transplantation.

OXYGEN DELIVERY

How is oxygen delivered to the patient?

- Oxygen delivery to the lungs depends on:
  - Patient airway
  - Concentration of inspired oxygen (FiO_2)
  - Adequate ventilation

- There are two key methods of delivery—variable and fixed performance devices.
- Variable devices:
  - Nasal cannulae
  - Face mask—a simple Hudson mask delivers an unreliable FiO_2 to the patient and its use should be avoided in the acute setting if at all possible
- Fixed performance devices (constant FiO_2):
  - Venturi mask
  - Reservoir bag—FiO_2 close to 0.7–0.8, mostly used in trauma
  - Continuous positive airway pressure (CPAP)—delivered by an airtight mask over the nose and mouth which provides a continuous positive pressure in the airways, thus splinting open alveoli and improving recruitment, reducing the work of breathing
  - Invasive ventilatory support

What is a Venturi connector?

- This is a reliable method of delivering a relatively constant FiO_2. The nozzle on the mask is designed to entrain air with oxygen and therefore delivers a specific FiO_2 depending on the nozzle used.
- It is essential, when using Venturi connectors, to ensure that the rate from the wall is the same as that printed on the connector.
- It relies on the Venturi effect—an example of Bernoulli's principle.
- Airflow through a tube with a constriction must speed up in the restriction, reducing its pressure and producing a partial vacuum. This vacuum encourages air to mix with the oxygen flow at a set rate, thereby setting the FiO_2.

How does a reservoir bag increase the FiO_2 given to a patient?

- The highest oxygen concentration that can be delivered on the ward is through a reservoir bag.
- As the flow of oxygen from the wall cannot match the flow generated by the patient, air mixes with each breath around the sides of the Hudson mask and through the holes in it.
- A mask with a reservoir bag must be close fitting and, with each breath, the extra air that cannot be supplied by the wall is supplied by the 100% oxygen in the reservoir bag, thus increasing the FiO_2.
- Despite this, a reservoir bag can still produce only around a 60%–70% FiO_2 as a result of imperfections in the fitting of the mask.

What are the potential complications of oxygen therapy?

- Absorption atelectasis—nitrogen is slowly absorbed, which splints the alveoli. High O_2 concentrations flush out the nitrogen and oxygen is absorbed rapidly, causing the alveoli to collapse.

- Pulmonary toxicity—oxygen can irritate the mucosa of the airways directly, leading to loss of surfactant and progressive fibrosis.
- Retinopathy is due to retrolenticular fibroplasia.
- There is a risk of fires and explosions.

POSTOPERATIVE ANALGESIA

What is the pain-relief ladder?

- This is a stepwise approach to controlling pain (WHO) where additional drugs are introduced until pain is fully controlled.
- The first step on the analgesic ladder is nonopioid drugs such as paracetamol or NSAIDs.
- If this is insufficient to control the pain, weak opioid drugs such as codeine and tramadol are added.
- The final step of the ladder involves the use of strong opioid drugs (e.g., Oramorph or morphine).
- At each step, the use of adjuvants (e.g., for anxiolysis) should be considered.
- If complete analgesia is not achieved with regular administration of drugs at one level, then the patient should move up one level.

What other drugs are used in conjunction with the analgesic ladder?

- Anxiolytics (e.g., diazepam)
- Antiemetics (e.g., cyclizine and ondansetron) to ease nausea and vomiting, especially with opioid drugs
- Gabapentin and amitriptyline—for neuropathic pain
- Steroids (e.g., dexamethasone and prednisolone) to improve the efficacy of analgesia, especially for the terminally ill patient

What is PCA and how does it work?

- Patient-controlled analgesia allows the patient to administer intravenous analgesia when needed and avoids waiting for nurses to give medication.
- The patient is given an initial loading dose to provide adequate analgesia.
- The patient then self-administers bolus doses—the minimum dose needed for analgesia consistently without producing side effects (usually 1 mg for morphine).
- There is a lockout interval when the pump will not administer a further dose, to prevent overdosing (usually 5 min).

What are the advantages and disadvantages of a PCA?

- Advantages:
  - It frees the nurses for other ward work.
  - It empowers patients to have control over their pain and helps to alleviate anxiety, which in turn reduces pain experience.

- It is immediate and effective.
- No injection is required, so there is no pain from the actual injection itself.
- Disadvantages:
  - The button can be accidentally pressed, delivering an unneeded dose of the medication.
  - Incorrect setup of loading dose and lock-out can lead to inadequate pain relief or overdose.

PRINCIPLES OF GENERAL ANAESTHESIA

What are the three components of general anaesthesia?

- Hypnosis (unconsciousness)
- Analgesia
- Muscle relaxation
- Each patient requires a balance of the three components depending on both patient and surgical factors:
  - A patient having a midline laparotomy will require muscle relaxation, large amounts of analgesia and hypnosis.
  - On the other hand, patients having a rigid cystoscopy may not need muscle relaxation.

What hypnotic agents are available?

- Intravenous agents—propofol, thiopentone, ketamine, etomidate:
  - Given as bolus to induce anaesthesia
  - Some (propofol) also used as infusion for maintenance of anaesthesia or sedation
  - Dose based on weight but also clinical effect—elderly/unwell will need less
  - Cause depression of airway reflexes, respiration and cardiovascular system
- Volatile agents—isoflurane, sevoflurane, desflurane, halothane:
  - Mostly used for maintenance of anaesthesia as irritant to the airway (sevoflurane and halothane are the exceptions)
  - Uncertain mechanism of action—likely at reticular activating system
  - Also cause depression of airway reflexes, respiration and cardiovascular system

What opioids are used in anaesthesia?

- A range of opioids with differing potency, onset times and duration of action is available.
- Most are subject to hepatic metabolism and renal excretion (accumulate in renal failure).

- Some (morphine/codeine) have active metabolites.
- They cause dose-dependent respiratory depression, as well as cardiovascular depression:
- Remifentanil—ultrashort-acting synthetic opioid:
  - Metabolism by plasma esterases which are unaffected by hepatic/renal disease
  - Used for intraoperative suppression of sympathetic stimulation
  - Does not provide any postoperative analgesia.
- Fentanyl—100 times potency of morphine:
  - Typically used at induction of anaesthesia
  - Can be used in PCA or as transdermal application for pain postoperatively
- Morphine—most commonly used drug for postoperative pain either as PCA or intermittent IV/oral doses

What drugs provide muscle relaxation under anaesthesia?

- Depolarising neuromuscular blockers (e.g., suxamethonium):
  - Short onset (45 s), short offset (4–5 min)
  - Causes depolarisation (muscles seen to twitch)
  - Noncompetitive blockade
  - Broken down by plasma cholinesterases
  - Abnormal cholinesterase activity and prolonged block (10 min–4 hr) for approximately 5% of population
- Nondepolarising neuromuscular blockers (e.g., atracurium, rocuronium, vecuronium)
  - Longer onset and offset (15–45 min), which are dependent on dose administered
  - Competitive blockade—actions overcome by increased acetylcholine at neuromuscular junction
  - Can be reversed by administering acetylcholinesterase inhibitors (e.g., neostigmine)

What is postoperative nausea and vomiting?

- It is nausea and/or vomiting within 24 hr of surgery.
- The aetiology is unclear but may be related to surgical, anaesthetic and patient factors.
- Patient factors include female gender, nonsmoker, previous history of PONV and history of motion sickness.
- Anaesthetic factors include use of volatile agents, large amounts of neostigmine, nitrous oxide and opioids.
- Surgical factors include duration of surgery and type (gynaecological and urological).

What mechanism controls the vomiting reflex?

- The vomiting centre is located in the medulla.
- The vomiting reflex may be triggered by any of five afferent pathways:
  - Chemoreceptor triggering zone
  - Vagal mucosal pathway in the GI tract
  - Neuronal pathways from the vestibular system
  - Reflex afferents from the cerebral cortex
  - Afferents from the midbrain

PULSE OXIMETRY

How does pulse oximetry work?

- Oxygenated and deoxygenated haemoglobin optimally reflect different wavelengths of incident light.
- The pulse oximeter uses two different light-emitting diodes at two wavelengths:
  - 660 nm (red light)—measures total amount of haemoglobin
  - 940 nm (infrared light)—measures oxygenated haemoglobin
- A percentage of saturated haemoglobin is calculated from a ratio of the two.
- The pulse oximeter then displays the percentage oxygen saturation of the arterial blood (SaO_2).
- A probe is attached to a finger or ear lobe.
- Some probes can also estimate pulse volume.

How do you interpret a pulse oximeter SaO_2 or ABG PaO_2 reading?

- SaO_2 and PaO_2 are meaningless without knowledge of the FiO_2 (concentration of inspired oxygen).
- A normal PaO_2 in room air (FiO_2 21%) is 12 kPa.
- The ratio of PaO_2 to FiO_2 should be around 0.6.
- A PaO_2 of 12 in a patient with a FiO_2 of 40% is clearly hypoxic (12/40 = 0.3). His PaO_2 should be 24.
- The PaO_2 has a nonlinear relationship to SaO_2, although the two are often confused.
- SaO_2 can be normal despite a low PaO_2 in acute pulmonary embolus, reinforcing the need for ABGs in acute respiratory failure.
- It must be remembered that pulse oximetry does not assess ventilation.
- End-tidal CO_2 and capnography must also be measured.

What does oxygen delivery depend on?

- Haemoglobin concentration
- Cardiac output
- Oxygen saturation (SaO_2)

- A drop in SaO_2 is picked up more quickly with pulse oximetry than with clinical observation for peripheral cyanosis:
  - SaO_2 must drop to 60%–70% before cyanosis is observed.
  - $DO_2 = CO \times [(1.39 \times Hb \times SpO_2) + paO_2 \times 0.003)]$.

What are the pitfalls and sources of error in pulse oximetry?

- Cold peripheries and poor tissue perfusion can lead to an inability of the pulse oximeter to get a reading.
- Abnormal pulses such as atrial fibrillation and tricuspid regurgitation can affect the reading because the signal is averaged over a number of heartbeats.
- Changes to Hb or pigments in the blood:
  - CO poisoning in fire victims and smokers (CO binds haemoglobin and changes its light reflectance properties to that of oxyhaemoglobin; thus, SaO_2 is reported as erroneously high despite a low O_2 saturation displaced by the CO.)
  - High bilirubin levels cause the pulse oximeter to underestimate the true SaO_2.
  - Methaemoglobinaemia
- Delay—SaO_2 is calculated over a number of heartbeats, so there is approximately a 20 s lag between physiological values and SaO_2 recording.
- Nail varnish prevents penetration of light and must be removed preoperatively.
- There can be electrical interference from diathermy.
- High ambient light can interfere with the incident light from the pulse oximeter.
- Movement/shivering can affect the signal.

What is methaemoglobin and how does its presence in the blood affect a pulse oximeter?

- Methaemoglobin (Met-Hb) has iron in a ferric state (Fe^{3+}) within the haem moiety instead of the ferrous state (Fe^{2+}), as in normal haemoglobin.
- Therefore, the Met-Hb molecule has a reduced oxygen-carrying capacity.
- It can be congenital—deficiency of Met-Hb-reducing enzymes (NADH methaemoglobin reductase) or acquired—result of nitrate pollution in the water supply or use of the local anaesthetic agent prilocaine.
- Treatment is by administration of a reducing agent such as methylene blue.

RESPIRATORY FAILURE

Define respiratory failure.

- An arterial pO_2 (at sea level, breathing air, at rest) < 8 kPa.
- There are two types:
  - Type 1—hypoxaemic respiratory failure:
    - Usually due to V/Q mismatch
    - Often associated with low $PaCO_2$ due to hyperventilation as a response to hypoxaemia

- – Caused by chest infection, PE, asthma, pulmonary oedema, ARDS, aspiration pneumonitis
- Type 2—hypercapnic respiratory failure/ventilatory failure
  - – Hypoxaemia with arterial PCO_2 exceeding 6.5 kPa
  - – Caused by hypoventilation
  - – Decreased central drive (e.g., opioids, anaesthetic agents, intracranial pathology, sleep apnoea)
  - – Impaired peripheral mechanism of breathing (e.g., airway obstruction, COPD exacerbation, restriction due to pain/obesity/ascites)
- Can also occur when patient with type 1 respiratory failure is exhausted by compensatory hyperventilation—a very bad sign

What are the indications for tracheal intubation?

- Airway obstruction
- Airway protection
- Unconscious patients or those with impaired laryngeal reflexes
  - Prevent soiling by blood or gastric contents
  - Airway toilet—facilitate aspiration of secretions/sputum
  - To facilitate mechanical ventilation
  - Anaesthesia
  - When muscle relaxation or mechanical ventilation is required
  - Prolonged surgery
  - Prone positioning

What is the aim of mechanical ventilation in intensive care? What harm can it cause and how is this minimised?

- The main principles are to maintain oxygenation and satisfactorily clear carbon dioxide.
- Ventilation can cause harm by:
  - Repeated opening and closing of alveoli (atelectrauma)
  - Overdistension of alveoli (volutrauma)
  - High pressure within alveoli (barotrauma)
- These can be minimised by:
  - Positive end-expiratory pressure (PEEP) to increase functional residual capacity (FRC)
  - Limiting tidal volumes to 6–8 ml/kg ideal body weight
  - Limiting peak airway pressures to <30 cm H_2O
- Oxygenation is mainly a function of inspired oxygen concentration and mean airway pressure and is improved by:
  - Increasing FiO_2
  - Increasing PEEP
  - Increasing inspiratory time (increases mean airway pressure)
  - Increasing inspiratory pressure in severe hypoxia

- Carbon dioxide elimination is mainly a function of alveolar ventilation and is improved by:
  - Increasing respiratory rate
  - Increasing tidal volume

Define a flail chest and describe the principles of managing a patient with a flail segment.

- This is disruption of chest wall integrity.
- A part of the bony thoracic cage is detached from the rest.
- This flail segment is able paradoxically to move inward on inspiration due to negative intrathoracic pressure.
  - At least two rib fractures are needed at two different places.
- It can occur secondary to thoracic trauma with multiple fractures involving several ribs.
- Problems include:
  - Hypoventilation (due to chest wall mechanics and pain)
  - Underlying pulmonary contusion or pneumothorax
- Management includes:
  - Supplementary oxygen (humidified if possible)
  - Satisfactory analgesia (can include opioids/intercostal nerve blocks/ epidural)
  - Chest drainage if required
  - Physiotherapy (aid clearance of secretions and re-expand atelectatic lung)
  - Continuous positive airway pressure (CPAP) or tracheal intubation if unsatisfactory arterial blood gases with preceding measures
  - Possible surgical fixation
- Complications include sputum retention, infection, poor nutrition (often due to gastric stasis).

What is CPAP and how does it improve oxygenation?

- CPAP is the application of positive airway pressure throughout all phases of respiration.
- Gas flow delivered must exceed peak inspiratory flow (can be up to 60l/ min).
- Gas is delivered to patient via nasal/face mask or hood.
- The seal must be such that patient can only breathe in from respiratory circuit.
- CPAP has several positive effects on ventilation:
  - It increases functional residual capacity by recruiting areas of atelectasis. This reduces work of breathing and improves oxygenation due to decreased shunt.
  - It increases pulmonary lymphatic flow—allows the lung to clear pulmonary oedema.
  - It improves mechanical function of the heart in cardiogenic pulmonary oedema to prevent further fluid buildup.

- Indications for CPAP include:
  - Hypoxaemic respiratory failure
  - Pulmonary oedema
  - Sleep apnoea

What are the risk factors for postoperative respiratory failure?

- Patient factors:
  - Pre-existing respiratory disease
  - Smoking
  - Obesity
  - Immunosuppression
- Surgical factors:
  - Emergency surgery
  - Thoracic/upper abdominal surgery

How do we monitor respiratory function?

- Respiratory rate
- Oxygen requirements (increasing FiO_2)
- Conscious level
- Blood gas analysis

What are the clinical indicators for failure of respiratory therapy?

- Increasing respiratory rate > 30/min
- Increasing oxygen requirements to maintain SaO_2
- Pa O_2 < 8 kPa
- $PaCO_2$ > 6.5 kPa with respiratory acidosis
- Dyspnoea/exhaustion/confusion or low GCS

SYSTEMIC RESPONSE TO SURGERY

How does the body respond to a surgical insult?

- Sympathetic nervous system activation due to pain and/or hypovolaemia:
  - Increase in cardiovascular output due to an increase in circulating adrenaline (tachycardia) and noradrenaline (peripheral vasoconstriction)
  - Aids activation of glycolysis in the liver and the renin–angiotensin–aldosterone axis
- Endocrine response:
  - ACTH production stimulated which, in turn, stimulates glucocorticoid release—predominantly cortisol (see following)
- Acute phase response:
  - Cytokines released by circulating monocytes and lymphocytes
  - Kinins, interleukins, TNF and interferons released—cause postoperative fever and further increase metabolic demand

- ACTH release further enhanced
- Clotting cascade activated
- Serum levels of acute phase proteins increase (CRP, fibrinogen, complement C3, ceruloplasmin and haptoglobin)
- Liver down-regulates albumin and transferrin production
- Vascular endothelium response:
  - Able to affect local vasomotor tone (via nitric oxide) and local coagulation
  - Can affect systemic response by modulation of platelet and leukocyte binding

What is the metabolic response to surgery or trauma?

- Ebb phase—reduced energy expenditure after injury for the first 24 hr and therefore a reduction in the metabolic rate
- Flow phase—dramatic increase in the metabolic rate and this catabolic state can last many days with associated negative nitrogen balance and impaired glucose tolerance:
  - Immediately after abdominal surgery, most patients are nil by mouth and therefore starvation and the response to trauma are both responsible for this catabolic state.
  - There is increased heat production in this phase, along with increased oxygen consumption and weight loss. The overall duration and increase in metabolic rate in the 'flow' phase depend on the type of stimulus:
    - 10% increase in elective surgical operations
    - 50% increase in polytrauma
    - 200% in major burns
  - Once the 'flow' phase has begun, correction of the underlying stimulus (e.g., controlling infection, correcting hypovolaemia, controlling pain) does not rapidly reverse the metabolic condition of the patient.
  - Finally, if recovery occurs, an anabolic phase occurs where the body replaces its fat and glycogen reserves and synthesises more protein.
  - Clearly this has a major implication for postoperative nutrition, where calculated daily required nutrition must take into account the extent and severity of the 'flow' metabolic phase of the patient.

How are lipids mobilised after trauma?

- Lipids are the principal source of energy after trauma.
- Lipolysis is stimulated by the sympathetic nervous system, ACTH, cortisol, decreased serum insulin levels and glucagon.
- Ketones are released and oxidised by all tissues except blood and brain.
- Free fatty acids and glycerol undergo gluconeogenesis in the liver to provide energy for all tissues.

How is carbohydrate metabolism affected by trauma?

- Insulin levels decrease and glucagon levels increase, mobilising glycogen stores and initiating glycolysis to create a transient hyperglycaemia.
- Increased glucocorticoid levels also result in insulin resistance of the tissues, thereby potentiating the effect.
- Glycolysis releases energy for obligate tissue (CNS, leukocytes and red blood cells—cells that do not require insulin for glucose transport).
  - This is a very important mechanism because in a serious injury or after major surgery, leukocytes can account for 70% of all glucose uptake.
- Body glycogen stores last for about 24 hr, after which blood glucose must be maintained by other methods:
  - Gluconeogenesis of lipid breakdown products
  - Gluconeogenesis of amino acids mobilised from protein breakdown

How is protein metabolism affected by trauma?

- Suppressed insulin levels encourage the release of amino acids from skeletal muscle.
- A three- to fourfold increase in serum amino acids is usually required after major trauma.
- The requirement reaches a peak at a week after injury, although it may continue for many days after this.
- In the absence of a constant exogenous supply of protein, the entire nitrogen requirement is gained from the skeletal muscle.
- The extent of the nitrogen requirement is directly proportional to the extent of injury (including trauma and sepsis) and the muscle bulk.
- Major protein loss results in endothelial dysfunction and atrophy of the intestinal mucosa, removing the barrier to translocation of pathogenic bacteria.
- A loss of over 40% of body protein is usually fatal.

Why is urine output often low in the first 24 hr after surgery?

- After trauma, the activation of the renin–angiotensin–aldosterone axis and the increase in ADH secretion lead to a retention of sodium and water at the expense of potassium.
- Although the total body sodium may be elevated, a dilutional hyponatraemia is not uncommon with an excess of serum ADH, leading to greater water than sodium retention.
- Furthermore, in catabolic cells with a degree of energy failure, sodium pumps are impaired, so sodium tends to drift into cells and thereby further decrease the plasma sodium concentration.

- This sodium and water retention leads to a low urine output (despite adequate filling) in the first 24 hr after surgery
- Although the water retention lasts for only 24 hr, the sodium retention may persist for much longer.
- A postoperative ileus promotes fluid extravasation into the gut lumen and intravascular depletion, leading to dehydration and further compounding the oliguria.
- The most common acid–base imbalance is a metabolic alkalosis because aldosterone promotes sodium retention at the expense of potassium. As potassium is excreted, so are H^+ ions in a cotransporter mechanism, leading to an alkalosis.
- In severe trauma, a metabolic acidosis can result due to increased production of lactic acid caused by poor tissue perfusion and anaerobic metabolism.

How might the systemic response to surgery be minimised?

- Preoperative factors:
  - Minimise fear and stress (informed consent and clear, concise explanation, pre-med anxiolytic if necessary) to reduce sympathetic activity
  - High-protein load preoperative nutrition; enteral feeding if possible before period of nil by mouth required for gastric emptying
  - Correction and control of preoperative infection
- Operative factors:
  - Good tissue handling
  - Minimally invasive surgery/minimal trauma
  - Shorten duration of anaesthesia
- Postoperative factors:
  - Correction of hypovolaemia
  - Prompt replacement of fluids and electrolytes
  - Transfusion for haemorrhage if necessary
  - Colloids for plasma loss
  - Correction of metabolic alkalosis/acidosis
  - Control of postoperative infection
    - Antibiotics
    - Enteral feeding as soon as possible to maintain gut mucosal barrier
    - Debriding wounds, draining pus, etc.
  - Effective pain control (reduces sympathetic activation and splinting/ hypoxia and their effects)
  - Correction of hypoxia
  - Increased arginine and glutamine intake can help improve nitrogen balance, encourage weight gain, wound healing and immune function
  - Trace elements such as zinc to improve wound healing

TRACHEOSTOMY

What are the types of surgical airways?

- There are three types of surgical airways:
  - Needle cricothyroidotomy with jet insufflation of oxygen
  - Cricothyroidotomy
  - Tracheostomy

How is jet insufflation of oxygen performed, and what is the main precaution to be considered?

- A large-bore intravenous cannula is passed through the median cricothyroid ligament.
- It is connected to a source of oxygen (e.g., jet ventilator/manujet) via a tracheal tube connector.
- The patient receives oxygen for 1 s and expires for 4 s.
- The patient is well oxygenated but poorly ventilated, leading to progressive hypercarbia.
- In consequence, its use should be limited to a 45 min period to allow time for a definitive airway to be established.

What are the indications for a tracheostomy?

- Airway obstruction (facial/neck/laryngeal trauma, head and neck tumours)
- Failed intubation/respiratory insufficiency
- Trauma to larynx
- Infection: acute epiglottis
- Long-term management of a ventilated patient (most common reason)
- Failed extubation in intensive care
- Chest injury (flail chest)
- Congenital (e.g., laryngeal cysts, tracheo-oesophageal anomalies)
- Bilateral vocal fold paralysis

What are the types of tracheostomies?

- Percutaneous and minitracheostomies
- Temporary and permanent
- Usually performed as an elective procedure due to the time taken; in the emergency setting, a cricothyroidotomy is quicker and safer to perform
- Percutaneous tracheostomy:
  - This can be done in the intensive care setting under local anaesthetic.
  - A 14G cannula is inserted with a guide wire with subsequent serial dilatation. Various types of tracheostomy sets are available for percutaneous tracheostomy.
  - The advantages include avoiding patient transfer and slightly reduced incidence of haemorrhage and infection.

- Minitracheostomy:
  - A small tracheostomy tube is placed through the cricothyroid membrane to aid bronchial toileting and aspiration of secretions.
  - This is not a definitive airway, because the tube is not cuffed.

How would you perform a tracheostomy?

For an elective tracheostomy:

- Position the patient supine with neck extended.
- Perform under general anaesthetic and intubation.
- Make a transverse incision 2 cm below cricoid cartilage.
- Deepen the incision and extend between strap muscles.
- Retract or divide thyroid isthmus.
- Recheck size of cuffed tube to be placed.
- Feel for first tracheal ring.
- Make a vertical incision through the second and third tracheal rings:
  - Damage to the first tracheal ring may result in subglottic stenosis; lower placement risks tracheo-innominate fistula.
- The anaesthetist should be asked to withdraw the endotracheal tube to above the incision and be ready to change the ventilator to the tracheostomy and then withdraw the endotracheal tube.
- Aspirate trachea.
- Insert tracheal dilator or cuffed tube to secure airway.
- Closure: skin edges are closed loosely, tapes to secure tube.

How would you manage a tracheostomy postoperatively?

- Nurse upright.
- Check for breath sounds on both sides of the chest and capnography trace.
- Check ventilator settings and tidal volumes.
- Confirm position with CXR.
- Suction as required.
- Use humidified oxygen
- Mucolytic agents are sometimes used.
- Monitor for bleeding and tracheostomy cuff leak.

What are the potential complications of performing a tracheostomy?

- Immediate:
  - Asphyxia
  - Pneumothorax
  - Haemorrhage or haematoma
  - Cricoid cartilage injury
  - Damage to the oesophagus

- Early:
  - Aspiration
  - Obstruction
  - Cellulitis
  - Tracheitis
  - Mucus plugging
  - Malpositioned tube
  - Creation of a false tract
  - Subcutaneous emphysema
- Late:
  - Delayed haemorrhage—usually secondary to tracheo-innominate fistula—occurs >48 hr postoperatively.
  - Vocal fold palsy
  - Atelectasis and bronchopneumonia
  - Tracheocutaneous or tracheo-oesophageal fistula
  - Subglottic stenosis
  - Tracheomalacia
  - Tracheal stenosis
  - Difficult decannulation

Which anatomical structure is at high risk of damage when a tracheostomy is performed on a child?

- The innominate vein is at high risk because it lies high on the trachea.

REFERENCE

1. *ATLS manual,* 8th ed. 2008. Standards and strategy for burn care. National Burn Care Review Committee (http://www.britishburnassociation.org/downloads/NBCR2001.pdf). Chicago, IL: American College of Surgeons.

3 Emergency Surgery

Elizabeth Ball, Nicole Keong, Dermot O'Riordan, C J Shukla, Tjun Tang, Colin Walsh and Stewart Walsh

CONTENTS

ACUTE LEG ISCHAEMIA

You are called to the emergency department. A 75-year-old man has been referred by his GP with sudden onset leg pain. What are you going to do?

- Take a history—when did the pain start, how severe is it, what makes it better, what makes it worse, what is the pain like, ever had it before, is it constant, does it radiate? Smoker? Heart problems? Previous leg surgery? Recent operations?
- Examine the patient—regular pulse? Pale leg? Pulses present?

His leg is pale and cool and you cannot feel any pulses below the femoral. What else do you need to know?

- Is sensation intact?
- Can he move his leg?
- Has he got pulses on the other side?

His leg is insensate and paralysed. He has a full set of pulses on the other side. What are you going to do?

- The presence of a full set of contralateral pulses implies that this is most likely an embolic rather than a thrombotic event.
- Sources include emboli secondary to cardiac arrhythmia, mural thrombosis, vegetations, cardiac tumours or from proximal aneurysms; arterial dissection.
- A paralysed, insensate leg indicates end-stage ischaemia. Assuming there is no fixed staining to indicate tissue death, revascularisation would be indicated.
- Options are a surgical embolectomy or thrombolysis.
- Given the presence of paralysis and loss of sensation, I would proceed immediately to a femoral embolectomy as his leg will not survive long enough for thrombolysis to work.

What is thrombolysis?

- This is a mode of therapy in which a clot is actively broken down—most commonly, pharmacologically although mechanical thrombolysis is occasionally an option. It differs from anticoagulation (e.g., with heparin), which simply prevents further clot formation and allows the body's inherent thrombolytic mechanisms to break down the existing clot.

- Most thrombolytic agents work by activating plasminogen, which then breaks down fibrin.
- Available agents include tissue plasminogen activator, streptokinase, urokinase, and alteplase.
- Their efficacy can be improved by direct intra-arterial administration and also by pulse-wave application of agent to the clot.
- Small clots may be lysed by mechanical means—thrombectomy catheters or pulsed jet lavage.

What is the half-life of streptokinase?

- Streptokinase has a biphasic half-life.
- There is an initial rapid half-life of 16 min and a slower half-life of 90 min.

What are the disadvantages of thrombolysis?

- It may take too long to salvage a severely ischaemic leg.
- There are several contraindications, including recent trauma/surgery, recent stroke, any intracranial bleed in the past, suspected dissection, thrombocytopaemia, known aneurysms, uncontrolled hypertension.
- There are high rates of reocclusion unless underlying culprit lesions are adequately treated.

You take this patient to theatre. What are you going to do?

- He needs to have a femoral embolectomy and fasciotomies as he is at high risk for compartment syndrome.
- Make the lower limb fasciotomies first, decompressing all four compartments of the lower leg and checking the viability of the muscle using diathermy. Living muscle will twitch. If all the muscle is dead, revascularisation is likely to result in a fatal washout of toxic metabolites.
- Assuming the muscle is viable, proceed to a femoral embolectomy.

Talk me through your approach to a femoral embolectomy.

- Make an axial incision over the femoral artery at the groin, commencing proximally at the inferior edge of the inguinal ligament.
- Then, identify and sling the common, profunda and superficial femoral arteries.
- Ensure that the patient has had 5,000 units of heparin.
- After the heparin has circulated for 2 min, clamp the arteries.
- Make a transverse arteriotomy on the anterior surface of the common femoral artery just proximal to the origin of the profunda femoris.

- Check the inflow; audible inflow is acceptable.
- Check for profunda backbleeding; if there is none, then pass a 3 Fogarty along the profunda and remove any clot.
- Then, check the superficial femoral artery for backbleeding and pass a number 3 Fogarty all the way to the ankle if possible. Inflate the balloon using gentle pressure and stop at the first sign of resistance. Extract the catheter slowly, controlling balloon inflation as this is done, removing distal embolus.
- Repeat the procedure until there are several consecutive passes free of clot, and then flush heparinised saline into the superficial femoral artery and reclamp. Recheck the inflow and the profunda back-bleeding.
- Close the arteriotomy with interrupted 5/0 prolene sutures.
- Warn anaesthetist prior to releasing clamps.
- If there are doubts about the patency of the distal runoff, an on-table angiogram may be performed.

How would you carry out the fasciotomies?

- The anterior incision is placed about two finger-breadths lateral to the anterior border of the tibia (avoiding the peroneal nerve) to access the anterior and lateral compartments.
- The posterior incision is placed about 2 finger breadths posterior to the medial condyle of the femur and medial malleolus (avoiding the long saphenous vein) to access the superficial and deep posterior compartments.

ACUTE PANCREATITIS

A 22-year-old woman complains of abdominal pain radiating to her back, nausea and vomiting. On examination she is tachycardic, tachypnoeic and in pain. The urine and pregnancy tests are negative. The WCC is 15, LFTs are mildly deranged and the amylase is 1275. How would you manage this patient?

- She has acute pancreatitis. I would resuscitate her with oxygen, IV fluids and opiate analgesia; insert a urinary catheter and consider a NG tube if antiemetics did not stop the vomiting.
- I would complete her Apache II scoring system for pancreatitis with ABGs, CRP and BMI.
- I would review her in 1 hr to assess the response to the fluid challenge, and if this was poor or she had a high Apache II score, contact HDU to escalate her care to a level 2 bed.

Following resuscitation, she rapidly improves and PCA analgesia controls her pain. What is the likeliest cause of her pancreatitis?

- The commonist causes of pancreatitis are gallstone disease, alcohol and ERCP.
- I would initially request an USS to look for gallstones.

- If this was negative and the history did not suggest alcohol intake, I would measure serum calcium and cholesterol levels and look for drug-related causes (e.g., steroids).

What scoring systems are used in pancreatitis?

- Glasgow, Ranson, and Apache II are widely used in the literature to predict severity.
- The Glasgow scoring system is completed 48 hr after admission.
- The Ranson criteria are primarily used in alcohol-induced pancreatitis.
- A high BMI and a high CRP (>150) are also indicators of severe pancreatitis.
- These scores can fail to identify some individuals with severe pancreatitis, so regular clinical assessment is needed to pick up patients who are not responding to resuscitation and to escalate their level of care.
- Patients with predicted severe pancreatitis should be monitored in a level 2 or 3 bed.

What are the components of the Glasgow score?

- Age > 55 years
- White cell count > $15 \times 10^9/l$
- PaO_2 < 60 mmHg (8 kPa)
- Serum lactate dehydrogenase > 600 units/l
- Serum aspartate aminotransferase > 200 units/l
- Serum albumin < 32 g/l
- Serum calcium < 2 mmol/l
- Serum glucose > 10 mmol/l
- Serum urea > 16 mmol/l
- A score of >3 indicates severe pancreatitis.

Do you routinely prescribe antibiotics in pancreatitis?

- No. Currently, there is no evidence to support use of antibiotics in pancreatitis, and it is not recommended in the British Society of Gastroenterologists Guidelines.

How and when would you feed this patient?

- There is no evidence to support keeping the patient nil by mouth to rest the pancreas.
- Enteral nutrition is the best method of feeding, because it maintains the gut barrier, and helps counteract the catabolic state better than TPN (total parenteral nutrition).
- In severe pancreatitis, patients may need NG or NJ feeding, depending on their ability to tolerate and absorb the feed.

After 48 hr, the patient scores 4 on the Glasgow system. She has deteriorated and an ITU opinion has been sought. They want her to have a CT scan before they admit her. What are your thoughts?

- If confident with the diagnosis from biochemistry and the history, then I would not carry out a CT scan at this stage.
- A CT scan is only beneficial after 5–10 days to detect local complications (collections, oedema, necrosis) and to determine severity using the Balthazar index.

What are the potential complications of severe acute pancreatitis?

- The complications can be divided into local or systemic, early and late.
- Local complications include necrosis (plus or minus superadded infection), sepsis, lesser sac collection, pseudocyst (late), disrupted pancreatic duct, pseudoaneurysm, bleeding, and diabetes (late).
- Systemic complications include SIRS, which can lead to respiratory failure, renal failure, GIT dysfunction/ischaemia, multiorgan failure, and death.

The patient continues to deteriorate and is transferred to ITU on day 3. A CT scan on day 5 shows 60% necrosis and a large pancreatic collection. How would you treat her?

- If she is stable, I would treat her conservatively, with radiological drainage of the collection, send material for MC+S to exclude infection and start antibiotics if the cultures are positive
- I would approach the necrosis with a percutaneous necrosectomy following a radiologically inserted left flank drain. It is important to leave the tract to mature for as long as possible.

A similar patient was admitted the same day, with gallstone-induced pancreatitis and deranged LFTs, which improved 24 hr later. How would you treat her gallstones?

- Ideally, I would offer her a laparoscopic cholecystectomy and laparoscopic USS of the CBD, or on-table CBD exploration during the same admission.
- If this was not possible because of theatre unavailability, I would aim to remove her gallbladder within 4 weeks of discharge.
- I would request an ERCP only if she had cholangitis or obstructive jaundice.

How would you treat a pseudocyst?

- If they are asymptomatic, these can be left alone.
- Otherwise, they can be drained endoscopically, laparoscopically, radiologically or by open cyst-gastrostomy, depending on anatomical constraints and patient preference.

- Endoscopic and radiological approaches have the advantage that they are less invasive, but the stents are still under development and can displace. If they displace into the stomach, they can easily be retrieved, but if they displace into the pseudocyst, then retrieval can be challenging.

ACUTE SCROTAL PAIN

A 12-year-old boy presents to A+E with a 3 hr history of severe right scrotal pain and two episodes of vomiting. His right hemiscrotum is swollen, red, warm and very tender to touch. What is the diagnosis and how will you confirm it?

- All acute scrotal pain is testicular torsion until proven otherwise.
- The diagnosis of torsion is clinical.
- All cases should be booked for an immediate scrotal exploration to confirm or exclude the diagnosis and to salvage the testicle.
- The role of diagnostic imaging (colour Doppler ultrasound) is confined to prepubertal boys in whom testicular torsion has been excluded on clinical grounds, to look for other pathology.
- Irreversible ischaemia begins after 6 hr of onset.
- Delaying surgery may result in resection of an ischaemic testicle.
- The differential diagnosis is torsion of a testicular appendage (hydatid of Morgagni)
  - 45%–50% of boys with an acute scrotum
- Other less common causes of an acute scrotum are epididymo-orchitis, idiopathic scrotal oedema, acute hydrocele, trauma and Henoch–Schönlein vasculitis.

What is the hydatid of Morgagni?

- It is an embryologic remnant of the cranial end of the Mullerian duct.
- It is present in 90% of males.

How does testicular torsion occur?

- The majority (90%) are due to congenital malformation of the processus vaginalis (bell-clapper deformity).
- Instead of the testis attaching posteriorly to the inner lining of the scrotum by the mesorchium, the mesorchium terminates early and the testis floats freely in the tunica vaginalis.
- Newborn infants can develop extravaginal torsion when the torsion occurs outside the tunica. The testes are usually necrotic at birth.

How would you perform the surgery?

- Make an incision (*say what you would do*)—paramedian, transverse, or midline.

- Divide the layers of the tunica to expose the testis.
- Untwist it and assess viability.
- If viable, evert the tunica (Jaboulay procedure).
- Perform three-point fixation of both testes using nonabsorbable sutures.

What are the long-term complications following torsion?

- Reduced fertility
- An ischaemia-reperfusion injury that damages the blood–testis barrier with resulting antisperm antibody production

ANASTOMOTIC LEAK

A 66-year-old female had an elective sigmoid colectomy for severe diverticular disease. On the fifth postoperative day, she is tachycardic, tachypnoeic, febrile and nauseated. Her abdomen is distended but soft and nontender on palpation. Her Hb is 9.6, WCC is 14.3, CRP > 250. How will you manage her?

- She has developed SIRS (systemic inflammatory response syndrome), and the likeliest cause is an anastomotic leak, as this is day 5 postop.
- Resuscitate her (ABCs, oxygen, IV crystalloid, catheterise), take a history, examine her and take an ABG.
- Repeat her observations, assess her fluid balance and review the history and operation note.
- Do not be falsely reassured by an empty drain; these can block.

Her O_2 Sats are 92% at FiO_2 0.4. She has bilateral basal crepitations. ABG shows pO_2 5.5, pCO_2 3.4, pH 7.3, BE – 5.0.

- She has type I respiratory failure and a metabolic acidosis.
- The most obvious diagnosis is a leak (need to exclude MI, PE).
- Start IV broad spectrum antibiotics, request a CXR, ECG and CT scan with oral and rectal contrast and ask for a critical care assessment.

Why do you want a CT scan?

- It is necessary to rule out a localised collection that can be radiologically drained.
- If her clinical condition deteriorates or she develops signs of peritonitis, book her for an urgent laparotomy.

The CT scan shows a large pelvic collection and a partial anastomotic dehiscence, with free fluid and air. You take her to theatre. What do you do?

- Drain collections.
- Peritoneal washout.

- Take down anastomosis and perform a Hartmann's procedure, leaving large pelvic drains in situ. Perform daily rectal washouts to prevent a stump blowout.
  - However, management should be guided by the status of the patient and the doctor's experience. Keep it simple and safe.
  - If leak is small (<1 cm), well vascularised with minimal contamination, consider a primary repair, covered with a loop ileostomy.

What are the causes of an anastomotic leak?

- Local factors—poor technique (tension, poor vascularity), local infection, previous radiation, missed proximal obstructing lesion, low anastomosis, >500 ml blood loss, peritonitis at initial operation
- General factors—BMI > 30, Crohn's disease, malnutrition, anaemia, steroids, diabetes, old age, arteriopath, smoking
- Anastomotic leak mortality rate: 7.5%
- Leak rates:
  - Intraperitoneal: 2.4%
  - Extraperitoneal (pelvic): 6%
  - Low anterior: 8%–10%

APPENDICITIS

A 23-year-old girl presents at 10 p.m. with a 2-day history of right iliac fossa pain, nausea and a low-grade pyrexia. How will you assess her?

- Take a history—GI/GU symptoms, last menstrual period, previous ovarian pathology, pregnancy.
- Examine her—RIF tenderness and peritonism.
- The classical signs on examination are:
  - Rovsing's sign—right lower quadrant pain with palpation of the left lower quadrant (suggests peritoneal irritation in the RLQ precipitated by palpation at a remote location)
  - Obturator sign—RLQ pain with internal and external rotation of the flexed right hip (suggests that the inflamed appendix is located deep in the right hemipelvis)
  - Psoas sign—RLQ pain with extension of the right hip (suggests that an inflamed appendix is located along the course of the right psoas muscle)
- Appendicitis is primarily a clinical diagnosis, but I would take bloods (raised WCC and CRP), do a pregnancy test and dip the urine to exclude a urinary tract infection.
  - The Alvorado scoring system is quoted in the literature as a diagnostic aid.
- If the patient is not septic and the diagnosis is in question, I would keep her on free fluids and observe her overnight.
- If she is not septic and I am certain about the diagnosis, I would start her on broad spectrum antibiotics and list her for theatre the next morning.

- If she is septic or peritonitic, I would start her on broad spectrum antibiotics and book her for theatre that evening.

What is the pathophysiology of acute appendicitis?

- Obstruction of the appendix lumen secondary to luminal blockage by fae-colith/worm/lymphoid aggregates leads to bacterial proliferation in the distal appendiceal lumen.
- Translocation into the appendix wall triggers inflammation, leading to vessel thrombosis, wall ischaemia, gangrene and perforation.

Your patient has rebound RIF tenderness, her WCC is 14 and she is not pregnant. Clinically, you feel she has acute appendicitis. Would you perform an open or laparoscopic appendicectomy?

- I would do a diagnostic laparoscopy in all females with suspected acute appendicitis as the diagnostic error is more than twice that of males (underlying gynaecological conditions).
- Two RCTs demonstrated the associated improved diagnostic accuracy after laparoscopy, which converts to a reduced hospital stay ± an improved quality of life (assessed 6 weeks after discharge from hospital).
- Laparoscopy pros:
  - Less pain, faster recovery, lower incidence of superficial wound infections (up to 15% with open surgery)
  - Ability to look for alternative pathology (mesenteric adenitis, ovarian cysts, cholecystitis, Meckel's diverticulum, terminal ileitis diverticulitis)
  - Easier if high BMI
- Laparoscopy cons:
  - Longer operating time (also learning curve to consider)
  - Increased cost
  - Physiological derangement of pneumoperitoneum
  - Damage to internal organs during port insertion
  - Threefold increase in intra-abdominal abscesses (*Cochrane Review*)

You do a laparoscopy and find a normal appendix and no other pathology. Would you remove the appendix?
Say what YOU would do, and why.

- Argument FOR removal:
  - There is a small incidence of appendicitis on histological examination of a macroscopically normal appendix.
  - It prevents the development of a diagnostic dilemma.
  - It is easy to remove a normal appendix with very low morbidity.
- Argument AGAINST removal:
  - All operative interventions are associated with some form of risk (adhesional small bowel obstruction, wound infection, etc.) and if the

appendix is normal at laparoscopy there needs to be a good reason to remove it.

- A pragmatic approach would be to remove the appendix only if it looks inflamed at laparoscopy and leave it if it looks normal.
- The patient must be clearly told the diagnosis made at laparoscopy and the procedure performed.
- The longer term sequelae of removing a normal appendix at laparoscopy remain unknown.

If on examination you found a mass in the RIF, how would this change your management?

- The differential diagnosis would be an appendix abscess, or Crohn's disease in a young girl.
- I would ask for a CT scan.
- If this showed an appendicular mass, I would treat her conservatively with antibiotics (risk of perforation has passed).
- I would not offer an interval appendicectomy.

A 12-year-old boy had an open appendicectomy 5 days ago. You are asked to see him in A+E with pyrexia, tachycardia and a pelvic mass. What do you do?

- It sounds like he has a pelvic abscess.
- I would resuscitate the child with IV fluids, oxygen and analgesia, take blood (including blood cultures), commence broad-spectrum antibiotics, and arrange an USS.
- I would review the operation note to see if the appendix was gangrenous or perforated and whether a faecolith was present.
- If USS showed a large collection, I would discuss with the radiologist on call whether this could be drained percutaneously.

What is your antibiotic policy in appendicitis?

- Once a diagnosis of appendicitis has been made, prescribe prophylactic IV broad-spectrum antibiotics.
- Patients should receive a single dose 30 min prior to surgery to protect against wound infection.
- If the appendix was perforated, I would prescribe a full treatment course over 5 days.

What do you do if you find a segment of terminal ileal Crohn's disease during an open operation?

- I would remove the appendix for two reasons—to prevent a future diagnostic dilemma and to get tissue that could confirm the diagnosis.
- I would carefully repair the base of the caecum, if necessary, to reduce the risk of fistula formation.

State clearly what you will do with the Crohn's segment.

- One option is to refer to Gastroenterology to start medical treatment.
- An alternative option is to resect with a primary anastomosis, as a proportion of patients will need a resection in the future due to failed medical management, particularly if there is a localised stricture.

You are asked to review a 32-week pregnant woman with right-sided abdominal pain and raised inflammatory markers. How will you assess her?

- The differential diagnosis is cholecystitis and appendicitis.
- The history of the pain would give some clues and a negative Murphy's sign may help exclude cholecystitis, but I would ask for an USS to look for an inflamed gallbladder and gallstones.
- I would also check with the midwife that there were no concerns regarding the pregnancy and that the foetal heartbeat was normal.

The USS shows a normal gallbladder. Would you ask for a CT to look at the appendix?

- A quick, accurate diagnosis should take precedence over concerns regarding ionising radiation, as a perforated appendix could be dangerous for both the mother and the baby.
- However, at this stage of pregnancy, I would be concerned that a CT might increase the risk of childhood hematologic malignancy.

You suspect appendicitis. What operation would you perform?

- I would do a diagnostic laparoscopy (safe in every trimester of pregnancy), with the patient in the left lateral decubitus position.
- I would access the abdomen in the subcostal region (both Hassan and Veress needle techniques are safe).
- The advantages of laparoscopy over open surgery are:
  - Decreased fetal respiratory depression due to diminished postoperative narcotic requirements
  - Diminished postoperative maternal hypoventilation
  - Shorter hospital stay
  - Decreased uterine irritability—less need for uterine manipulation compared to open surgery

BLUNT CHEST TRAUMA

You are called to a 55-year-old male car driver in Resus. He has been involved in a head-on collision with an articulated truck. He is hypoxic with an SpO$_2$ of 90% on room air. His blood pressure is 80/60. What could be causing his hypoxia?

- Hypoxia is the commonest manifestation of moderate to severe chest trauma.
- The hypoxia is due to mechanical factors resulting in reduced gas exchange surface, reduced ventilation and reduced cardiac output.
- Examples of chest trauma are rib fractures, simple/tension/open pneumothorax, haemothorax, pulmonary contusion, blood flow shunt through nonventilated lung and blast lung.

How do blast injuries produce hypoxia?

- Combination of diffuse pulmonary contusions, pneumothoraces, pulmonary haemorrhage and arteriovenous fistulae resulting in air emboli

How can blunt chest trauma compromise cardiac output?

- Through two means:
  - General—hypovolaemia (e.g., aortic transection, hilar injury)
  - Cardiac—tamponade, contusion, ischaemia, infarction, valve disruption

How do you assess patients with thoracic injuries?

- Follow ATLS principles.
- During the primary survey, evaluate neck (airway obstruction, neck injury or tracheal deviation), chest wall (symmetry of expansion, open wounds, flail segment, rib or sternal fractures), pleura (pneumothorax, haemothorax), lung (blast, contusion), heart (bleeding, tamponade, contusion), mediastinum (air or blood), bullet entry and exit wounds, objects transfixing thoracic cavity.
- Obtain a chest x-ray during or immediately after the primary survey.

This patient's chest x-ray is normal. He has no clinical signs of major thoracic trauma. He is still hypotensive and hypoxic despite 2 l of warmed Hartmann's solution, and clinically unstable. What are you going to do now?

- Take him to theatre for a laparotomy as the most likely source of blood loss is within his abdomen (consider laparoscopy).
- He is haemodynamically unstable so should not have a CT scan or other investigations until the haemorrhage is controlled.

At laparotomy his peritoneal cavity and retroperitoneum are normal. Now what?

- No intra-abdominal source of blood loss is found.
- Make a pericardial window from below to rule out cardiac tamponade.
- If that is normal, do a thoracotomy.

Other lines of questioning:

- *Indications/contraindications to emergency room thoracotomy*
- *Operative approaches to control severe thoracic haemorrhage*

BOERHAAVRE SYNDROME

A 36-year-old male with learning difficulties is admitted to the emergency department with sepsis and dehydration. The carers report he has been vomiting for the past 24 hr. On examination he is febrile, tachycardic and has surgical emphysema in his neck. What is the diagnosis?

- Boerhaave syndrome is a full thickness tear of the oesophageal wall secondary to vomiting.
- The classical presentation of Boerhaave syndrome is a constellation of symptoms known as Mackler's triad—vomiting, lower thoracic pain and subcutaneous emphysema.
- These signs, however, are not always found, particularly if there has been a delay in presentation.

What is the most likely position of the tear?

- The left posterolateral wall of the lower third of the oesophagus, 2–3 cm above the gastro-oesophageal junction.
- Other common sites are the upper thoracic area and the subdiaphragmatic region.
- It is thought that the tear is due to a sudden rise in intraluminal pressure that occurs during vomiting as a result of muscle incoordination that causes failure of relaxation of the cricopharyngeus muscle.

How would you initially manage this patient?

- Resuscitate the patient with oxygen, IV fluids, and analgesia, request a CXR and start broad-spectrum antibiotics and antifungal treatment.
- A CT thorax with oral contrast will confirm the diagnosis and provide information regarding the extent of mediastinal and pleural contamination and presence of an ongoing leak. Alternatively, an oral water-soluble contrast study could be performed.

What are the treatment options?

- Oesophageal rupture has an extremely high mortality, particularly if there is delay in diagnosis and treatment.
- Treatment is aimed at repair of the oesophageal perforation and drainage of pleural and mediastinal sepsis, and it depends on the size of the perforation, the degree of contamination and the duration of the symptoms.

- Surgery can be performed through an open (left thoracic or transabdominal incision) or thoracoscopic approach.
- An on-table OGD should be performed to localise the perforation accurately.
- Primary repair is appropriate if the diagnosis is made within 24 hr and the perforation is small.
- In the presence of extensive contamination and larger perforations, the hole is closed over a T-tube to create an oesophagocutaneous fistula.
- A venting gastrostomy and feeding jejunostomy should also be considered alongside mediastinal and pleural drains after extensive lavage.
- Nonsurgical management may be appropriate for selected cases with minimal mediastinal contamination, using an endoscopic covered stent.
- Delayed presentation with well-contained collections can be managed with radiological drainage, PEG for gastric decompression and a jejunal extension for enteral feeding.

CELLULITIS

A 56-year-old diabetic on the ward presents with a hot, swollen right lower leg 5 days after an elective right hemicolectomy. What would you do?

- Take a history and perform a full examination (looking for signs of infection, demarcation, abscesses, diabetic ulcers, skin trauma/IV access and regional lymphadenopathy) and review the charts.
- Take bloods for FBC, CRP, U+Es, Glc and blood cultures if septic (high WCC and CRP will indicate systemic upset; baseline creatinine will help guide antibiotics if indicated).
- The differential is DVT and cellulitis.

This patient had a venflon removed from his right foot 2 days ago and is now pyrexial. How would you treat him?

- The likely diagnosis is cellulitis, but I would exclude other causes of a postop pyrexia (e.g., anastomotic leak, lower respiratory tract infection, wound infection, DVT/PE, MI), and swab the venflon site.
- Simple cellulitis can be treated on an outpatient basis with oral antibiotics; however, I would treat this patient with IV antibiotics. He has systemic signs of sepsis and is a diabetic.
- I would mark the demarcation of the cellulitis and monitor for progression on treatment; this may indicate a necrotising fasciitis which would need emergency debridement.

What bacteria typically cause cellulitis?

- *Streptococcus pyogenes* and *Staphylococcus aureus*
- Immunocompromised patients can become infected from opportunistic organisms (*Pseudomonas, Proteus*) and anaerobes.

How is cellulitis classified?

- I: no systemic toxicity
- II: significant comorbidity
- III: significant systemic upset
- IV: necrotising fasciitis

What antibiotics would you prescribe?

- I would consult hospital antimicrobial guidelines:
  - First line—PO flucloxacillin (narrow-spectrum active against staph and strep); PO erythromycin or clarithromycin if allergic
  - Second line—IV flucloxacillin and benzylpenicillin. PO clarithromycin or IV teicoplanin if allergic (if this is associated with a diabetic ulcer, I would change to IV Co–Amoxiclav—broader spectrum cover)
  - Third line—IV benzylpenicllin and ciprofloxacin (discuss with microbiology)

When would you consider surgical intervention?

- Cellulitis associated with an abscess requires surgical drainage of the source of infection for adequate treatment.
- Clinical concerns for necrotising fasciitis include crepitus, circumferential cellulitis, necrotic-appearing skin, rapidly evolving cellulitis, pain disproportional to physical examination findings, severe pain on passive movement.
- If necrotising fasciitis was suspected, I would resuscitate the patient, start him or her on broad-spectrum antibiotics and take the patient straight to theatre for debridement of necrotic tissue and fasciotomy.
- I would plan a second-look operation in 24 hr to debride further tissue as necessary.

DAMAGE CONTROL LAPAROTOMY

What is a damage-control laparotomy (DCL)?

- This is an abbreviated or staged laparotomy where the operation is rapidly terminated.
- The patient is physiologically unstable on the operating table, and there is not time to repair the effects of trauma formally.
- The surgeon quickly controls life-threatening bleeding and bile/faecal contamination, followed by correction of abnormal physiology on ITU.
- A laparotomy is converted to a DCL when the patient starts to develop the lethal triad of
  - Hypothermia
  - Acidosis
  - Coagulopathy
    - This requires regular communication with the anaesthetist.

When do you consider the need for DCL?

- Any patient with acidosis, hypothermia and/or coagulopathy
- Inability to achieve haemostasis (e.g., liver or major venous injury [requiring packing])
- Time-consuming procedure in an unstable patient (usually >90 min)
- Associated life-threatening injury in second anatomical location
- Planned reassessment of abdominal contents (e.g., bowel ischaemia)
- Inability to close abdomen due to visceral oedema or abdominal compartment syndrome

What factors predict the need to pack early for severe intra-abdominal haemorrhage?

- Coagulopathy
- Hypotension (systolic BP < 70 mm Hg) for >70 min
- pH < 7.2
- Serum lactate > 5 mmol/l
- Hypothermia (temperature < 34°C)
- Injury severity score > 35
- Transfusion > 4 l of blood

What are the stages of DCL?

- Decision to perform DCL
  - Ideally made within a few minutes of starting the procedure
- Damage control procedure
  - Haemorrhage or definitive surgical control
    - Packing
    - Direct arterial ligation, vascular shunts and balloon catheter tamponade
  - Contamination limiting
    - Stapling bowel ends without definitive repair
    - Occlusion with umbilical tape, suture or towel tag ligation
    - Bowel anastomosis and diversion delayed until reoperation
  - Temporary closure
    - Towel clips
    - Sandwich technique
    - Bogota bag
- Restoration of physiology
  - Correction of hypothermia (essential for enzyme function, especially in coagulation cascade—core temp > 35°C for coagulation)
    - Passive rewarming
      - Bair Hugger
      - Warmed fluids
      - Humidified ventilator gases

- – Active rewarming
    - – Lavage of thoracic/abdominal cavity
    - – Gastric and bladder lavage
- • Correction of coagulopathy
    - – Aim to achieve INR < 1.25
- • Optimise oxygen delivery and improve tissue perfusion to reduce lactate to <2.5 mmol/l
- • Planned definitive surgery within 24–48 hr
    - • Second relook procedure
    - • Removal of packs
    - • Haemostasis
    - • Restoration of GI continuity/stoma
    - • Debridement of necrotic tissues
- • Abdominal wall reconstruction if required
    - • Composite or vicryl mesh
    - • Rectus sheath lateral release

DIVERTICULITIS

A 55-year-old patient presents with left iliac fossa pain, fever and a fullness in the LIF. How would you manage him?

- • Differential diagnosis is diverticular disease or a carcinoma.
- • First, resuscitate (IV fluids, analgesia, HDU input as needed).
- • Take a history (red-flag symptoms and previous episodes, smoking), examination (LIF peritonism), bloods (FBC, U+E, Glc, blood cultures, G+S) urinalysis and a CXR (free air indicating a perforation).
- • Confirm diagnosis with CT scan with oral and IV contrast.

How is acute diverticulitis classified?

- • Hinchey classification:
- • Grade I—inflammation of pericolic fat or pericolic abscess
- • Grade II—pelvic or distant abscess (pus in pelvis)
- • Grade III—generalised purulent peritonitis (pus everywhere)
- • Grade IV—generalised faeculent peritonitis (poo everywhere)

This patient has grade II disease. How will you treat him?

- • Conservatively—provide clear fluids, antibiotics to cover anaerobes (*Bacteroides fragilis, Clostridium*), aerobes (*Escherichia coli, Klebsiella, Proteus, Streptococcus* and *Enterobacter*) (e.g., Co–Amoxiclav).
- • If the abscess is greater than 4 cm, I would arrange percutaneous CT-guided drainage.
- • Laparoscopic washout is an alternative, depending on my experience and speciality.

How would your management plan change for grade III and IV disease?

- Initially, I would arrange for NBO, IV antibiotics (tazocin; tigecycline if penicillin allergic).
- The next stage depends on experience and speciality (*again, say what YOU would do and then offer alternatives*).
- The ideal therapeutic option is a one-stage procedure (resection, intraoperative lavage of the colon and primary anastomosis) in selected patients.
  - It avoids morbidity/mortality associated with a stoma and its reconstruction.
  - It is contraindicated in faecal peritonitis, septic shock, unstable patients, chronic steroid therapy and high ASA grade.
  - A protective ileostomy is associated with lower rates of anastomotic leak and wound infection.
  - Diverticulitis in young patients has an aggressive and fulminant course and 40% need early surgery for complications; consider one-stage procedure in these patients.
- Hartmann's procedure is the standard technique; however, a high percentage of patients will not undergo further surgery, leaving them with a permanent stoma.
- Laparoscopic peritoneal lavage is a safe alternative in experienced hands for grade III disease.

How would your management change if the patient was 75, a heavy smoker and in AF with grade III disease?

- In an unstable patient, I would do the simplest operation—Hartmann's procedure, pelvic lavage and placement of large pelvic drains.

ECTOPIC PREGNANCY

A 35-year-old woman presents to the emergency department with a 6 hr history of severe lower abdominal pain. She is tachycardic and hypotensive. She reports a positive home pregnancy test 1 week earlier. What is the differential diagnosis?

- This presentation in a woman of reproductive age is a ruptured ectopic pregnancy until proven otherwise.
- Other possible aetiologies include miscarriage of an intrauterine pregnancy, ovarian cyst accident (rupture, torsion or haemorrhage) or nongynaecological causes (acute appendicitis, UTI, renal calculus, other GI disease).

What will you do?

- Establish large-bore intravenous access, start IV fluids, send blood for a full blood count, urea and electrolytes and cross match for four units.

- The period of amenorrhoea should be ascertained and an urgent urinary pregnancy test undertaken (current dipstick pregnancy tests are sensitive at b-hCG levels of approximately 25 IU/l) to confirm pregnancy.
- The gynaecology team should be notified immediately in cases of suspected ectopic pregnancy.
- Notify theatres and the anaesthetic team.
- Contemporary standard of care is a diagnostic laparoscopy (to confirm the diagnosis) proceeding to laparoscopic salpingectomy or salpingostomy for tubal ectopic pregnancy.
- Assuming a healthy contralateral tube, salpingectomy of the affected tube is usually performed.
- Laparotomy may occasionally be indicated for haemodynamically unstable women with life-threatening hypovolaemia.
- Surgical specimens should be sent for histopathological examination to confirm ectopic pregnancy and exclude molar pregnancy.

What is an ectopic pregnancy?

- A fertilised ovum is implanted outside the uterine cavity.
- The rate of ectopic pregnancy is 1%–2% of all pregnancies.
- Heterotopic pregnancy (the coexistence of an ectopic pregnancy with an intrauterine pregnancy) is very rare (1 in 10,000–50,000 spontaneous conceptions), but is significantly more common (up to 1%) following assisted conception such as IVF.

What are the risk factors for ectopic pregnancy?

- Previous ectopic pregnancy
- IVF pregnancy (4%–5% risk)
- Known fallopian tubal disease
- Previous pelvic inflammatory disease
- Current progesterone contraceptive use (progesterone-only pill, intrauterine device) and smoking

Where do ectopic pregnancies usually occur?

- 95% develop in the fallopian tube.
- Rarer sites include interstitial ectopic (the proximal portion of the tube as it enters the uterine angle, associated with a high rate of catastrophic haemorrhage), ovarian, cervical, caesarean scar and abdominal ectopic pregnancy.

What imaging can help confirm the diagnosis?

- Transvaginal ultrasonongraphy—empty uterus, adnexal mass (may contain gestational sac or foetal pole) and free pelvic fluid

- At bhCG levels of ≥1500 IU/l an intrauterine gestation would expect to be seen.

Are there any nonoperative options for an ectopic pregnancy?

- Early ectopics (b-hCG ≤ 3000–5000 IU/l) without evidence of rupture can be managed medically with methotrexate on an out-patient basis.
- In very select cases in asymptomatic women, expectant management may be considered, as some ectopics will resolve without treatment ('tubal abortion').

EPIGASTRIC STAB WOUND

A 22-year-old man arrives in the emergency department with a single stab wound in his epigastrium. His heart rate is 100 beats per minute and his blood pressure is 105/80. What injuries could he have sustained?

- Thoracic—cardiac tamponade, pneumothorax, haemothorax, great vessel injury
- Abdominal—liver laceration, splenic laceration, perforated viscus, great vessel injury, mesenteric laceration

How will you assess the patient?

- Follow ATLS principles.
- During primary survey look for features of pneumothorax, haemothorax, cardiac tamponade, intra-abdominal haemorrhage and peritonitis.
- Obtain a chest x-ray for pneumothorax, haemothorax, mediastinal widening (great vessel injury), pneumoperitoneum and pneumomediastinum.
- Perform a FAST scan for intra-abdominal free fluid.

His chest x-ray demonstrates a pneumoperitoneum while the FAST scan shows some free fluid in Morrison's pouch. What are you going to do now?

- He is tachycardiac with free gas and fluid in his abdomen. He needs a laparotomy.

What are the general principles of a trauma laparotomy?

- Give antibiotic prophylaxis.
- Keep the patient warm with warming devices on the extremities and upper body.
- Use a full length midline incision from xiphisternum to symphysis pubis.
- Prep and drape the torso so that a thoracotomy or other extended incisions can be made.
- Have two wide-bore suckers and large abdominal packs available.
- First priority is to locate the source and stop the bleeding.

There are 2 l of blood in his abdomen. No source is immediately apparent. How will you proceed?

- Four-compartment packing, then assessment of each quadrant in turn
- Right upper quadrant—bleeding from liver, IVC, lesser omentum, duodenum, pancreas, right adrenal, right kidney or retrohepatic veins
- Left upper quadrant—bleeding from splenic laceration, left lobe liver, stomach, diaphragm, pancreas, left adrenal, left kidney
- Assessment of infracolic compartment by lifting omentum and transverse colon out of abdomen, moving small bowel laterally, packing to left and right of small bowel mesentery—bleeding from bowel, mesentery, retroperitoneum
- Small bowel lifted out and pelvis packed—bleeding from fractures, pelvic vessels or organs
- *Other lines of questioning:*
  - *Evidence of functioning contra-lateral kidney prior to nephrectomy*
  - *Approach to localising an occult bowel perforation at laparotomy*

FEMORAL HERNIA

You are asked to see a 73-year-old woman who has presented with vomiting for the last 2 days. She has been admitted with possible gastroenteritis. What will you do?

- Take a history: When did the vomiting start? How often? Passed flatus or faeces? Has she any pain? Any previous abdominal surgery? Recent change in bowel habit or weight loss? Any blood per rectum? Any other medical problems?
- Examine her: heart rate, blood pressure, temperature? Is she dehydrated? Is there obvious abdominal distension? Any abdominal scars? Any visible peristalsis? Signs of peritonism? Any palpable abdominal mass? Any groin swelling? Conduct per rectum and per vaginal exams.
- She should have a full blood count, urea and electrolytes, an ECG and a plain abdominal x-ray.

She has a virgin abdomen with a palpable tender left groin swelling. What is the most likely diagnosis?

- An obstructed left groin hernia. Given her gender and age, this is likely to be femoral although it could be inguinal.

How would you differentiate femoral from inguinal hernias clinically?

- Inguinal hernias generally lie above and medial to the pubic tubercle, whilst femoral hernias lie below and lateral to the tubercle.

- In nonobstructed hernias, inguinal hernias are generally soft, reducible and have bowel sounds, whilst femoral are generally firm, irreducible and lack bowel sounds.

Which is more common in women: femoral or inguinal hernia?

- Although inguinal hernia is more common in females, femoral hernia is the most common type of hernia to present as an emergency with incarceration and strangulation.

Why are females more likely to develop femoral herniae?

- Normally, ileopsoas and pectineus muscle acts as a barrier to development of hernia. Aging atrophy of muscle mass and a wide pelvis in women make them prone to develop femoral hernias.

What structures comprise the femoral ring?

- Anterior—inguinal ligament
- Medial—lacunar ligament
- Posterior—ileopectineal ligament, pubic bone and fascia over pectineus muscle
- Lateral—thin septum and femoral vein

How will you manage this patient?

- She will need intravenous access and fluid resuscitation, antibiotics, analgesia and DVT prophylaxis.
- Pass an NG tube and consent her for an urgent surgical exploration.

Outline your surgical approach.

- Supine position
- A modified Pfannenstiel inscision two finger-breadths above inguinal ligament (modification of McEvedy's inscision) can be used to convert to a laparotomy.
- The external oblique is divided vertically at the lateral edge of rectus sheath (lateral to rectus).
- The rectus muscle is retracted medially and the preperitoneal plane is entered.
- The inferior epigastric artery may have to be sacrificed.
- Blunt dissection in preperitoneal plane exposes femoral canal and access to femoral ring from above.

How will you release the constriction?

- Blunt dissection with artery clip, or divide inguinal ligament or divide lacunar ligament (risk of injury to accessory obturator artery).

What other approaches can be used for elective femoral herniae?

- Lockwood (low approach): used in elective hernia repair; use mesh plug to close the ring and approximate inguinal ligament to ileopectineal ligament
- Transinguinal approach (Lothiessen): through posterior inguinal wall (less favoured)

How will you decide if the small bowel caught in the hernia is viable?

- Three Ps—presence of **p**ulse, **p**eristalsis and **p**ink colour

GROIN ABSCESS

You are asked to see a 37-year-old man in the emergency department with a swelling in his left groin. What is the differential diagnosis?

- Can be related to any of the structures in the groin
- Skin (sebaceous cyst, abscess), fat (lipoma), muscle and fascial layers (inguinal or femoral hernia), vein (saphena varix), artery (femoral artery aneurysm), nerve (Schwannoma), lymph node, psoas bursa or abscess

What will you do with the patient?

- Take a history: How long has he had the lump? How did he notice it? Is it painful? Does it come and go? Is it getting bigger? Has he ever had one before? Any other lumps?
- Check vital signs.
- Examine the site, size, shape, consistency, borders, overlying skin, surrounding skin, fluctuance, expansility, transilluminability, reducibility, auscultate (bruit or bowel sounds).
- Check for generalised lymphadenopathy and examine the leg for skin lesions.

The lump is 4 cm, tender, hot and fluctuant. He has a temperature of 38°C. He attends the local methadone clinic. What is the most likely diagnosis?

- The most likely diagnosis is a groin abscess secondary to intravenous drug use.
- The most important differential is femoral artery pseudoaneurysm.

What are you going to do?

- He needs analgesia and IV broad spectrum antibiotics.
- I would arrange an urgent duplex scan of his groin (out of hours if necessary) to rule out a pseudoaneurysm.
- If the scan shows that the collection is separate from the artery, then he needs an incision and drainage of the abscess with packing of the cavity.

Your FY2 sees the patient before you do and takes him straight to theatre to incise and drain the abscess. The theatre staff have called you to report that there is torrential bleeding from the wound. Now what?

- Tell the FY2 to apply direct pressure to the wound and then go straight to theatre.
- First priority is to get proximal control as this sounds like an infected pseudoaneurysm.
- Make a left iliac fossa incision, enter the extraperitoneal space, sling and clamp the left external iliac artery.
- Once proximal control is established, make an axial incision along the line of the left femoral artery in the groin.
- Attempt to identify and clamp the superficial and profunda femoris branches (usually a mass of granulation tissue and fibrosis).
- If the groin vessels cannot be dissected out, ligation of the external iliac is the only option.

How will you revascularise his leg?

- Synthetic bypasses invariably become infected.
- IV drug users do not generally have any usable veins.
- In about 50% of cases, collateral circulation will keep the leg alive long term, though with short distance claudication.
- Overall, the most appropriate option is simple ligation and then above-knee amputation if the leg proves nonviable in the next 24 hr.
- Finally, fill in an incident form.

GUNSHOT WOUNDS

A 22-year-old man is hit in the arm by a single bullet fired from a handgun. What is the difference between high- and low-velocity bullets?

- High-velocity bullets have a velocity > 300 m/s. They are fired by rifles or machine guns.
- Low-velocity bullets have a velocity < 300 m/s and are fired by handguns or shotguns.

How does a bullet cause injury?

- Bullets injure by transferring energy into body tissues.
- The energy is determined by the kinetic energy equation (ke = $\frac{1}{2} mv^2$).

What types of injury might this patient sustain in his arm?

- There may be injury to soft tissue, tissue, vessels, nerves and bones.
- The severity of the wound depends on whether the bullet strikes bone.

- If the bullet passes through without hitting bone, there is only a small transfer of energy and it may only cause a small wound.
- If the bullet strikes bone, much greater energy transfer results, leading to a large wound and greater tissue destruction.

How will you evaluate the patient?

- Follow ATLS principles.
- Look for life-threatening injuries.
- Consider antibiotics and tetanus.
- Assess the wound extent and the tissues that have been damaged.
- Rule out major vascular injury.
- Determine the need for surgery.

Would you ever consider nonoperative management of these wounds?

- Yes, provided that the patient presents within the first 24 hr, is systemically well and is available for follow-up/reoperation

What types of wound are suitable for nonoperative management?

- Entry and exit wounds < 1 cm maximum diameter
- Soft tissue injury only
- No involvement of body cavities
- No involvement of major neurovascular structures
- No gross contamination at presentation

Assuming this man's wound is suitable, outline your nonoperative management plan.

- Clean and dress the wound.
- Check tetanus status and immunise if necessary.
- Administer antibiotics—IV benzylpenicilin × 24 hr, then oral penicillin V for 5 days.
- Watch for signs of infection, compartment syndrome or vascular compromise.
- Splint the wound with an incomplete cast if fracture is present.
- Plan for wound review at 5 days or earlier if there are complications.

HEAD INJURY

A 25-year-old man arrives in the emergency department following a fall from 15 feet onto concrete. He is moving all four limbs. His blood pressure is 110/70 and his heart rate is 80 beats per minute. He is not opening his eyes to voice. What will you do?

- Assess him according to ATLS protocol.
- Check his airway, breathing and circulation whilst maintaining C spine immobilisation.
- Insert two large-bore intravenous cannulae; give 1 l warmed Hartmann's solution.
- Send bloods for FBC, U+E, amylase, clotting, Glc, group and save.
- Request a portable chest and pelvic x-ray.

His primary survey is clear, including normal pelvic and chest x-rays. He has a laceration over his occiput with a boggy underlying haematoma. His GCS is 13. What will you do?

- The patient has a head injury and needs an urgent CT scan.
- Whilst waiting for the CT, I would complete the secondary survey to look for other injuries, given the nature of the fall.
- Failure to treat serious injuries in other body regions promptly (e.g., ruptured spleen) may result in hypotension and secondary brain injury due to reduced cerebral perfusion pressure.

What is cerebral perfusion pressure (CPP), and what physiological changes affect it?

- CPP = MAP—ICP.
- MAP = 1/3 pulse pressure + diastolic pressure.
- Decreasing ICP or increasing MAP should increase CPP.
- BP is not equivalent to blood flow/oxygen transfer, and the brain may be ischaemic despite an adequate CPP of >70 mmHg.

What is the Monroe–Kellie doctrine?

- Intracranial pressure (ICP) is related to the balance between the volume of blood, brain and CSF in the skull.
- If brain volume increases (e.g., cerebral oedema), in order to maintain a normal ICP, the blood, CSF or both must decrease in volume.

What are the causes of raised ICP?

- Surgical:
  - Extradural haematoma—classic lucid interval
    - Arterial injury stripping pericranium away from the skull (mass effect increases ICP)
  - Subdural haematoma—tearing of dural bridging veins
    - Indicates underlying cortical damage
    - Increased ICP due to mass effect

- Subarachnoid haemorrhage—result of direct contusional injury
    - Impaired CSF reabsorption and cerebral oedema due to hypoxia increase ICP
- Contusions—rapid deceleration of brain against inside of skull vault (classically a coup contrecoup injury)
    - Swelling of bilateral contusions, leading to reduced GCS
    - Size often underestimated by initial CT scan
    - Mass effect due to bleeding and oedema increasing ICP
- Diffuse axonal injury—shearing of white against grey matter
    - Fibre disruption and permanent brain injury
    - ICP increased by generalised oedema
- Medical:
    - Electrolyte imbalance (causes cerebral oedema)
    - Ischaemia (CVA)
    - Infection (meningitis)

What are the symptoms of raised ICP?

- Decreased conscious level
- Headache
- Nausea and vomiting

What are the clinical and CT signs of raised ICP?

- Clinical signs:
    - Dilated pupil, unreactive to light—suggestive of third nerve palsy
    - Defect in lateral gaze due to paralysis of lateral rectus muscle—traction injury on the sixth cranial nerve
    - Fall in GCS
    - Papilloedema
- CT signs:
    - Extradural haematoma—localised convex haematoma (strips dura away from the skull, respects suture lines) ± midline shift
    - Subdural haematoma—thin sheet of blood overlying cortex, ± midline shift
    - Subarachnoid haemorrhage—blood in the subarachnoid space, extending into ventricles in a large bleed—increasing risk of hydrocephalus
    - Loss of grey/white differentiation—suggestion of acute ischaemia

Why does the pupil dilate in raised intracranial pressure (ICP)?

- The optic nerve is pushed against the free edge of the tentorium by a haematoma.
    - This is a sign of impending tentorial herniation (coning).
- In some cases the opposite pupil can be dilated (false localising sign).

What will you do for your patient?

- Intubate the patient to provide a definitive airway and transfer to the CT scanner to look for a focal haematoma amenable to drainage.
- Medical management:
  - Nurse at 30° (taking care to immobilise C-spine)
  - Mild hypothermia
  - Mild hyperventilation to keep the pCO_2 around 4.5 kPa
  - Mannitol bolus after discussion with neurosurgeon
  - Consider loading with phenobarbitone/benzodiazepines to control seizures
  - Increase CPP by raising MAP with inotropes (dopamine, adrenaline)

His CT scan demonstrates cerebral oedema only and the neurosurgeons advise conservative treatment in your intensive care unit. What options are available to measure his intracranial pressure?

- Invasive methods:
  - External ventricular drain in the anterior horn of the lateral ventricle— gold standard
  - Brain parenchymal ICP transducer through a cranial access device (usually referred to as a 'bolt')
- Noninvasive methods:
  - Transcranial Doppler can be used to measure velocity in the middle cerebral artery and derive a 'pulsatility index' that may correlate with ICP.

INTUSSUSCEPTION

A 2-year-old girl is brought to A+E with abdominal pain, vomiting, and inconsolable crying. The paediatricians have asked you to see her. What do you do?

- Take a history—nature of the pain (colicky/constant), type of vomit (gastric/bilious), diarrhoea/bloody stools, recent coryzal illness.
- Examine her after analgesia—general signs of dehydration and sepsis, abdominal distension, peritonism, palpable mass.
- Request an AXR to look for small bowel obstruction.

She is recovering from a chest infection. The pain is colicky. Her bowels have not moved since the pain started. She is tachycardic and pyrexial, and the AXR suggests small bowel obstruction. What is the likely diagnosis and how will you treat her?

- This sounds like intussusception.
- I would resuscitate the child with intravenous dextrose saline and analgesia, and arrange an abdominal USS to look for a mass in the ileocaecal region.

- Target or doughnut sign on transverse section.
- Pseudokidney sign (bowel within bowel) on longitudinal section.
- If confirmed and she was not peritonitic, I would arrange reduction using either an air enema or hydrostatic reduction, under USS or fluoroscopic guidance.
  - The success rate is around 80%.
- If two enemas had failed or she was peritonitic, this needs to be treated surgically—initial laparoscopy to confirm diagnosis, with resection of any lead point and nonviable small bowel.

What is the recurrence rate?

- The average recurrence rate is 5%.

What are the causes of intussusception?

- Primary (idiopathic):
  - Patient is 6 months to 3 years of age; there is no pathological lead point.
  - Hypertrophy of Peyer's patches drags the neighbouring bowel wall.
  - The most common site is ileocolic but it can happen anywhere in the bowel.
- Secondary:
  - Patient is 3 years or older; there is an identifiable lead point—Meckel's diverticulum, polyp, appendix, foreign bodies, lymphoma
- Intussusceptum—proximal invaginating bowel
- Intussuscipiens—distal receiving intestine

Are you aware of any predisposing factors for intussusception?

- Recent viral illness
- Henoch–Schonlein purpura
- Cystic fibrosis
- Coeliac disease

LAPAROSCOPIC INJURY

What injuries can occur during laparoscopic port insertion?

- Injuries to viscera (mainly bowel and bladder) and vessels can occur.
- The risk is increased in patients with adhesions and if blind trocar entry is attempted.

What vascular injuries can occur?

- Both superficial (e.g., inferior epigastric) and deep vessels (e.g., aorta) are at risk.
- Major vessel injury occurs in 0.05% to 0.5% of initial trocar insertions.

- Major vessel injury usually is immediately identifiable due to visible bleeding and haemodynamic instability.

You are undertaking a laparoscopic appendicectomy on a 17-year-old girl. Umbilical port insertion and establishment of a pneumoperitoneum are uneventful but when you insert a 5 mm trocar suprapubically, you lose vision and there is immediate heavy bleeding visible in the camera lens. Her blood pressure drops suddenly to 80/40. What are you going to do?

- Inform the anaesthetic team that there is heavy bleeding and that you are converting to an open case.
- Tell the theatre team to open a laparotomy and a vascular set.
- The most likely site of injury is the iliac vein, followed by omental vessels, cava and aorta.
- Given the likely sites, a midline laparotomy will be performed.
- If a major vessel is injured, control the bleeding with pressure and ask for assistance from a vascular surgeon (*unless you are a vascular surgeon— then say what you would do*).
- Major arterial injuries need to be repaired without tension and with precise intima-to-intima apposition.
- Major venous injuries may also need tension-free repair, though sometimes ligation may be the safer alternative.

How does bowel injury after trocar insertion present?

- It may present immediately with obvious spillage of bowel contents at laparoscopy, but more commonly as a delayed presentation in a patient failing to improve after surgery.
- Diagnosis can be difficult, especially as findings such as a pneumoperitoneum are expected after a laparoscopic procedure.
- Patients with evolving peritonitis should have a repeat laparoscopy or an open exploration together with bowel repair.

How does an air or gas embolus present during a laparoscopic case?

- These occur when intra-abdominal pressure exceeds intravenous pressure and communication between the abdominal cavity and a large vein results in gas being forced along a pressure gradient into the venous circulation.
- Sufficiently large gas boluses may trigger cardiovascular collapse by interfering with right ventricular function.
- The patient will have a machinery type heart murmur, hypotension and hypoxia.

How do you treat a gas embolus during laparoscopic surgery?

- Stop insufflation.
- Vent the abdominal cavity.

- Place the patient in a left lateral position with head down.
- Place a central line into the right ventricle and aspirate gas bubbles.

LIVER LACERATION

A 65-year-old male fell off a ladder and is brought to A+E. On examination, he is tachycardic and hypotensive with a large bruise over the right lower chest wall. He is very tender over his RUQ. When you arrive, he has been resuscitated, and his BP has improved. A CXR and pelvic XR are normal, and a FAST scan shows some free fluid in the abdomen. How will you manage this patient?

- Firstly, I would check that the initial resuscitation is complete (ABCs, oxygen, analgesia, warm IV crystalloid fluids) and that large-bore cannulae have been placed and routine bloods taken (including group and save).
- I would review the A+E notes and ask for a catheter to be placed. I would then take an AMPLE history and confirm from the paramedics how far he had fallen. I would also look for obvious long bone trauma, given the nature of the fall.
- With the bruising over the right side of the chest, a normal CXR and initial hypotension, I suspect he has a liver injury.
- Because he has responded to the resuscitation and is maintaining his blood pressure, I would ask for an urgent CT scan with contrast. However, he has obviously lost at least 1–2 l of blood, and I will want to keep a close eye on his observations, with a low threshold for operating if he deteriorates.

Why would you not take the patient to theatre?

- He is stable and has responded to the resuscitation.
- A CT scan will grade the degree of liver trauma.
- Small lacerations can be successfully managed conservatively, without the need for a laparotomy.
- A CT scan will identify other injuries that may need definitive treatment and help plan surgery/call other colleagues for help.

How are liver injuries classified?

- Use the liver injury scale from the American Association of Surgery for Trauma (AAST).
- There are six grades of liver trauma:
  - Grades I–IV classify lacerations or subcapsular haematomas, increasing in percentage of the liver involved.
  - Grades V and VI correspond to major vascular injuries and hepatic avulsion and are associated with high mortality.
- The majority of grade I–III lacerations can be managed conservatively, if the patient is stable.

His CT scan shows a grade III liver laceration and no other internal injuries. How will you manage him?

- I would monitor him in a critical care unit, with strict bed rest and hourly observations.
- There should be serial abdominal examinations, ideally by the same surgeon, to assess for peritonism/abdominal distension.
- Serial FBCs look for a drop in haematocrit or haemoglobin, indicating a further bleed.
- Transfuse as necessary.

During transfer to HDU, the patient becomes cold, clammy and hypotensive. What do you do?

- The patient is now unstable and needs an immediate laparotomy to control the bleeding from the liver laceration.
- I would take the patient straight to recovery and call the anaesthetist and theatre team to prepare a theatre.
- Following the principles of a damage-control laparotomy, I would make a long midline laparotomy incision, remove blood clots, pack all four quadrants of the abdomen and then wait for the anaesthetist to resuscitate the patient.
- Once the patient had been stabilised, I would carefully remove the packs from the three 'normal' quadrants to check that there were no hidden injuries causing blood loss and then repack them.
- If the only source of bleeding is coming from the liver bed, I would repack the liver, using a sandwich technique, placing packs over and under the liver, and then close the skin.
- I would then call the local liver unit and arrange transfer of the patient.

Are you aware of any techniques that can be used to repair a damaged liver?

- The Pringle manoeuvre can be performed for up to 1 hr to control the bleeding and assess the damage.
- A venovenous bypass (common femoral vein to axillary vein) can be done for venous injury.

LOWER GASTROINTESTINAL BLEED

A 70-year-old gentleman arrived in A+E shocked, after a couple of a large PR bleeds. How would you manage him?

- Resuscitate the patient—patent airway, high-flow oxygen, large-bore IV access, take bloods for FBC, U+E, coagulation studies, group + save and cross-match, give warmed one l Hartmann's solution, insert urinary catheter.

- Examine the patient to elicit abdominal tenderness and signs of shock, assess severity of bleeding, and perform a PR. Ask about drug and past medical history and review old notes.
- Review in 30–60 min to assess response to resuscitation and estimate degree of blood loss:
  - <200 ml = no effect on HR/BP
  - 800 ml = drop in BP of 10 mmHg, increase in HR of 10 bpm
  - 1500 ml = could induce shock
- If there is evidence of ongoing or aggressive bleeding, I would transfuse two units to maintain the blood pressure and ask for an anaesthetic opinion to consider HDU care.
- If there was a coagulopathy (INR > 1.5) or thrombocytopaenia (<50), I would talk to the haematologist on call about whether the patient needs beriplex, FFP, platelets or vitamin K.

Which patients are at risk for developing a lower GI bleed?

- Patients taking aspirin, NSAIDs and anticoagulants (e.g., warfarin)
- History of previous rectal bleeding, pelvic irradiation, colonoscopy or polypectomy in the previous 2 weeks
- Patients with liver cirrhosis, ulcerative colitis and Crohn's disease, and symptoms suggestive of colorectal cancer
- Of patients with a fresh PR bleed 11% will have a massive upper GI bleed
- 80%–85% stop spontaneously
- Overall mortality of 2%–4%

What are the causes of lower GI bleeding?

- Diverticular disease—17%–40%
  - Acute, painless, arterial in nature, occurs at the dome or neck of a diverticulum, stops spontaneously in 80%; 25% rebleed within 4 years
- Angiodysplasia—9%–21%
  - Majority in right colon, often multiple, bleed due to coagulopathy, red circumscribed mucosal lesions (1 mm–3 cm) at colonoscopy
- Colitis (ischaemic, chronic, IBD, radiation): 2%–30%
  - Sudden, often temporary, reduction in mesenteric blood flow resulting from episodes of low BP/vasospasm—occurs at watershed areas of the colon (splenic flexure and rectosigmoid junction) and mainly affects elderly with atherosclerosis
  - Present with abdominal pain followed by PR bleed/bloody diarrhoea; usually self-limiting but has increased risk of mortality
- Neoplasia and postpolypectomy bleeds: 11%–14%
  - Delayed bleeding can occur up to 2 weeks postprocedure
- Anorectal disease (haemorrhoids, rectal varices): 4%–10%

- Upper GI bleeding: 0%–11%
- Small bowel bleeding: 2%–9%

The patient stabilises after two units of blood, and his blood pressure returns to normal, although he continues to pass small amounts of fresh blood PR. What do you do?

- Consider an urgent colonoscopy (diagnostic yield of 89%–97%), provided the patient remains stable.
- Current recommendations advise giving bowel prep in acute LGIB, as it improves diagnostic yield and decreases the risk of perforation.
- Bleeding lesions can be injected, coagulated, clipped or band ligated.

The patient has another large PR bleed on the ward and becomes hypotensive. He needs another two units of blood to stabilise him. What would you do now?

- Arrange mesenteric/CT angiography, which can detect bleeding at a rate of >0.5–1 ml/min, and is 100% specific, with 47% sensitivity in the acute setting.
- There is the possibility of controlling the bleeding with an endovascular coil or embolisation and to identify the bleeding point if the patient needed surgery.

When would you operate on patients with a massive rectal bleed? What would you do in theatre?

- Surgery is the last resort—only in unstable patients with fulminant bleeding or recurrent bleeding without localisation of the bleeding source.
- I would first do an OGD to exclude a massive upper GI bleed and a proctoscopy to look for haemorrhoidal bleeding.
- Blind segmental colectomy is associated with unacceptably high rates of morbidity (rebleeding rate up to 75%) and mortality (up to 50%).
- I would attempt intraoperative colonoscopy, using the appendix to wash out the colon and to localise the bleeding source, and hope to identify a bleeding point. If this were negative, I would attempt small bowel enteroscopy, as bleeding can come from the small bowel. Directed segmental resection has low morbidity, mortality (4%) and rebleeding rates (6%).

What risk factors predict a severe course or a rebleed?

- HR > 100 bpm, BP < 115 mmHg systolic, syncope
- A second PR bleed within the first 4 hr of admission
- More than two active comorbidities
- Aspirin

MESENTERIC ISCHAEMIA

A 60-year-old woman in AF presents with acute abdominal pain. Your foundation doctor (FY2) tells you that her abdomen is soft and, because there are ECG changes, he is referring her to the medics. What do you do?

- I would be concerned that the patient has mesenteric ischaemia. I would want to assess the patient thoroughly myself.
- Patients classically present with severe central abdominal pain out of proportion with the clinical signs, which is often resistant to opioid analgesia. They are often not peritonitic.
- I would check the history for a possible embolic source, such as a recent MI/CVA, cardiac arrhythmia and peripheral vascular disease.

What are the causes of mesenteric ischaemia?

- Occlusive and nonocclusive
- Thrombotic causes:
  - Arterial embolism (64%)
  - Arterial thrombosis (27%)
  - Mesenteric venous thrombosis:
    - Primary (protein C/S/antithrombin III deficiency, factor V Leiden)
    - Secondary (portal hypertension, pancreatitis, trauma and the OCP)
- Nonocclusive mesenteric ischaemia (NOMI) results from low flow states (e.g., severe vasoconstriction due to reduced cardiac output in shock [sepsis, cardiac shock, hypovolaemia])

How will you manage the patient if you suspect mesenteric ischaemia?

- Firstly, I would resuscitate the patient with oxygen, IV fluids and opioid analgesia, and take routine bloods including gases and blood cultures. If the patient were septic, I would start the sepsis bundle and prescribe broad-spectrum antibiotics.
- A raised WCC, amylase, lactate and metabolic acidosis point toward the diagnosis, although these can be late findings. Plain AXR is rarely helpful, but may show thumb-printing from mucosal oedema.
- If the patient is not peritonitic and the diagnosis is uncertain, I would ask for a CT scan (mesenteric venous gas, pneumatosis intestinalis and fat stranding).
- If the patient is peritonitic and fit for surgery, I would take him or her immediately to theatre for a diagnostic laparotomy.
- Elderly patients with multiple comorbidities are unlikely to survive surgery (overall mortality is 90%), so I would have a frank discussion with the patient and family about the two options: surgery (which may not be curative) or keeping the patient comfortable.

What will you do at laparotomy?

- Establish the diagnosis and check for pulsation in the mesenteric vessels and viability of the duodenum, jejunum and small bowel.
- An embolus usually lodges distal to the origin of the middle colic and pancreaticoduodenal branches of the SMA, sparing the stomach, duodenum and proximal jejunum.
- A thrombosis occurs at the origin of the SMA, and only the stomach and duodenum are spared.
- In the vast majority of cases, ischaemia is extensive, the abdomen is closed and the patient is palliated on the ward.
- If a resection is performed, successful reperfusion will release free radicals, causing an inflammatory response which can lead to multiorgan failure.

When would you consider nonsurgical treatment? How would you manage it?

- Peritonitis was absent or there were nonocclusive causes.
- The underlying condition should be treated and cardiac output optimised with inotropes.
- Papaverin infusion is sometimes used; phosphodiesterase inhibitor increases mesenteric flow.
- Intra-atrterial thrombolysis can be used for mesenteric venous occlusion, but only if there is no evidence of bowel infarction. These patients need long-term anticoagulation because of high recurrence rates.

NECROTISING FASCIITIS

It is 1 a.m. A 65-year-old diabetic male presents with a painful red swelling in his right thigh and groin. He is pyrexial, hypotensive and dehydrated. How will you treat him?

- Resuscitate the patient with oxygen and IV fluids and take baseline bloods, BM, urinalysis and arterial gases.
- Take a history and examine the patient.
  - Check for trauma, IV drug use, symptoms of bowel obstruction.
- Consider differential diagnosis—cellulitis/abscess/necrotising fasciitis/strangulated hernia.

What is necrotising fasciitis?

- It is polymicrobial infection of skin and fascia with necrosis of subcutaneous tissue, sparing the underlying muscle.
- It can progress rapidly to severe sepsis, multiorgan failure and death.
- Primary necrotising fasciitis is due to bacterial entry from mild skin trauma.
- Secondary necrotising fasciitis is due to prior infection (e.g., deep abscess/visceral perforation).

- Risk factors are diabetes, immunosuppression, steroids, old age, malnourishment and renal failure.

What are the clinical signs?

- Erythema, swelling, and pain
- Warning signs: dusky blue skin, crepitus (indicating gas in the tissues), patchy areas of necrosis, bullae and signs of systemic sepsis

How would you confirm the diagnosis?

- Blood tests: leucocytosis, acidosis, deranged clotting, hypoalbuminaemia, abnormal renal function
- Imaging: soft tissue gas on x-ray or CT (if the patient is stable)
- Stab incision over crepitus releases murky fluid from skin.

How would you treat the patient?

- IV broad spectrum antibiotics are used against *Streptococcus,* Gram-negative aerobes (*E. coli* and *Pseudomonas*), anaerobes (*Bacteroides*):
  - Start with augmentin/metronidazole initially and consult with the microbiologist on call.
- Take patient to theatre following initial resuscitation (may need HDU/ITU) because this is a life-threatening emergency.
- Incise down to deep fascia; debride all nonviable tissue.
- Take back in 24 hr for a second look and further debridement.
- Some studies report the benefit of hyperbaric oxygen (controversial and not widely used).

NEEDLESTICK INJURY

You are sitting in the theatre coffee room when you get called to say that your ST5 has just had a needlestick injury. He was operating on a previous IV drug user. What do you do?

- Check what happened. Was it a clean needle/blade or had it already been used during the operation?
- Tell the SpR to encourage free bleeding.
- Wash with soap or chlorhexidine.
- Do not scrub/suck the wound.
- Send the ST5 to Occupational Health.
- Report the incident via local guidelines.

- Report to the Health Protection Agency (anonymous national surveillance scheme).

What will Occupational Health do?

- Take blood for storage (proves not infected at the time).
- Check whether Hep B booster is needed.
- Counsel regarding:
  - Risks of seroconversion
  - Risks in this incident
  - Safe sex
  - No blood donation
  - No work restrictions
  - HIV/HCV/HBV follow-up blood tests

What are the risks of seroconversion?

- 0.3%: percutaneous needlestick from HIV-infected patient
- 0.1%: mucocutaneous contamination from HIV-infected patient
- 0.5%–1.8%: percutaneous needlestick from HCV-infected patient
- 30% (for nonimmune individual): percutaneous needlestick from Hbe Ag positive patient

The anaesthetic FY2 has helpfully taken blood from the patient whilst he was still asleep. What do you test it for?

- It has to be discarded.
- Blood can only be taken from the source with his consent.
- There must be a pretest discussion prior to HIV testing:
  - The same tests as done for blood donors
  - Confidentiality
  - Decision to take blood not based on perceived risk of positive result; patient can decline
- Blood not to be taken by the exposed member of staff

How do you prevent needlestick injuries?

- Surgery performed by most experienced members of surgical team (includes scrub staff)
- Standard universal precautions
- No-touch technique (pass blades and needles in kidney dish)
- Never resheath a needle
- Safety-shielded venous and arterial cannulae
- Safe disposal of sharps

If the patient was known to have HIV, what extra measures should your SpR take?

- Postexposure prophylaxis started within 1 hr of injury
  - Twenty-eight days of tenofovir/emtricitabine, ritonaivir/lopanovir and antiemetic
  - May need time off work due to drug side effects
  - Named patient basis as not licensed
- Can be started within 72 hr of exposure, but less effective

PAEDIATRIC TRAUMA

An 8-year-old boy was hit by a car travelling at 35 miles per hour. He was thrown to the pavement and hit a tree. He was alert and oriented at the scene and complained of left upper abdominal pain. He is brought to A+E with a cervical collar on a spinal board. How will you manage this child?

- According to ATLS principles (ABCs with C-spine control with simultaneous resuscitation), two cannulae should be inserted and bloods send for FBC, U+Es, Glc and urgent cross match. Consider venous cut-down or intraosseus infusion if the child is shocked and unstable.
- Assess GCS and examine for life-threatening injuries.
- Take AMPLE history, review of ABCs after resuscitation and complete secondary survey. The cervical spine should be kept immobilised till the cervical injury has been ruled out—may need CT scan to do this if distracting injuries are present.
- Decreased GCS or suspicion of raised intracranial pressure or spinal injury warrants a CT scan of brain and spine as per the NICE guidelines and appropriate intervention or referral.
  - If GCS < 8, child should be intubated and ventilated.
- CT scan of the abdomen and thorax with IV contrast is the gold standard investigation in a stable child following trauma.
- Breslow tape helps guide fluid and drug dosage.

How much fluid will you give to this child?

- The fluid requirement is guided by the haemodynamic stability.
- Two boluses of 20 ml/kg of normal saline may be given.
- If the child remains hypotensive, I would then give 10 ml/kg of packed RBCs.

What is the principle of management of solid organ injury in paediatric patients?

- If the child is stable or responds to resuscitation, conservative management is routine, with IV fluids, blood transfusion if needed, daily FBCs and bed rest.
- The only indication for surgery is failure to respond to resuscitation, ongoing blood loss or presence of hollow viscus injury.

What is the 'seat belt sign'?

- Bruises or abrasions on the anterior abdominal wall due to the restraint of a seat belt. It is more common with a lap belt than a traditional seat belt with three-point restraint.
- It often indicates an underlying visceral injury—duodenual transection, mesenteric haematomas, retroperitoneal injuries and lumbar spine fractures (chance fractures).

A 12-year-old boy hits the kerb whilst riding his bike and flips over, landing on the handle bars. What are the possible injuries?

- Transection of the duodenum
- Duodenal haematoma
- Pancreatic trauma—amylase may not be raised in early stages

PENETRATING CHEST TRAUMA

A 23-year-old woman arrives in A+E following an assault. She has multiple stab wounds to both sides of her praecordium and arrested in the ambulance 2 min before reaching hospital. What are you going to do?

- An immediate thoracotomy must be done.

Why?

- Likelihood of cardiac injury or major intrathoracic bleed
- Pre-hospital cardiac arrest with < 10 min CPR
- In hospital cardiac arrest

What might you find?

- Cardiac tamponade
- Massive haemothorax
- Haemomediastinum

Tell me how you will do it…

- Antisepsis, scalpel and Gigli saw; clamshell thoracotomy at the level of the fifth interspace

She has a tamponade—now what?

- Open the pericardial sac along the long axis of the heart, evacuate the clot, start cardiac massage.

There is a hole in her right ventricle—what now?

- Finger over the hole, get a foley catheter, insert it and temporarily close the defect with vertical mattress sutures consult local cardiac unit.

What would make you abandon the procedure?

- Visible air in the cardiac vessels
- Irretrievable injury such as massive haemomediastinum from aortic disruption
- Unable to fill the heart after 5 min
- No spontaneous cardiac rhythm after 10 min
- Unable to sustain a systolic BP of >70 or a palpable carotid pulse after 15 min

PENETRATING NECK TRAUMA

You are the consultant general surgeon on call at a district general hospital and are called immediately to attend the emergency department to assess a 31-year-old male who has sustained a stab wound to the left side of his neck. What are your thoughts regarding initial management as you rush down from your office?

- Assess and resuscitate patient according to ATLS principles.
- Undertake airway management with supplementary oxygen—may need endotracheal intubation depending on the site and severity of the injury.
- Consultant anaesthetist should be present and intubate if there is respiratory difficulty, depressed level of consciousness or expanding neck haematoma.
- Assess breathing and look for tension pneumothorax/haemothorax.
- If this is an active haemorrhage, consider cautious external compression (beware of prolonged compression over carotid arteries).
- Assess haemodynamic status—the physiology will dictate further management.
- If the patient is unstable, radiological or surgical intervention may be necessary to control bleeding.
- If there is a pulsatile or rapidly expanding haematoma, after intubation I would consider taking the patient directly to theatre for a neck exploration:
  - This may need input from vascular and radiological colleagues, depending on subspeciality and experience.
- If the patient is stable, I would perform a secondary survey, take history and conduct a full examination.
- I would take a history—important points are mechanism of injury, size of weapon, amount of bleeding, neurological status (including drop in GCS) and evidence of impending airway compromise (e.g., stridor).
- I would perform an examination—hard and soft signs can be indicative of vascular injury, crepitus, haemoptysis, hoarseness, bubbling in the wound.

Can you tell me about the zones of the neck, in relation to neck trauma?

- Zone I—clavicles to cricoid cartilage
  - Contents—proximal carotid, subclavian and vertebral arteries, oesophagus, trachea, thoracic duct, brachial plexus, spinal cord and upper lung
- Zone II—cricoid cartilage to angle of mandible
  - Contents—carotid and vertebral arteries, jugular veins, larynx, oesophagus, trachea, vagus and recurrent laryngeal nerves, spinal cord
- Zone III—angle of mandible to base of skull
  - Contents—pharynx, distal carotid and vertebral arteries, parotid, cranial nerves

What are the triangles of the neck?

- Posterior triangle
- Anterior triangle (subdivided into submental, digastric, carotid and muscular)

What are the borders and contents of the triangles of the neck?

- Posterior triangle:
  - Borders:
    - Anterior–posterior border of sternocleidomastoid
    - Posterior–anterior border of trapezius
    - Inferior—clavicle
  - Contents:
    - Muscles (floor of triangle)—splenius capitis, levator scapulae, scalenus medius (scalenus anterior), (serratus anterior)
    - Nerves—branches of cervical plexus, spinal accessory nerve (travels from one-third of the way down posterior border of sternocleidomastoid to trapezius), trunks of brachial plexus
    - Other—lymph nodes (occipital/supraclavicular), subclavian artery, transverse cervical and suprascapular vessels
- Anterior triangle:
  - Borders of anterior triangle:
    - Midline
    - Posterior border of sternocleidomastoid
    - Ramus of mandible
  - Contents:
    - Muscle—suprahyoid muscles (digastric, stylohyoid, mylohyoid, geniohyoid)
    - Strap muscles (thyrohyoid, sternothyroid, sternohyoid)
    - Nerves—recurrent and external laryngeal nerves (from vagus nerve)
    - Vagus nerve (in carotid sheath), ansa cervicalis, hypoglossal nerve

- – Vessels—common carotid artery and bifurcation, branches of external; internal jugular vein
- – Other—thyroid gland, parathyroid glands, submandibular gland, trachea and oesophagus

What are the hard and soft signs indicative of vascular injury?

- Hard signs:
  - Active external bleeding
  - Rapidly expanding cervical haematoma
  - Absent carotid pulse
  - Bruit or thrill
- Soft signs:
  - Bleeding from neck wound or pharynx
  - Ipsilateral Horner's sign
  - Deficit of the superficial temporal artery pulse
  - Dysfunction of cranial nerves IX–XII
  - Widened mediastinum
  - Fractures of the skull base and temporal bone
  - Fractures and dislocation of the cervical spine

If the patient was stable, what diagnostic tests would you request?

- Request lateral C-spine—evidence of undetected emphysema.
- Request chest x-ray—widened mediastinum or pneumomediastinum, pneumothorax, haemothorax, tracheal deviation.
- Consider bronchoscopy/laryngoscopy for airway injuries.
- Request CT neck—to assess structures in neck including oesophageal and vascular injury.
- Consider angiography for zone I and III injuries.

How would you surgically manage zone I, II and III injuries?

- Zone I injury—stable:
  - Diagnostic workup as described previously; CXR important
  - Unstable—urgent exploration in theatre with help available if needed
  - Principles of surgery:
    - – Sternotomy to obtain proximal control for all vessels (including right subclavian, innominate vessels), except injury lateral to left midclavicular line (then needs left anterolateral thoracotomy)
    - – Left subclavian artery approached using a trapdoor incision
- Zone II injury:
  - Exsanguinating, shocked or those with an evolving stroke should go straight to theatre for exploration.
  - Those not exsanguinating or without an evolving stroke can be observed in a critical care area.

- Soft signs are not an indication for angiography or surgery in this group.
- Repeated physical examination is as sensitive for vascular injury as angiography.
- Zone III injury:
  - Exsanguinating patients require immediate haemorrhage control.
  - This is often due to branches of the external carotid.
  - Surgical access is very difficult.
  - Thus, even in unstable patients, radiological embolisation is preferred.
  - Patients with an evolving stroke require immediate exploration to rule out an internal carotid artery injury.
  - Stable patients should be managed as for zone II.

PENILE FRACTURE

A 27-year-old man attends your A+E department at 11 p.m. presenting with a swollen, bruised penis that occurred during sexual intercourse. What is the differential diagnosis?

- Penile fracture (a corporal tear of the tunica albuginea of the penis)
- Rupture of suspensory ligament of the penis
- Bruising from rupture/trauma to a superficial vein

What in the history would point to/away from a fracture of the penis?

- Forcible bending of the erect penis, often associated with an audible snap and then immediate detumescence and a large haematoma (often called the aubergine sign), pointing toward a fracture
- If there was no detumescence or a delayed one, then a penile fracture is less likely. If this is the case and I am unsure, ultrasound or MRI performed on the next day would confirm a diagnosis.

What other features are relevant?

- Haematuria can occur in about 10% of cases and is associated with a concomitant urethral injury.

How would you manage him?

- Admit patient and ensure he is voiding satisfactorily.
- Do not catherise him.
- If he is voiding and there is extravasation of urine into subcutaneous tissues (due to a urethral injury) or an expanding haematoma, he will need the urgent attention of the urologist. It is therefore advisable to review the patient regularly to ensure that there is no expanding haematoma.
- Inform the on-call urologist and list patient for repair of the fracture.

- Previously, patients used to be managed conservatively, but this was associated with a high rate of erectile dysfunction. As a result, some surgeons advocated immediate repair (i.e., in the middle of the night). Evidence from a large retrospective case series suggests that this is unnecessary. Thus, the patient can wait for his operation until the next morning.
- The principles of repair include degloving the penis and repair of the corporal defect and urethra.

PERFORATED DUODENAL ULCER

A 55-year-old lady is seen in the emergency department with heartburn after starting steroids and NSAIDs 1 week ago to manage a flare-up of rheumatoid arthritis. She complains of sudden-onset epigastric pain that has been getting progressively worse over the past 36 hr. An erect chest radiograph does not reveal any free intra-abdominal air under the diaphragm. Despite this, you strongly suspect she has a perforated peptic ulcer. How accurate are plain radiographs in detecting pneumoperitoneum?

- It can be possible to detect 1 ml of free air on an erect chest radiograph or decubitus view (can be more sensitive at detecting free air).
- The absence of subdiaphragmatic air on an erect chest radiograph does not exclude a perforated peptic ulcer. In approximately 10%–30% of cases, free intra-abdominal gas is not demonstrated on an erect chest radiograph.
- A CT scan of the abdomen with IV and oral contrast is the most definitive investigation. This will also exclude pancreatitis as a potential alternative diagnosis.

The CT scan showed a thickened duodenum with locules of free gas and a collection in the right iliac fossa, confirming your suspicions of a perforated duodenal ulcer. How would you proceed?

- I would initially resuscitate the patient with IV fluids, analgesia, broad-spectrum antibiotics, IV proton pump inhibitor therapy, and a urinary catheter and, if possible, pass a nasogastric tube.
- In a fit, healthy patient with clinical signs of peritonitis, surgery is the preferred treatment option.
- I would start laparoscopically if the patient were not haemodynamically compromised. Profoundly septic, medically unfit, hypotensive patients would find it difficult to tolerate the further drop in blood pressure on creation of a CO_2 pneumoperitoneum, and in these circumstances it would be safer to approach repair of the ulcer via an upper midline incision.

How will you repair the ulcer?

- Small (<0.5 cm) perforated duodenal ulcers on the anterior wall can be repaired either laparoscopically or at open surgery.

- An interrupted primary closure with an absorbable suture should be performed with a superimposed omental patch.
- If there were no omentum in close proximity that could be mobilised to plug the defect, I would utilise the falciform ligament. This is more difficult at open surgery, as the ligament is often incorporated and divided within the incision.
- Lavage and eradication of peritoneal soiling is a vital part of the surgical management in all cases of perforated peptic ulcers.
- Larger ulcers are not considered appropriate for laparoscopic repair. Meta-analysis comparing open with laparoscopic repair found a higher leak rate in repairs performed laparoscopically.

At the time of surgery, you find a large friable perforated duodenal ulcer that is too large to close with a patch. What are your options?
Say what YOU would do (depends on your surgical expertise).

- A young, fit patient with a large friable perforated ulcer in the first part of the duodenum should be considered for a distal gastrectomy with Roux-en-Y gastrojejunostomy reconstruction.
- If distal gastrectomy is not appropriate (patient or surgeon factors) an alternative is to fire a stapler proximal to the ulcer, to exclude the area from gastric contents, and close the perforation over a Foley catheter to create a controlled fistula. A gastrojejunostomy will then need to be constructed to establish gastrointestinal continuity.
- If the patient was in extremis and damage limitation surgery needed, simply closing the defect with a purse string around a Foley catheter to create a controlled fistula is another option.

You find a perforated gastric ulcer at laparoscopy. How will you close it?

- Primary closure with omental patch is still appropriate.
- However, biopsies must be taken to exclude malignancy.
- Definitive radical resection of the stomach should be delayed until biopsies prove malignancy, the patient has been staged and they have been discussed at an MDT.

Is there a role for conservative management of perforated peptic ulcers?

- Yes, if the patient is clinically well with no evidence of haemodynamic instability or peritonitis, and a CT scan shows there is no ongoing leak.
- The patient should be placed nil by mouth with a nasogastric tube on free drainage and started on IV antibiotics and a proton pump inhibitor.
- Intra-abdominal collections may need radiological drainage.

PERIANAL SEPSIS

A 30-year-old male presents to A+E with severe anal pain and a tender perianal swelling. How will you manage him?

- I would take a history—duration of symptoms, pain with defecation, rectal bleeding, fever, previous surgery for perianal sepsis—and ask about diabetes and Crohn's disease.
- Examination is often limited by pain. I would look for a well-defined painful lump or an area of induration and check whether the skin over the lump was necrotic.
- If this was the first presentation, I would book the patient for an incision and drainage of the abscess. If there were a history of recurrent abscesses or fistulas, or a suspicion of Crohn's disease, I would order a gadolinium contrast MRI to delineate the extent of the sepsis and look for horse-shoeing.

What would you do in theatre?

- I would perform a rectal exam and a rigid sigmoidoscopy to exclude malignancy and look for an obvious internal opening. If there were suspicions about Crohn's disease or HIV, I would send tissue to pathology and microbiology.

What *YOU* do next depends on *YOUR* training and expertise and whether *YOU* suspect a fistula:

- For a noncolorectal surgeon, a simple incision and drainage is safest in the acute stage and avoids damaging sphincters.
- For a colorectal surgeon, discussion could involve performing a fistulotomy for low fistulas (if present) or inserting a loose draining Seton. The patient must have been consented preoperatively for possible incontinence to flatus and liquid stool.

What is the microbiology of perianal sepsis?

- Skin organisms—the abscess should not recur.
- Gut organisms—it is likely that there is an underlying fistula and the patient will get recurrent abscesses.

What is Goodsall's rule in relation to perianal fistulas?

- If the external opening is anterior to the transverse anal line, the track runs directly to the internal opening in the anal canal.
- If the external opening is posterior to the transverse anal line, the track curves backward to the posterior midline.

How would you manage someone with perianal Crohn's disease?

- In the acute setting, I would order an MRI scan to delineate the nature of sepsis, perform an incision and drainage and refer to my gastrointestinal and colorectal colleagues for definitive management.

A colorectal trainee can place a loose Seton.

- Skin tags should be left alone.
- I would optimise the medical management of the Crohn's disease with steroids/azathioprine/infliximab where indicated; often fistulas will heal.
- Patients may need a defunctioning stoma to allow complex fistulas to heal, and, in some cases, resection of the diseased bowel will also improve fistulas.

POSTOPERATIVE FEVER

You are asked to review a 60-year-old man 3 days following an endovascular repair of his abdominal aortic aneurysm. He is now febrile at 38.2°C. What do you do?

- Assess the patient (basic ABCs).
  - Check pulse to exclude AF. Is patient cold and clammy or sweaty to touch?
  - Is pain controlled, or has pain recently increased?
  - Look at the patient for obvious source of sepsis—reduced air entry, infected groin wounds, cloudy urine, DVT, cellulitis around venflon sites, etc.
  - Check pulses in legs after AAA repair.
  - Ask about bowel habits—rectal bleeding/diarrhoea (? ischaemic colitis).
- Review the chart—is this a new spike or has patient been septic overnight?
  - Is he hypoxic, tachycardic and hypotensive (i.e., is this SIRS)?
- Start resuscitation if needed.
  - Give O_2, IV fluids if low urine output or clinically dehydrated, take bloods for blood cultures from all lines, swab wounds and lines, etc., CXR and ECG.
- Review notes—PMHx, drug history, operation notes/problems during operation.
- Review results of tests.

What are the common causes of postoperative fever?

- Seven Cs: Cut, Chest, Cannula, Catheter, Central line, Collection, Clot
- Immediate—endocrine crises—thyrotoxicosis, Addisonian crisis
- Days 0–2—atelectasis, reaction to implanted material (e.g., vascular graft)
- Days 3–5—UTI, bronchopneumonia
- Days 5–7—wound infection/abscess, anastomotic leak
- Day 7–10—deep vein thrombosis
- Any time—line sepsis, transfusion reaction, drug reaction

What is SIRS?

- Systemic inflammatory response syndrome
- Any two of:
    - Heart rate > 90 beats per minute
    - Temperature < 36°C or > 38°C
    - White cell count < $4 \times 10^9/l$ or > $10 \times 10^9/l$
    - Respiratory rate > 20 breaths per minute or $PaCO_2$ < 32 mmHg
- This is caused by cytokine release in response to trauma, inflammation or infection.
- The SIRS criteria are nonspecific and must be interpreted within the clinical context.

What is the difference between SIRS and sepsis?

- SIRS is triggered by trauma, inflammation or infection leading to organ dysfunction, organ failure and possibly death.
- SIRS has many potential triggers.
- Sepsis is a physiological state of SIRS in the presence of known infection.

What conditions can cause SIRS?

- Conditions are broadly divided into infectious and noninfectious.
- Noninfectious causes include burns, bleeding, trauma, pancreatitis and ischaemia.
- Other causes include complications of aortic aneurysms, adrenal insufficiency, drugs, pulmonary embolus and cardiac tamponade.

What complications can SIRS lead to?

- End-organ damage:
    - Acute lung injury
    - Acute kidney injury
    - Multiorgan dysfunction syndrome
    - Shock

RUPTURED ABDOMINAL AORTIC ANEURYSM

A 52-year-old male hypertensive smoker is referred to A+E with left loin-to-groin pain which began suddenly about 3 hr ago. He is pale and sweaty. His heart rate is 100 beats per minute and his blood pressure is 110/80. Urinalysis is normal. What is the differential diagnosis?

- A leaking abdominal aortic aneurysm often masquerades as renal colic on first presentation.
- Ninety percent of renal colic patients have blood in their urine on dipstick.

- The patient's blood pressure is a little low with a narrowed pulse pressure.
- Given the absence of haematuria in this patient, the main concern is a leaking AAA. Other possibilities include renal colic, pyelonephritis, pancreatitis, mesenteric ischaemia.

Define an aneurysm.

- An arterial aneurysm is a segmental dilation of the vessel wall to 1.5 times its normal diameter or, in the case of the aorta, to greater than 3 cm in diameter.

How will you exclude the possibility of a leaking aneurysm?

- A portable ultrasound in the emergency department may demonstrate the presence of an aneurysm, but cannot determine whether or not it has leaked.
- A contrast-enhanced CT scan is required to exclude a leaking AAA in a stable patient. A CT will also help plan a possible endovascular repair of a leaking aneurysm.

An emergency department ultrasound reveals an 8 cm abdominal aortic aneurysm. What are you going to do?

- Given the presentation, relative hypotension and tachycardia, it is likely that this AAA has leaked.
- The patient should be resuscitated—oxygen, two large-bore IV cannulae, bloods (including a cross-match and renal function), a urinary catheter and an ECG.
- Warn theatres, critical care and anaesthetic teams that there is a patient with a likely leak.
- He is relatively stable, so he should undergo CT to (1) confirm diagnosis and (2) evaluate suitability for endovascular repair.

What features on the CT scan suggest a leak?

- The primary signs of a leak are periaortic stranding, a retroperitoneal haematoma and extravasation of contrast.
- The posterior pararenal and perirenal compartments are the most common locations for retroperitoneal haematomas in leaking AAAs.
- More subtle indications of impending leak include the draped aorta, discontinuity of intimal calcification, a high attenuating crescent due to haematoma in the wall or mural thrombus.

The CT scan shows a small retroperitoneal haematoma. There are no vascular surgeons in your hospital. What will you do now?

- Outcomes following elective and emergency major vascular surgery are better in high-volume centres.

- Contact the vascular surgeon on call at the local vascular referral centre and arrange for the transfer of the patient. Also arrange for the CT images to be transferred to the receiving hospital.

Are there any special instructions that you will give the paramedic crew transferring the patient?

- It is important to avoid over-resuscitating the patient.
- Accept low blood pressure readings as long as the patient is alert and oriented.
- Administering large volumes of fluids to achieve normal blood pressure readings may simply result in disruption of the clot at the leak site, exacerbating the bleeding.

Can you explain the pathophysiology of aneurysm formation?

- In cases of degenerative aneurysms, the aneurysm wall is characterised by reduced elastin content, increased collagen production and degradation, inflammation and imbalances between matrix metalloproteinases and their inhibitors.
- Some patients have a genetic predisposition, particularly in Marfan's or Ehler–Danlos type IV.
- The risk of degenerative aneurysm formation is increased by smoking, age, male gender, COPD, hypertension and family history.

Do any factors increase the risk of rupture?

- In addition to size, other independent predictors of rupture include current smoking, higher mean blood pressure and lower FEV1.
- A rapid expansion rate and an unfavourable aneurysm morphology may also predict rupture.

SIGMOID VOLVULUS AND PSEUDO-OBSTRUCTION

A 78-year-old man presents with acute abdominal distension. What are you going to do?

- Take a history: When did he notice the distension? Is it coming and going? Has he had it before? Is he vomiting? When did he last pass faeces or flatus? Does he have pain? What is the history of previous surgery? Has he noticed any recent alteration in bowel habit? Blood or mucus per rectum? Is he taking any medications? Does he have any other major illnesses?
- Examine the patient: Is he tachycardiac, tachypnoeic, pyrexial, hypotensive? Is he dry? How marked is the distension? Does he have any features of peritonitis? Any hernias, scars? PR examination: Is there a mass? Is there an empty ballooned rectum?

- Establish intravenous access, take bloods (full blood count, urea and electrolytes, group and save), start IV fluids and organise an abdominal x-ray.

The abdominal x-ray shows a coffee bean-shaped loop of bowel pointing toward the right upper quadrant. What is the diagnosis?

- Sigmoid volvulus typically presents with massive abdominal distension, absolute constipation and a coffee-bean shadow concave to the left.
- If the diagnosis is in doubt, it can be confirmed using a CT scan or contrast enema, which demonstrates a bird's beak deformity with nonpassage of contrast proximally. Gastrograffin should be used rather than barium due to the risk of perforation of ischaemic bowel.

Now what?

- The volvulus needs to be decompressed.
- If the patient already has peritonitis, then he needs a laparotomy.

Why can it not be left and treated with 'drip and suck'?

- Spontaneous detorsion is uncommon.
- The volved segment behaves as a closed loop obstruction with accumulation of gas and fluid raising the intraluminal pressure, leading to compromised circulation in the intestinal wall, intestinal wall necrosis, sepsis and death.

How will you treat the volvulus?

- If the patient has no features of bowel ischaemia, I would decompress it with a flexible sigmoidoscope and flatus tube.
  - This is successful in about 75% of cases with a 2.5% complication rate.
- The risk of recurrence is >90% with detorsion alone, so a definitive procedure should be considered once the patient has been adequately resuscitated.

You resuscitate the patient and place him on the emergency list for definitive treatment the next day. What operation will you undertake?

- He needs a sigmoid colectomy. Provided that the volvulus has been reduced and he is otherwise well, a primary anastomosis may be feasible. This avoids the potential morbidity of a second operation to reverse a temporary colostomy.

What if you found infarcted perforated sigmoid colon?

- In that case, I would undertake a Hartmann's procedure, as there will be localised contamination placing the anastomosis at increased risk of leakage.

Suppose the caecum had perforated due to the obstruction. What would you do?

- In that situation, I would do a subtotal colectomy with an end-ileostomy in the right iliac fossa.

What would you do if you found an obstructing sigmoid cancer instead of the expected volvulus?

- Assuming the rest of the colon was viable, I would proceed to a sigmoid colectomy with an end colostomy. If the proximal colon was damaged, then I would proceed with a subtotal colectomy and end-ileostomy.

SPLENIC TRAUMA

A 23-year-old woman fell off a horse, landing on her left side. A CXR shows left rib fractures 10–12. She is tachycardic but not hypotensive. How would you treat her?

- Resuscitate according to ATLS principles (ABCs with C spine control, O_2 and analgesia), two large-bore IV cannulae, slow Hartmann's infusion (normotensive), bloods (FBC, U+E, G+S, pregnancy test, amylase, LFTs), C spine and pelvic x-ray.
- Take a history—AMPLE (allergies, medication, past medical history, last meal, events surrounding trauma).
- Perform an examination—head to toe, including PR.
- There is concern about splenic trauma; consider FAST scan in A+E.
- Then proceed to a contrast CT scan if stable.

What are the symptoms and signs of splenic injury?

- Left upper quadrant pain (capsular stretching)
- Peritonitis (extravasated blood)
- Kehr's sign—left shoulder tip pain due to blood irritating diaphragm
- Associated injuries—low left rib fractures, bruising of lateral chest and abdominal wall

How do you grade splenic trauma?

- Use the AAST (American Association of Surgery in Trauma) classification.
- Grades I–III classify lacerations or subcapsular haematomas, increasing in percentage of the spleen involved (10% to >50% haematoma, 1 to >3 cm laceration).
- Grade IV corresponds to a laceration involving segmental or hilar vessels, with >25% devasculariation of the spleen.

- Grade V corresponds to a completely shattered spleen, or a hilar injury that devascularises the spleen.

This patient has a grade III injury. How would you treat her?

- Conservatively. This is a blunt injury, and she is haemodynamically stable (as long as there is no free blood in the abdomen and minimal other injuries.)
- Perform serial abdominal exams, daily FBC and order strict bed rest for 4–7 days.
- There is a low threshold for operating if the patient becomes unstable/Hb drops.
- If initial management is successful, obtain a follow-up ultrasound scan at 5 days to document nonprogression of splenic injury.
- A postdischarge CT scan is advised 6 weeks after injury to confirm complete healing.

You take her to the ward, and her BP drops to 70/30. What do you do?

- Resuscitate with fluid and blood and arrange an emergency laparotomy.
- At laparotomy, I would pack all four quadrants, and suction blood with a cell saver.
- Confirm source of bleeding and assess splenic damage.
- If the patient stabilises, I would consider spleen-conserving measures:
  - Topical agents (e.g., fibrin glue)
  - Mattress pledgeted sutures
  - Vicryl mesh wrap
  - Argon beam coagulation
- If the patient remains unstable, I would remove the spleen:
  - Divide lienorenal ligament to deliver spleen into wound.
  - Compress vascular pedicle between finger and thumb.
  - Enter lesser sac, palpate the splenic artery and ligate it.
  - Separate the left colic flexure from the spleen.
  - Divide the gastrosplenic ligament and short gastric vessels.
  - Double-tie and divide the splenic pedicle, whilst avoiding the tail of the pancreas.
  - Place a drain in the splenic bed and consider passing an NGT.

The patient becomes septic on the ward on day 3. What are the causes?

- Those relating to surgery in general include:
  - Surgical site infection (wound and lines), DVT, UTI, atelectasis, pneumonia
- Those relating to splenectomy include:
  - Abscess in splenic bed, bowel injury missed at laparotomy, pancreatic injury during surgery, small bowel obstruction, acute gastric dilatation
- OPSI

What changes are seen on a blood film after splenectomy?

- RBC morphology changes to include the appearance of Howell–Jolly bodies and Pappenheimer granules.
- Occasionally, there are erythroblasts.
- WBCs are increased and there is a marked left shift in the differential count.
- Platelet count rises to >1000 × 10^9/l at 7–14 days.

What is OPSI?

- This is flu-like prodromal illness followed by headache, fever, malaise, coma, adrenal haemorrhage and circulatory collapse.
- It affects 2% of trauma splenectomies (risk is greatest if performed during infancy).
- It occurs usually within 2 years of operation.
- Mortality rate is high: 50%–90%.
- It is due to encapsulated bacteria:
  - *Pneumococcus* (50%)
  - *Meningococcus*
  - *Escherichia coli*
  - *Haemophilus influenzae*

What is the postoperative treatment after emergency splenectomy?

- The treatment is vaccination against encapsulated bacteria (*Streptococcus pneumoniae, Haemophilus influenzae* type B and *Neisseria meningitidis*) > 14 days postop, and an annual flu vaccine.
  - Usually given 2–3 weeks postop
  - Prevents OPSI
- Duration of penicillin prophylaxis is debatable. Some surgeons advocate lifelong prophylaxis, whereas others suggest a shorter interval of around 2 years, with a low threshold for antibiotic treatment in the advent of any infection. Infants are recommended to continue to take it until adulthood. Most prescribe Penicillin V.
- Use of a Medic-Alert bracelet
- Splenectomy patient card in wallet

SWALLOWED FOREIGN BODY

You are asked to review a 7-year-old boy who is brought to A+E by his parents after he swallowed a coin. What do you do?

- Take a history:
  - How long ago did he swallow the coin?
  - Was it witnessed?
  - How large was the coin?

- Has the child been vomiting, drooling or complaining of difficulty swallowing or speaking? Is there chest or abdominal pain?
- Perform an examination:
  - Airway—signs of obstruction (coughing, wheezing, stridor)
  - Oropharynx—bleeding, trauma
  - Abdomen—peritonism (bowel obstruction/perforation)
- Obtain two plain XR views from larynx to abdomen:
  - To confirm that a coin has been swallowed
  - To locate the position of the coin
  - To look for evidence of perforation and bowel obstruction

The child says he swallowed the coin yesterday and is now complaining of epigastric pain. The x-rays show a 50p coin lodged in the upper oesophagus. How will you manage the child?

- Any foreign body with sharp edges, or a blunt foreign body lodged in the oesophagus for more than a day, needs to be removed endoscopically to prevent perforation.
- If the coin has been there for <24 hr, it can usually be removed using a Foley catheter, under fluoroscopic guidance and sedation, in the Trendelenberg position.
  - A lubricated catheter is passed through the nose until distal to the coin.
  - A balloon inflated with 5 ml air and gently retracted to base of tongue.
  - Traction is stopped and patient is encouraged to cough out the coin.
- If this fails, formal endoscopic removal is warranted.
- Take a repeat x-ray to check that there was only one swallowed coin.
- Children with distal oesophageal coins may be safely observed for up to 24 hr before an invasive removal procedure, as most will spontaneously pass.

How would your plan change if the coin were in the stomach?

- If the child was asymptomatic, I would discharge the child and ask him to return in 7 days for re-evaluation, or sooner if symptoms develop (nausea, vomiting, abdominal pain, rectal bleeding).
- Objects > 5 cm will not pass through the second part of the duodenum in a child under 2 years of age.
- There is no need for parents to sift through stools.
- A bulk laxative may help decrease intestinal transit time so that the object is passed more quickly.
- Emetic agents (e.g., ipecac) should not be used.

What if the child has swallowed a battery?

- Children most commonly swallow button batteries.
- Batteries lodged in the oesophagus can cause serious injury within 2 hr of ingestion.

- Therefore, the child should be x-rayed immediately and if the battery is lodged in the oesophagus, immediate removal is indicated regardless of when the child last ate.

What are the narrowest points in the GI tract that you should be aware of when assessing ingestion of foreign bodies?

- The narrowest and least distensible part of the gastrointestinal tract is the cricopharyngeus muscle at the level of the thyroid cartilage.
- This is followed by the pylorus, the lower oesophageal sphincter and the ileocaecal valve.
- Most objects that pass through the throat should pass through the anus as well.
- In general, foreign bodies below the diaphragm should be left alone.

TENSION PNEUMOTHORAX

A 43-year-old male pedestrian has been hit by a car. He is alert and talking. His heart rate is 100 beats per minute, his blood pressure is 90/60 and he feels breathless. The pulse oximeter reads 91% on air. His right hemithorax is not moving on respiration and is hyper-resonant to percussion. What is the most likely diagnosis?

- Tension pneumothorax

Explain the pathophysiology of a tension pneumothorax.

- It usually occurs secondary to perforation of lung or airway surface allowing movement of air into the pleural space.
- Unidirectional airflow into the pleural cavity occurs during inspiration.
- It cannot then escape during expiration as tissue acts as a flap valve.
- Progressive accumulation of air in the pleural space collapses the ipsilateral lung and pushes the mediastinum into the opposite hemithorax, causing hypoxia.
- Mediastinal shift + increased intrathoracic pressure = reduced venous return, reduced cardiac filling and reduced cardiac output.

How will you treat it?

- Immediately decompress with a cannula placed in the right midclavicular line, second interspace, just above the upper border of the rib below
- Then place an intercostal drain with an underwater seal.

Talk me through the placement of an intercostal drain.

- Take verbal consent from the patient and check and mark the correct side.
- Place drain in the triangle of safety—edge of pectoralis major, the lower border of the second rib and the midaxillary line, between the second and fifth interspaces.

- Infiltrate the area with 20 ml of 1% plain lignocaine.
- Make a 2 cm transverse incision along the upper border of the rib below to avoid the neurovascular bundle.
- Use blunt dissection with an artery forceps to work through the intercostal muscles and into the pleural cavity.
- Insert a finger through the tract and sweep around the pleural cavity.
- Remove the trocar from a large-bore drain and introduce it using artery forceps.
- Drains for air should be placed toward the apex and anteriorly in supine patients.
- Drains for blood should be placed basally and posteriorly in supine patients.
- Secure the drain, place a purse-string suture and attach to an underwater seal.
- Perform a chest x-ray to check drain placement.

TOXIC MEGACOLON

A 28-year-old male presents with abdominal pain and bloody diarrhoea with mucus. He is pyrexial and disorientated, with abdominal tenderness and distension. What will you do?

- I would resuscitate the patient with oxygen, IV fluids and analgesia, send bloods for FBC, U+E, CRP, LFTs and cultures and take an ABG.
- I would then take a history—known diagnosis of ulcerative colitis or Crohn's disease, family history of inflammatory bowel disease and whether the patient was taking steroids.
- I would examine the patient, looking for peritonism and other systemic features of inflammatory bowel disease, perform a rectal exam and check for tachycardia and hypotension on the observation chart.
- I would insert a catheter and an NG tube, ask for an abdominal x-ray, ask the nurses to send a urine and stool sample and start broad-spectrum IV antibiotics.

The abdominal x-ray shows a dilated transverse colon measuring 9 cm. His WCC is 18. What is the diagnosis?

- Acute colitis is diagnosed using Truelove and Witt's criteria (more than six bloody stools, Hb < 10.5, ESR > 30, temp > 37.8°C, HR > 90).
- Toxic megacolon is diagnosed if there is:
  - >6 cm transverse colonic dilatation
  - Any three of fever, tachycardia, leukocytosis, anaemia
  - Any one of dehydration, altered mental status, electrolyte abnormality or hypotension
- The microscopic hallmark is inflammation extending beyond the mucosa.

What are the causes of toxic megacolon?

- Ulcerative colitis
- Crohn's disease

- Pseudomembranous colitis
- Infectious colitis

What is the prognosis of toxic megacolon?

- It is good if there is no perforation (mortality rate of 2%–4%).
- The mortality rate is up to 20% if there is a perforation.
- With UC, a proctocolectomy is curative.

How would you manage the patient?

- There are three goals of treatment:
  - Reduce colonic distension to prevent perforation.
  - Correct fluid and electrolyte disturbances.
  - Treat toxaemia and precipitating factors.
- Joint care with gastroenterologists is vital, and I would ask for a review by the critical care team.
- The initial resuscitation involves:
  - Aggressive fluid and electrolyte replacement
  - Broad-spectrum intravenous antibiotics
  - Stopping all medications that may affect colonic motility (narcotics, antidiarrhoeal agents)
  - NBM with parenteral nutrition
  - An NG tube to assist GI decompression
  - DVT prophylaxis
- If the patient is not peritonitic and has been on steroids, I would ask for a CT scan to exclude a local or contained perforation.
- The patient needs daily abdominal examination (ideally by the same doctor), abdominal x-rays and blood tests (FBC, U+Es and CRP).
- I would start IV steroids.
- Cyclosporine could be given as second-line treatment if the patient is not responding, and this may obviate the need for urgent colectomy, allowing more controlled semielective surgery (significant side effects: renal and neurological complications).

When would you operate and what would you do?

- I would operate if there was:
  - Free perforation (fivefold increase in mortality to 20%)
  - Massive haemorrhage needing six- to eight-unit transfusion
  - Increasing toxicity and progression of colonic dilatation
  - Improvement after 24–72 hr of maximal medical therapy
- A stool frequency of more than eight per day or CRP > 45 mg/l at 72 hr predicts the need for surgery in 85% of cases (Travis criteria).
- Steroids can mask abdominal signs.
- I would perform a subtotal colectomy:

- The patient is very ill and therefore I want to do the quickest and safest procedure.
- A subtotal colectomy preserves the possibility for an ileo-anal anastomosis.
- I would leave a long rectal stump and preserve the IMA to aid delayed reconstruction.

TRAUMA IN PREGNANCY

A healthy 26-year-old woman, 31 weeks' pregnant in her first pregnancy, is brought by ambulance to A+E following a motor vehicle accident at 60 km per hour. On arrival, her BP is 80/40 and her pulse is 110 beats per minute. What general principles should be considered in the resuscitation of obstetric patients following major trauma?

- Multidisciplinary management involving emergency physicians, surgeons, anaesthetists, obstetricians and neonatologists is essential.
- Ideally, pregnant trauma victims should be managed in major trauma centres to allow provision of appropriate medical expertise.
- Primary assessment (ABCs) should be undertaken as in nonpregnant patients, with emphasis on potential intracranial, intra-abdominal and pelvic injury.
- Maternal hypovolaemia should be aggressively treated; hypotension can compromise the uteroplacental blood flow and foetal well-being.
- Supplemental oxygen is recommended in pregnancy, even if intubation is not required.
- Once the mother has been stabilised, a prompt assessment by a senior obstetrician is necessary to assess gestational age, foetal well-being and evidence of obstetric complications.
- Foetal viability should be confirmed by ultrasound as soon as practically possible in the assessment of pregnant trauma victims.
- Vaginal examination and speculum examination are indicated if there is suspicion of preterm labour or abruption.
- Finally, resuscitation of pregnant women should be undertaken at 15° left lateral position (or with a rolled towel under the spinal board) as there is a risk of aortocaval compression from the gravid uterus in women lying supine, with a consequent risk of foetal hypoperfusion.

What obstetric risks are associated with blunt trauma in pregnancy?

- Placental abruption (in up to 40% of severe trauma cases)
- Preterm labour
- Preterm premature rupture of membranes
- Uterine rupture (<1% of severe trauma)
- Direct foetal injury (head trauma, fractures or intracranial haemorrhage) and foetal death

- Obstetric complications may occur immediately at the time of impact or may be delayed for several hours after the incident, making ongoing surveillance imperative for women involved in significant motor vehicle accidents.

What physiological changes of pregnancy are pertinent to the case presented here?

- An increase in cardiac output of 1–1.5 l/min and a 50% increase in maternal blood volume. The increase in red cell mass is less pronounced, resulting in a physiological dilutional anaemia of pregnancy.
- An increase in maternal heart rate by 10–15 bpm in the third trimester and a physiological fall in BP in the second trimester, with a gradual increase to prepregnancy levels toward term.
- The blood flow to the uterus is 600 ml/min at term; there is potential for catastrophic haemorrhage if the uterine vasculature is disrupted.
- These changes can mask the severity of maternal injury, and significant changes to vital signs in pregnancy may be associated with more critical hypovolaemia and shock than in the nonpregnant patient.

What laboratory investigations are indicated?

- Full blood count, urea and electrolytes, coagulation profile (including fibrinogen if severe hypovolaemia is suspected) and cross match
- Rhesus status (Rhesus negative pregnant women require prophylactic anti-D administration following blunt trauma in accordance with local guidelines.)
- Urinalysis (pelvic fracture may be associated with haematuria.)
- 'Kleihauer test' (to assess for a foeto–maternal haemorrhage)

What is the role of radiological investigations in obstetric trauma?

- Necessary radiological investigations should not be deferred because of concern for foetal radiation exposure.
- No single diagnostic procedure delivers a radiation dose sufficient to threaten the well-being of a foetus in mid- to late gestation.
- Plain x-rays pose minimal radiation exposure.
- Although CT exposes the foetus to 2–5 rad (20–50 mGy) of radiation, animal studies indicate foetal malformation risk only at thresholds exceeding 10 rad (100 mGy), particularly at more vulnerable early gestational ages.

Discuss the effects of pregnancy on surgical exploration.

- Diagnostic laparoscopy can be safely performed at all stages of pregnancy; after 20 weeks the uterine fundus reaches above the level of the umbilicus, so port placement needs to be adjusted accordingly.
- Pregnancy causes elevation of the diaphragm, and chest tube placement is generally one to two spaces higher than in nonpregnant patients.

- At gestations ≥ 24 weeks, foetal monitoring intraoperatively and postoperatively should be considered. Concomitant caesarean section ± hysterectomy may be required.
- Pregnancy itself is a significant risk factor for venous thromboembolism and adequate thromboprophylaxis is recommended postoperatively.

UPPER GASTROINTESTINAL BLEED

A 73-year-old man presents as an emergency with severe bleeding per rectum and an Hb of 7. After initial resuscitation, a colonoscopy was negative. He had another rectal bleed on the ward overnight. How will you manage him?

- Up to 15% of patients with rectal bleeding actually have a source in the upper GI tract (oesophagus, stomach, duodenum). Therefore, if no lower GI source is found, I would arrange an OGD in the first instance
- All patients with an upper GI bleed should be managed in accordance with the Scottish Inter-Collegiate Guideline Network 2008 guidance[1] as the British Society of Gastroenterology guidance is now outdated and the BSG has adopted the SIGN guidance.
- I would resuscitate the patient (ABCs), ensure oxygen and wide bore intravenous access with warmed Hartmann's fluid running, check that blood had been taken for clotting, group and save and cross match blood and repeat FBC and U+E.
- I would review the history and examine the patient, paying particular attention to use of nonsteroidal anti-inflammatory drugs, anticoagulants, history of peptic ulcer disease and indigestion, alcohol intake, signs of chronic liver disease, and assess the observation chart to look for hypotension and tachycardia/tachypnoea.

You arrange an urgent OGD which shows a bleeding gastric ulcer. How can you control the bleeding?

- All actively bleeding sources, visible vessels and ulcers with adherent clot should be treated in the first instance with endoscopic therapy.
- Endoscopic therapy should include dual rather than single modalities. Treatment should comprise a minimum of 13 ml injection of 1 in 10,0000 adrenaline and either heater probe or endoclipping.
- Repeat endoscopy ± endotherapy should be considered in those patients with a suboptimal initial endoscopy.
- There is insufficient evidence that pre-endoscopic treatment with proton pump inhibitors in acute upper GI bleeding affects clinical outcome.

Are you aware of any scoring systems to assess risk in these patients?

- The Rockall scoring system.
- This scores a patient based on age, degree of systemic shock, comorbidity, endoscopic diagnosis and presence of major stigmata of recent haemorrhage.

- Patients with an initial Rockall score of 0 should be considered for either discharge or an early discharge with an outpatient follow-up as they have an extremely low risk of death or rebleeding.
- Patients with an initial Rockall score of ≥1 should be considered for an early upper GI endoscopy. Those with a full Rockall score of <3 have a low risk of rebleeding and should be considered for an early discharge and outpatient follow-up.

What are your treatment options if the patient has a significant rebleed after the initial endoscopy?

- Repeat endoscopy
- Coeliac and mesenteric angiogram with radiological arterial embolisation (This obviously depends on local availability and resources but is an excellent option in high-risk surgical patients. In order to visualise the source of bleeding, the rate of bleeding must be at least 1 ml/min.)
- Surgery

Discuss your management if the source of bleeding is found to be oesophageal varices.

- Initial resuscitation should be performed, as previously stated.
- Pre-endoscopic treatment with terlipressin can be used.
- Endoscopic therapy with variceal band ligation or cyanoacrylate injection could be undertaken.
- Failure to control variceal bleeding endoscopically requires temporary balloon tamponade followed by transjugular intrahepatic portosystemic shunting (TIPSS).
- Oesophageal transection is becoming a historical surgical operation for the treatment of bleeding oesophageal varices as this is so rarely performed nowadays that few surgeons have the expertise.

URINARY RETENTION

Your FY1 calls just as you are about to scrub for an appendicectomy to inform you that he has seen a 65-year-old man referred from the A+E department with acute urinary retention. What do you want to ascertain over the phone?

- The most important immediate information is:
  - The residual volume (<800 ml = acute retention, >800–1000 ml = chronic retention)
  - Renal function
  - Symptoms or signs of sepsis
  - Previous urological surgery and urinary symptoms

He was catheterised, and the residual volume was 1.2 l. What further information do you need?

- His current and baseline renal function
- The colour of urine on catheterisation (blood, clots, pus. etc.)

His creatinine was 300 (baseline was 65 nmol/l 3 months ago). How will you manage him on the ward?

- Monitor hourly urine output. If he diureses and passes a large volume (>200 ml/hr for 6 hr or more), I would start IV fluid replacement (50%–100% of the hourly urine output).
- Perform daily renal function tests, monitoring worsening renal failure and low K.
- Daily assessment of body weight ensures gradual loss of third space fluid accumulated over time.
- Lying and standing BP—postural drop due to dehydration would prompt fluid replacement.

If his residual volume was 250 ml but his serum creatinine was 300 nmol/l, how would you manage him?

- This is not acute urinary retention (unless the patient has a reduced bladder capacity/compliance—e.g., after pelvic radiotherapy or chronic inflammation such as TB).
- An urgent USS is necessary, as well as a digital rectal examination to feel for pelvic malignancy and a PSA level.
- The patient should remain catheterised to monitor urine output, with strict input and output fluid balance assessment and daily U+Es. A renal team input may also be necessary.

The USS showed bilateral hydronephrosis. What next?

- This would depend on the results of the rectal exam and PSA. If these are normal, then a noncontrast CT is essential to identify the cause and the level of the ureteric obstruction.
- If these are grossly abnormal (e.g., PSA > 100 ng/ml) and pathognomonic of prostate cancer, then commence treatment for prostate cancer and involve the urologist and/or the oncologist.

UROLOGICAL TRAUMA

A 35-year-old man falls over while drunk and attends A+E. He was referred to you with microscopic haematuria. What investigations would you request?

- This would be determined by the history/mechanism of injury and his signs/observations.
- If the mechanism is minor, with no abnormal clinical signs (bruising/ecchymoses in the flank, tachycardia, hypotension), then no investigations are needed and the patient can be discharged without follow-up.
- If there is a serious mechanism of injury (e.g., fall from a height, assault and/or adverse signs of flank ecchymoses, hypotension [SBP < 90 mmHg or tachycardia]), then after resuscitation, I would request an urgent contrast CT to identify and grade the injury.

If he had been kicked in the loin by a horse and presented with frank haematuria and tachycardia, how would you manage him?

- I would resuscitate him and request a four-phase CT (precontrast, arterial phase, venous phase, collecting system phase).
- These phases are important as they show enhancement (sign of viable tissue), arterial leaks, and urinoma/collecting system defects, which are all important for grading renal trauma.

Can you describe the grading and its relevance in renal trauma?

- The AAST classification grades renal trauma into five main grades. This guides management.
  - Grade 1—contusion or nonexpanding subcapsular haematoma, no laceration
  - Grade 2—nonexpanding perirenal haematoma; cortical laceration < 1 cm deep without extravasation
  - Grade 3—cortical laceration > 1 cm without urinary extravasation
  - Grade 4—laceration: through corticomedullary junction into collecting system; vascular: segmental renal artery or vein injury with contained haematoma, or partial vessel laceration or vessel thrombosis
  - Grade 5—laceration: shattered kidney; vascular: renal pedicle injury or avulsion

How would you manage this man if his CT urogram showed viable renal tissue, with contrast enhancement and some minor urinary extravasation?

- This is a grade 3 injury.
- Admit patient, resuscitate, commence antibiotics (e.g., IV Augmentin) to reduce risk of infection of urinoma.
- Prescribe bed rest for 48 hr; repeat imaging to ensure no expansion of haematoma and/or urinoma. If he spikes a temperature or drops his Hb/blood pressure, then repeat CT scan.
- If his urinoma is expanding, then it may need draining with stent placement.
- If the patient remains stable, he needs an outpatient renogram in 3 months to look at residual split kidney function.

What are the complications of renal trauma?

* Delayed bleeding
* Post-traumatic hypertension
* Urinoma and perirenal abscess

REFERENCE

1. Management of acute upper and lower gastrointestinal bleeding—A national clinical guideline. http://www.sign.ac.uk/pdf/sign105.pdf

BIBLIOGRAPHY

Davies, John M., Michael P. N. Lewis, Jennie Wimperis, Imran Rafi, Shamez Ladhani and Paula H. B. Bolton-Maggs. British Committee for Standards in Haematology. 2011. Review of guidelines for the prevention and treatment of infection in patients with an absent or dysfunctional spleen: Prepared on behalf of the British Committee for Standards in Haematology by a working party of the Haemato-Oncology Task Force. *British Journal of Haematology* November: 1365–2141.

Working Party of the British Society of Gastroenterology, Association of Surgeons of Great Britain and Ireland, Pancreatic Society of Great Britain and Ireland, Association of Upper GI Surgeons of Great Britain and Ireland. 2005. UK guidelines for the management of acute pancreatitis. *Gut* 54: iii1–iii9.

4 General Surgery

Elizabeth Ball, Pankaj Mishra, Dermot O'Riordan, C J Shukla, Tjun Tang, Thomas Tsang, Colin Walsh and Stewart Walsh

CONTENTS

ANAL FISSURE

A 36-year-old woman has been referred to your clinic with severe anal pain after defecation. How will you assess her?

- Take a history: How long does the pain last? Is there associated rectal bleeding? Has there been a change in bowel habit or other 'red flag' symptoms?
- Examine the patient, looking for an anal fissure, a sentinel skin tag (which may indicate a chronic fissure) and haemorrhoids.

The patient has a sentinel tag, but it is too painful for her to tolerate a rectal examination. You suspect an anal fissure. What do you do now?

- I would start her on laxatives and recommend a sitz bath to prevent the fissure recurring and to make defecation less painful.
- I would treat the fissure with topical GTN 0.2% for 6 weeks and see her in clinic in 8 weeks' time. This heals 60%–70% of fissures, but 25% of patients experience severe headaches.
- If she could not tolerate the GTN, I would switch her to Diltiazem 2%. The aim is to relax the internal sphincter tone.

She comes to see you 3 months later. The GTN cream has not worked and she is still experiencing severe pain and bleeding. What will you do now?

- I would list her for an EUA and inject Botox into the internal sphincter on either side of the fissure (total dose of 50 units), which heals 70% of fissures.
  - Complications of injection include transient incontinence, haematoma, pain and sepsis.
- If this did not work, I would consider a lateral sphincterotomy, after counselling the patient about the risk of permanent incontinence to flatus (30%) and faecal soiling (10%). This will cure 85% of patients.

Botox therapy did not work, and she had a lateral sphincterotomy. However, she comes back to see you in 2 years with a recurrent fissure. What are your treatment options?

- She needs to have anal manometry and an endoanal ultrasound.
- Patients with high resting pressures may benefit from a repeat lateral sphincterotomy in the opposite lateral quadrant.
- If the resting pressures are low, she may benefit from an anal advancement flap.

ASEPSIS AND ANTISEPSIS

Can you define asepsis, antisepsis and sterilisation?

- Asepsis—prevention of the introduction of bacteria to the surgical field
- Antisepsis—destruction of pre-existing bacteria in the surgical field
- Sterilisation—complete destruction of all viable micro-organisms, including spores and viruses, by heat, chemicals or irradiation.

What are the principles of asepsis?

- Patient factors:
  - Hair removal on day of surgery
  - Preoperative bowel preparation (where indicated)
  - Prophylactic intravenous antibiotics (where indicated)
- Surgical team factors:
  - Scrubbing with disinfectant
  - Choice of skin prep
  - Wearing sterile gowns and gloves
  - Draping to surround the sterile field
  - Sterile instrumentation and no-touch technique

Do you routinely wear masks and visors in theatre?
This comes down to personal choice. With either choice, you need to be able to explain your reasons.

- Wearing masks in theatre is not compulsory, unless you are working in an ultraclean theatre, inserting prosthetic implants or using standard universal precautions. Few bacteria are discharged from the mouth and nose during breathing. Most surgeons wear masks to protect themselves from blood-borne viruses and bodily fluids.
- Visors are used to protect the wearer's mucous membranes from blood-borne viruses and other bodily fluids.
- Some surgeons work on the principle that every patient may have a blood-borne virus and routinely wear a mask, visor and double-glove.

How is surgical equipment sterilised?

- The majority of surgical instruments and drapes are sterilised using an autoclave (saturated steam at high pressure), at 134°C, a pressure of 2 atm for a holding time of 3 min. This kills all organisms including viruses and heat-resistant spores. The steam penetration is monitored with the Bowie–Dick test, which should be checked prior to every operation.
- Dry-heat sterilisation is used for moisture-sensitive instruments and those with fine cutting edges. The tools are heated to 160°C for 1 hr.
- Ethylene oxide is a highly penetrative gas used to sterilise heat-sensitive equipment (rubber, electrical equipment), and it will kill vegetative bacteria, spores and viruses.
- Gamma irradiation is used in industry to sterilise large batches of single-use items such as catheters and syringes.

What are the differences between chlorhexidine and povidone-iodine?

- Chlorhexidine:
  - Good against *Staphylococcus aureus,* moderate activity against Gram-negative bacteria, some activity against pseudomonas, poor activity against spores, fungi and viruses
  - Nontoxic to skin and mucous membranes
  - Inactivated by soap and pus
  - Acts by disrupting bacterial cell walls
  - Persistent with a long duration of action, up to 6 hr
  - Two solutions:
    - Four percent in detergent 'Hibiscrub'—scrubbing up
      - Rapidly active, persists with cumulative effect, even under gloves.
    - Half a percent in alcohol–skin prep
      - MUST be air-dried prior to using diathermy, and pooling can cause skin irritation and is potentially flammable.
- Povidone–iodine:
  - Good broad-spectrum activity against Gram-positive and Gram-negative bacteria, spores, fungi and viruses including HIV and Hep B (bactericidal)
  - Easily inactivated by organic material (blood, faeces, pus)
  - Must be used at optimum freshness
  - Acts by oxidation and substitution of free iodine
  - Does not have a prolonged effect when used for scrubbing

What do you use for skin prep?
This is a matter of personal choice, and you need to be able to explain why you use your solution. You need to be aware of the recent publications discussing this. You should also be aware of NICE guidance CG74 (Surgical Site Infection).

- Chlorhexidine-alcohol provides superior clinical protection in clean-contaminated surgery.[1,2]
  - This is possibly due to more rapid action and persistent activity despite exposure to bodily fluids.

BENIGN SKIN LESIONS

A 76-year-old man comes to your clinic with a raised greasy plaque on his back. What is the likely diagnosis and treatment?

- This sounds like a seborrhoeic keratosis, also known as a senile wart.
- Senile warts are a benign overgrowth of the basal epidermis and produce a grey/brown hypertrophic greasy plaque, more common on the back, face and hands. They can itch and bleed.
- They can be picked off, but will reform.
- They are familial (autosomal dominant) and can be a sign of visceral malignancy—more likely with sudden onset of multiple keratoses (Leser–Trelat sign)—and rarely transform into SCC.
- I would liaise with a dermatologist because they need excising with curettage or cryotherapy as the keratosis lies above the level of the surrounding normal epidermis. They can also be left alone at the patient's request as they are benign.

A 67-year-old male presents with a raised lesion on his cheek with a central 'horn'. What is your diagnosis and management?

- This sounds like a keratoacanthoma. It is a self-limiting rapid overgrowth of hair follicle cells, with a central keratin plug.
- They are associated with sun exposure, coal, tar and visceral and laryngeal malignancy and are commonly seen on the face and dorsum of the hand (sun-exposed parts of the body). They are more common in males.
- They spontaneously regress, but can leave a deep scar.
- Treatment:
  - Nonsurgical—leave alone if asymptomatic, particularly in the young.
  - Surgical—excise to confirm the diagnosis, exclude an SCC (particularly in the elderly) and prevent scar formation. I would liaise with my plastic surgical colleagues if a flap was needed for skin closure.

What is Bowen's disease?

- This is a premalignant intraepidermal cancer.
- It is slow growing and presents as a thickened brown/pink plaque with flat papular crusted clusters that can mimic eczema.
- It is commonly seen on the trunk and legs and is not usually seen at sites of sun damage.

- It should be excised with a 5 mm margin.
- Histologically, it resembles SCC, but this is limited to the epidermis. It will develop into SCC if not excised. The condition is associated with subsequent development of visceral malignancies, usually 5–7 years later, particularly if the area of skin affected has never been exposed to the sun.
- When seen on the penis, vulva or oral cavity, it is known as erythroplasia of Queyrat.

A 22-year-old girl presents with multiple cutaneous soft nodules and brown patches on her skin. What is the most likely diagnosis, and how would you classify the disease?

- This sounds like neurofibromatosis (von Recklinghausen's disease). Patients present with multiple neurofibromas, more than six café-au-lait patches, axillary freckling and Lisch nodules on the iris. It is familial (autosomal dominant) and is present at birth.
- Patients can develop acoustic neuromas, and there is a 5%–10% risk of malignant change. A neurofibroma is a hamartoma—an overgrowth of neural tissue.
- There are four types of neurofibromatosis. The first is type I, with the features already mentioned. Type II is associated with neurofibromas in the central nervous system, which can damage the cranial nerves. Type III is schwannomatosis, which is very painful and very rare. Type IV has plexiform neurofibromas, which are infiltrative lesions on the head and neck, have a higher risk of malignant transformation and a rapid metastatic spread.

What complications can neurofibromata give rise to?

- Pressure effects (e.g., spinal cord and nerve root compression)
- Deafness involving the eighth cranial nerve
- Sarcomatous transformation—only in VRD
- Intra-abdominal effects—obstruction, chronic gastrointestinal bleed
- Skeletal changes which can cause pseudoarthrosis, kyphoscoliosis

How would you classify benign pigmented skin lesions?

- These develop from melanocytes in the epidermis and dermis.
- Epidermal lesions include lentigo and café-au-lait patches. Lentigo are skin patches with an increased number of melanocytes. There are three types: simplex (young and middle aged), senilis (elderly) and solar (after sun exposure).
- Dermal lesions include blue naevi and a Mongolian blue spot.
- This is a blue/grey pigmented lesion over the sacrum.

- A halo naevus is surrounded by an area of depigmented skin which regresses, leaving a small scar.

BREAST INFECTION

A 25-year-old breast-feeding mother presents in A+E with a hot, painful breast. What is the likely cause, and how will you manage her?

- Lactational mastitis occurs in 5% of breast-feeding women, most common in the first month and during weaning.
- Take a history and examine patient (breasts and axillae)—check for cracked nipples, problems with milk flow, breast pain, systemic sepsis.
- If systemically well/no obvious abscess, treat with oral broad-spectrum antibiotics (Co-Amoxiclav or Erythrocymycin against *S. aureus*) and encourage breast-feeding.
- If septic, admit for IV broad-spectrum antibiotics and arrange an USS-guided drainage of any abscess cavity under local anaesthetic.

A 40-year-old woman presents with a painful, red mass close to her nipple. What is the cause and how will you treat her?

- This is periductal mastitis (associated with heavy smoking):
  - Polymicrobial—aerobic and anaerobic bacteria
  - Present with periareolar inflammation/mass/abscess
- Take a history and examine the patient—check for smoking history, previous abcess/surgery, skin necrosis.
- Treat with USS-guided drainage under local anaesthetic.
  - Rescan and drain every 2–3 days until resolution.
  - Formal surgical drainage is done only when skin thinning/necrosis occurs.
  - If septic, give broad spectrum antibiotics.
- Any woman > 35 years needs a mammogram after resolution to exclude DCIS (ductal carcinoma in situ).
- Encourage the patient to stop smoking (high recurrence rate, can get fistulae).

A 70-year-old woman presents with a hot, red, painful breast. What is the likely cause and how will you treat her?

- Consider inflammatory cancer until proven otherwise.
  - Locally advanced breast cancer spreads through dermal lymphatic vessels, giving erythematous appearance to whole breast.
- Take a history and perform a triple assessment.
  - Clinical examination (breast mass, peau d'orange, axillary nodes)

- Mammography, ultrasound and core biopsy
- Review results in MDT, arrange staging CT/bone scan and give neoadjuvant chemotherapy.

CHEMOTHERAPY

What classes of chemotherapeutic agents do you know?

- Phase-dependent drugs:
  - Kill cells at a lower dose
  - Act within a specific phase of the cell cycle
  - Examples include methotrexate and vinca alkaloids (vincristine, vinblastine)
- Non-phase-dependent drugs:
  - Kill cells exponentially with increasing dose
  - Equally toxic for cell within the cell cycle or G0 phase
  - Examples include alkylating agents (cyclophosphamide, cisplatin), 5-flurouracil and anthracyclines (e.g., doxorubicin)

How do chemotherapeutic agents work?

- Modes of action include:
  - Bleomycin, which inhibits DNA polymerase, causing breakage of single stranded DNA
  - Doxorubicin, which inhibits RNA synthesis by intercalating between DNA base pairs
  - Cisplatin which inhibits DNA synthesis by cross-linking DNA strands
  - Methotrexate, which inhibits dihydrofolate reductase
  - Vinca alkaloids, which bind to tubulin and inhibit the metaphase of mitosis

What side effects occur with chemotherapeutic agents?

- Some side effects occur with many cytotoxic agents:
  - Nausea and vomiting
  - Bone marrow toxicity
  - Gastrointestinal toxicity
  - Alopecia
  - Gonadal effects
  - Hyperuricaemia
- Some side effects are specific to particular drugs:
  - Pulmonary fibrosis—bleomycin
  - Haemorrhagic cystitis—cyclophosphamide
  - Cardiomyopathy—doxorubicin
  - Hepatic damage—methotrexate
  - Skin pigmentation—5-flurouracil

How do alkylating agents work?

- They react with DNA to form covalent bonds, causing single-strand or double-strand DNA breaks and cross linking.
- They are used for haematological and solid malignancies.
- There is a steep dose–response curve.
- Examples include chlorambucil, mitomycin C.

What are the heavy metal agents and how do they work?

- Cisplatin (nephrotoxic), carboplatin and oxaliplatin
- Activated intracellularly to form reactive intermediates that form covalent bonds with nucleotides from DNA cross links

What are the antimetabolite agents?

- They resemble naturally occurring purines, pyrimidines and nucleic acid.
- They inhibit key enzymes involved in DNA synthesis and incorporate into RNA and DNA to cause strand breaks.
- They act at the S-phase of the cycle.
- Examples include methotrexate, 5-fluorouracil, gemcitabine.

What are the aims of chemotherapy?

- Inhibit one or more processes involved in cell division.
  - Cells die by apoptosis.
- Treat advanced (metastatic) cancer.
  - Best response may be reduction in tumour volume; this may palliate by prolonging survival or improving symptom control.
- Cells can develop resistance from acquired mutations.
  - Treatment for early primary cancer as an adjunct to surgery.
- It is routinely offered to those at high risk of recurrence after surgery (bowel, breast cancer).
  - Neoadjuvant treatment for a localised cancer before planned surgery (rectal, breast), allowing for more conservative surgical resection.

What are the limitations of chemotherapy?

- Cell proliferation mechanisms affect normally dividing and cancer cells.
- Selectivity toward cancer cells is seen as some tumours are highly proliferative compared with normal cells (e.g., lymphoma) or defective in their ability to repair DNA and therefore cannot repopulate
- Therapeutic ratio (toxic dose and therapeutic dose) for a drug should be close to 1, so that damage to normal tissues is self-limiting.
- Drug-induced damage to normal tissue that is rapidly dividing (bone marrow, GI mucosa) can be life threatening.

Are any malignancies fully curable with chemotherapy?

- Tumours curable with chemotherapy include teratoma, seminoma, high-grade non-Hodgkin's lymphoma, Hodgkin's lymphoma and Wilm's tumour.
- Chemoresistant tumours include melanoma, renal cancer, hepatoma, cholangiocarcinoma.

How is chemotherapy delivered?

- Combination:
  - Use different classes for broader coverage of activity and reduce risk of resistant subclones
  - For example, in the CMF regime, all have single-agent activity against breast cancer, but combined the response rate is two to three times higher.
- High dose
  - Give on steeper part of sigmoid dose–response curve.

CIRCUMCISION

An anxious mother is referred to your clinic by her GP requesting a circumcision for her 2-year-old who has an irretractable foreskin. What are the indications for circumcision in the UK?

- The British Association of Paediatric Urologists has stipulated criteria for indications for paediatric circumcisions in order to reduce the routine circumcision rates. These include:
  - Balanitis xerotica obliterans (BXO), causing pathological phimosis (occurs in 1.5% of boys)
  - Severe recurrent balano-posthitis (this has to be genuine infection and not minor redness or irritation) (i.e., greater than or equal to three to four per year (occurs in 1% of boys)
  - Recurrent febrile UTIs (urinary tract infections) with an abnormal urogenital tract
  - Traumatic foreskin injury which cannot be salvaged
- Religious circumcision is not funded by the NHS in England and Wales.
- The following are NOT indications of circumcision:
  - Nonretractile foreskin (physiological phimosis)
  - Preputial adhesions
  - Preputial pearl of smegma
  - Paraphimosis (for which reduction is recommended)

At what age does the foreskin become retractile?

- Preputial construction is complete by 16 weeks' gestation. Epithelia lining the prepuce and glans are contiguous and adhesions between the two are physiological.

- Almost all boys have a nonretractile foreskin at birth.
- During the first 3–4 years epithelial debris (smegma) accumulates and separates glans from prepuce (erections).
- 90% are retractile at 3 years and <1% have nonretractile foreskin at 17 years.

What symptoms and signs will help you decide if this boy would benefit from a circumcision?

- These would include if the patient has had balanoposthitis (not minor redness), UTIs with an abnormal renal tract, difficulty passing urine and a BXO/tight phimosis on clinical examination.
- This is ascertained by gentle retraction of the foreskin and if the constriction is not at the tip, (physiological phimosis), there is a 'flower-petal' appearance
- In pathological phimosis, the constriction is at the tip.

What are the specific issues to cover in consenting for a circumcision?

- The risks/complications include:
  - Bleeding (1.5%)
  - Ooze (36%)
  - Infection (8.5%)
  - Urinary retention
  - Meatal stenosis
  - Excess or inadequate skin removal (and need for revision)
  - Urethral or glans injury (urethrocutaneous fistula, ischaemia of distal penis)

Are there any alternative treatment options?

- Topical steroids (0.05%–1%, bd, 20–30 days)
  - Success rate of 67%–95%
- Preputioplasty—may not be cosmetically acceptable

How would you perform a circumcision?

- Supine position, IV antibiotics if current balanitis, penile block
- Prepuce retracted and glans beneath cleaned; preputial adhesions broken down using a probe (may need a dorsal slit)
- Foreskin divided between two clips to 5 mm below the corona, with a circumferential incision around the penis at the same level, and skin excised
- After careful haemostasis, ridge of skin below corona and free edge of remaining foreskin opposed with interrupted Vicryl Rapide
- Sexually active men to be advised to refrain from intercourse for 2–3 weeks.
- Foreskin sent for histology if BXO or carcinoma is suspected

CLINICAL GOVERNANCE

What is clinical governance?

- It is a framework through which NHS organisations are accountable for continually improving the quality of their services and safeguarding high standards of care by creating an environment in which excellence in clinical care will flourish.
- It was introduced by the government in 1998 to restructure change within the NHS.
- The chief executive of a hospital trust is now responsible for creating an environment in which effective changes can be made to achieve high-quality care and he or she can be held accountable if this is not provided.
- For surgeons, clinical governance aims to ensure that:
  - There are systems in place to monitor quality of clinical practice and that they are functioning well.
  - Clinical practice is reviewed and improved as a result.
  - They continue to meet national standards as issued by the professional bodies.

What are the seven pillars of clinical governance?

- Clinical effectiveness—the degree to which the organisation ensures that 'best practice' is used (e.g., evidence-based medicine).
- Risk management—having systems to monitor and minimise risk to staff, patients and visitors.
- Clinical audit—the systematic critical analysis of the quality of clinical care
- Education and training—ensuring that support is available to enable staff to be competent at their jobs and to develop their skills to be up to date (includes CPD [appraisal and revalidation]).
- Staffing and staff management—ensure effective working conditions and promote culture of learning and responsibility.
- Information use—systems in place to collect and analyse information on service quality.
- Patient experience and public involvement—ensuring that individuals have a say in their own treatment

This can be summarised in the mnemonic SPARE IT.

What is an audit?

- An audit is a process used by clinicians to improve patient care by assessing clinical practice, comparing against accepted standards and making changes if necessary.

What is an audit cycle?

- Collect data.
- Assess conformity of data to a predetermined standard.

- Gather and feedback results.
- Update standards if necessary.
- Intervene to promote change.
- Set standards.
- Close the loop and repeat.

What are the benefits of clinical audit?

- Identifies and promotes good practice and can lead to improvements in service delivery and outcomes for users
- Can provide the information that you need to show others that your service is effective (and cost effective) and thus ensure its development
- Provides opportunities for training and education
- Helps to ensure better use of resources and, therefore, increased efficiency
- Can improve working relationships, communication and liaison between staff, between staff and service users and between agencies
- The overall aim of clinical audit is to improve service user outcomes by improving professional practice and the general quality of services delivered

CLOSTRIDIUM DIFFICILE

An 83-year-old lady admitted with a UTI develops diarrhoea on the ward. How will you manage her?

- As she is likely to have been given antibiotics for her UTI, she probably has developed *Clostridium difficile* diarrhoea.
- She needs to be isolated within 2 hr of the onset of diarrhoea, gloves and aprons used for all contact, and hand washing with soap and water before and after each contact (wash away spores)—not alcohol gel.
- Take a history, examine her and review her observation and drug charts.
- Ask the nurses to collect a stool specimen and send it to microbiology.
  - Must take shape of container, > 1/4 full, Bristol Stool Chart 5–7.

What is *Clostridium difficile*?

- Gram-positive, anaerobic, spore-forming bacillus that causes antibiotic-associated diarrhoea and colitis
- One of the most common nosocomial infections
- Produces two toxins:
- Toxin A is an enterotoxin, and toxin B is a cytotoxin. Both play a role in the pathogenesis of *C. difficile* colitis in humans.

How is it diagnosed?

- Clinically—watery diarrhoea, abdominal cramping, pyrexia and dehydration; rarely with fulminant life-threatening colitis; suspect in any patient with diarrhoea who received antibiotics within previous 2 months or after 72 hr of hospitalisation

- Stool testing (three tests available)—toxin gene (PCR), glutamate dehydro-genase EIA (GDH) and toxin enzyme immunoassay (EIA)—NOT suitable as stand-alone test
- Start with PCR or GDH:
  - If negative, no further test is needed.
  - If positive, do EIA; if both are positive, *C. difficile* is likely; reporting is mandatory.
  - If second test is negative, *C. difficile* could be present; no mandatory reporting.
- Endoscopically—pseudomembranes (raised yellow plaques) ranging from 2 to 10 mm in diameter and scattered over the colorectal mucosa (14%–25% mild disease, 87% patients with fulminant disease)

What is the cause of *C. difficile* colitis?

- *C. difficile* is present in 2%–3% of healthy adults. Colonisation occurs by the faecal-oral route.
- Antibiotic use suppresses normal bacterial colonic flora, allowing prolifera-tion of *C. difficile* and release of toxins that cause mucosal inflammation and damage.
- The most common antibiotics are cephalosporins, ampicillin and amoxi-cillin. It is also caused by macrolides (erythromycin, clarithromycin) and other penicillins.
- *C. difficile*-associated diarrhoea has a mortality rate of 25% in frail, elderly patients. Independent predictors of mortality are age 70 years or older, severe leukocytosis/leukopenia and cardiorespiratory failure.

How would you treat this patient?

- For moderate disease, use metronidazole: bactericidal, dose-dependent. Oral is the preferred route. *C. difficile* remains in colonic lumen without invading the colonic mucosa.
- For severe disease, use vancomycin: faster symptom resolution, inhibits cell wall synthesis. Vancomycin is poorly absorbed and therefore there are high concentrations within the intestines and few adverse systemic effects.
- For NBM patients, use IV metronidazole: excreted into bile; exudation from the inflamed colon results in bactericidal levels in faeces. IV vancomycin is ineffective.

What do you know about Department of Health targets for *C. difficile* infection?

- Outbreaks should be reported as a SIRI (serious incident requiring investigation).
- All trusts should have policies for antibiotic prescribing, protocols for diagno-sis of diarrhoea, isolation and enhanced nursing care and cleaning protocols.

• DoH asked NHS to reduce *C. difficile* infections by 17% in 2012/2013, following 30% reduction from 2007/2008 to 2010/2011, with a targeted maximum rate of 8.5 cases per 10,000 population.[3] The SHA is accountable.

COMMON BILE DUCT STONES

A 50-year-old man has been admitted as an emergency under your care with a history of right upper quadrant tenderness and altered liver LFTs. How will you manage him?

• Review the history—known gallstone disease, previous episodes of cholecystitis, previous biliary surgery, drug and alcohol history.
• Perform full clinical examination—general (signs of dehydration, jaundice, sepsis), RUQ peritonism, Murphy's sign, Charcot's triad.
• Review the blood tests—WCC, amylase, CRP, clotting and LFTs and urinalysis.
• Resuscitate the patient with IV fluids, analgesia and broad-spectrum IV antibiotics if there are signs of sepsis/cholangitis.
• Arrange an urgent USS to look for gallstones and a dilated biliary tree.

The USS shows multiple small gallstones, a slightly dilated intrahepatic duct and a 7 mm CBD. He is not septic. His LFTs return to normal over the next 24 hr. You suspect he has passed a CBD stone. What is your next management step?

This depends on your expertise and what YOU would do as a consultant. UGI/ HPB trainees would be expected to talk about surgical CBD exploration. Other trainees should probably discuss preop imaging and treatment.

• Discuss with the patient the two treatment options, depending on the patient's fitness for surgery:
  • MRCP to confirm that CBD is clear, followed by laparoscopic cholecystectomy
  • Laparoscopic cholecystectomy and on-table cholangiogram or laparoscopic USS, proceeding to CBD exploration and stone extraction if necessary

What are the risk factors for having CBD stones?

• Age > 55 years
• Bilirubin > 30
• CBD dilatation on USS (70% chance of stones)
  • Less than 5% chance of having CBD stones at time of surgery for a nonjaundiced patient with normal diameter CBD at USS

If the USS shows multiple small gallstones and a stone in the CBD, how will your management change?
There are two options—say what YOUR preference is.

- ERCP to evaluate CBD—remove stones/sphincterotomy/place stent, followed by laparoscopic cholecystectomy.
  - ERCP will clear the duct of stones, making surgery simpler, but it is not without risk.
- Option if not fit for surgery (may be definitive treatment).
  - Laparoscopic cholecystectomy and on-table cholangiogram or lap USS, proceeding to CBD exploration and stone extraction if necessary
    - Complications of bile duct leakage and tube displacement
    - Needs surgical expertise and special theatre equipment

Expect to discuss what you would do if a stone was found at surgery but you did not have skills for CBD exploration.

What are the advantages and disadvantages of these options?

- Preop ERCP ensures that the CBD is clear of stones prior to surgery, but it has complications, including a small mortality risk.
- Laparoscopic cholecystectomy and CBD exploration require surgical expertise and special equipment.
- There is no evidence of a difference in efficacy, morbidity or mortality when ERCP is compared to laparoscopic CBD stone extraction, but surgery has a shorter stay, because the patient is treated in one admission.

How would you perform a lap CBD exploration?

There are two approaches:

- Transcystic—small stones < 7 mm and fewer than three stones
  - Can only remove stones below insertion of cystic duct as cannot retro-flex into common hepatic duct
- Direct supraduodenal CBD exploration—large stones and multiple stones
  - Avoid if small-calibre CBD due to risk of stenosis.
- A longitudinal dochotomy is made with hooked scissors avoiding the bile duct arteries at 3 and 9 o'clock.
- Stones are extracted via endoscope or a basket.
- Completion cholangiogram is performed and the hole is closed. If it is too large to close, leave a T-tube.
- Do T-tube cholangiogram in 5–7 days; tube is clamped if it is clear and there is free flow into duodenum. Remove in OPD in 6 weeks' time.

COLONIC CANCER

A 56-year-old man presents in your rapid access clinic with intermittent diarrhoea for 5 weeks. His GP has noted that his Hb is 11 g/dl. The history is otherwise noncontributory. Abdominal and rectal examinations are unremarkable. How will you investigate him?

- Patients with suspicious symptoms or a proven colorectal cancer should be investigated with a total colonoscopy, CT colonography or barium enema.

- Balance between gold-standard investigation, waiting list for procedure and patient fitness.
- A colonoscopy must see the ileocaecal valve but carries risks of perforation and bleeding from polypectomies and biopsies.
- CT colonography picks up 6 mm polyps and is becoming a standard investigation, replacing barium enema.
- Barium enema shows 'apple-core' stricture and may pick up polyps.
  - False positive (1%) and false negative (7%) results can occur, but are more common in sigmoid and caecum. No longer first-line test.

What symptoms are considered low risk for colorectal cancer?

- Patients with no iron deficiency anaemia, no palpable rectal or abdominal mass
- Rectal bleeding with anal symptoms and no persistent change in bowel habit (all ages)
- Rectal bleeding with an obvious external cause (e.g., anal fissure) (all ages)
- Change in bowel habit without rectal bleeding (<60 years)
- Transient changes in bowel habit, particularly to harder or decreased frequency of defecation (all ages)
- Abdominal pain as a single symptom without signs and symptoms of intestinal obstruction (all ages)
- Soreness, discomfort, itching, lumps, prolapse or pain

What symptoms are considered high risk for colorectal cancer?

- Rectal bleeding with a change in bowel habit to looser stools or increased frequency of defecation persisting for 6 weeks (all ages)
- Change in bowel habit as in the preceding without rectal bleeding and persisting for 6 weeks (>60 years)
- Persistent rectal bleeding without anal symptoms (>60 years)
- Palpable right-sided abdominal mass (all ages)
- Palpable rectal mass (not pelvic) (all ages)
- Unexplained iron deficiency anaemia (all ages)

What is the natural history of colon cancer?

- The majority of colonic cancers arise from pre-existing adenomatous polyps.
- In 50% of cases, cancers arise on the left side and on 25% on the right.
- In 5% of cases, there are synchronous lesions.

What evidence is there that the majority of colonic cancers arise from pre-existing polyps?

- Prevalence of adenomas correlates well with that of carcinomas.
- Average age of adenoma patients is 5 years younger than patients with carcinoma.

- Sporadic adenomas are histologically identical to FAP adenomas, which are unequivocally premalignant.
- Large adenomas are more likely to display cellular atypia than small polyps.
- Adenomas are found in up to one-third of colons resected for colorectal cancer.
- The incidence of colorectal cancer has fallen with a screening programme involving colonoscopy and polypectomy.

What is the genetic basis of colon cancer?

- APC (adenomatous polyposis coli) gene mutations
  - Occur early in 60% of all adenomas and carcinomas
- K-ras mutations (induce cell growth)
  - Occur later in large adenomas and carcinomas
- p53 mutation (involved in DNA repair and induction of apoptosis)
  - Later, in invasive colonic cancers
  - Accompanied by invasion

What risk factors are known for colonic cancer?

- Lifestyle factors can be a risk.
  - Risk decreases with physical exercise, dietary fibre, calcium, garlic, nonstarchy vegetables and pulses.
  - Risk increases with obesity, red meat, processed meat, alcohol, animal fat and sugar.
  - Long-term smoking is associated with a relative risk of between 1.5 and 3.0.
- Predisposing conditions:
  - Long-standing ulcerative colitis and Crohn's disease
  - Previous gastric surgery (controversial association)—possible due to altered bile acid metabolism after gastrectomy and vagotomy
  - Previous ureterosigmoidostomy

At colonoscopy, your patient is found to have a large fungating tumour in his caecum. Biopsies confirm invasive adenocarcinoma. His staging CT suggests localised disease. What will you do?

- Consent him for a right hemicolectomy.

What are the principles of surgery for colorectal cancer?

- The tumour must be radically excised with the vascular pedicle and accompanying lymphatic drainage.
- In an unfit patient, limited resection can be performed.
- Mechanical bowel prep is no longer indicated.
- There is no evidence for routine pelvic drain placement.
- Perform open or laparoscopic surgery, depending on surgical training and expertise.

- Elective operative mortality should be <5%.
- Wound infection rate should be <10%.
- Overall leak rate should be <4%.
- Extent of bowel resection depends on tumour site.
- Ascending colon cancers right hemicolectomy (divide ileocolic and right colic arteries at SMA, and branch of middle colic artery may also need to be divided).
- Descending colon cancers left hemicolectomy (divide IMA).
- Splenic flexure cancers—two options:
  - Extended right hemicolectomy—divide middle colic and ascending branch of left colic artery
    - Will also remove associated lymphatic drainage
    - Less ischaemia as ileum is well vascularised
  - Left hemicolectomy—divide IMA and left branch of middle colic
  - Anastomosis is needed between right colon and rectum (difficult to make tension free).

You undertake a right hemicolectomy. How do you fashion your anastomosis?

Say what YOU do, and why. There are two options: stapled or hand sewn.

- Appositional hand-sewn serosubmucosal anastomosis
  - Mesenteric defects not closed
  - Best results in literature (leak rates of 0.5%–3%)
- Stapled anastomosis
  - 'Functional end to end' for right hemicolectomy
  - Check the staple line for bleeding
  - Close defect with linear stapler
- No consistent difference in leak rates between two techniques

How does colon cancer spread?

- Direct—longitudinally, transversely and radially
- Radial spread is the most important (may involve ureter, duodenum, etc.)
- Lymphatic—from paracolic nodes to the para-aortic nodes (30% skip a tier of nodes)
- Rare for a colonic cancer that has not breached muscle wall to have lymph node metastases
- Blood-borne—most common site is the liver by the portal venous system (50%); other sites include lung (10%), ovary, adrenals, bone, brain, kidney
- Transcoelomic—via subperitoneal lymphatics or viable cells shed from serosa of tumour resulting in malignant ascites

What is the survival rate for colon cancer?

- The 5-year relative survival rate is currently in the region of 50% and has improved over the last 30 years from a figure of around 20% in 1971.

What do you know about the staging of colon cancer?

- Two main classifications—Dukes' and TNM
- Dukes' staging—based on specimen histology:
  - A: invasive carcinoma not breaching the muscularis propria; 85% 5-year survival
  - B: invasive carcinoma breaching the muscularis propria, but not involving regional lymph nodes; 67% 5-year survival
  - C1: invasive carcinoma involving the regional lymph nodes (apical node negative)
  - C2: invasive carcinoma involving the regional lymph nodes (apical node positive); 37% 5-year survival
  - D: distant metastases
- TNM staging:
  - T1: tumour invading submucosa
  - T2: tumour invading muscularis propria
  - T3: tumour invading into subserosa
  - T4: tumour perforating visceral peritoneum/direct invasion
  - N0: no regional lymph node metastasis
  - N1: metastasis in one to three pericolic or perirectal lymph nodes
  - N2: metastasis in four or more pericolic or perirectal lymph nodes
  - N3: metastasis in any lymph node along the course of a named vascular trunk
  - M0: no distant metastases
  - M1: distant metastases

CUSHING'S SYNDROME

A 50-year-old patient has been referred to your clinic with a recent onset of hirsutism, weight gain, easy bruising and weakness in the arms. On examination you see striae, a round face and hump on the upper back. What is the likely diagnosis?

- Cushing's syndrome

What is Cushing's syndrome?

- It is the signs and symptoms that develop after exposure to high levels of circulating glucocorticoids (cortisol).
- The clinical features include obesity, hirsutism, proximal muscular weakness, striae and bruising, hyperpigmentation, increased incidence of bone fractures and hypokalaemia.

What are the causes of Cushing's syndrome?

- ACTH dependent:
  - Pituitary microadenoma (Cushing's disease)

- Ectopic secretion
  - Small-cell lung cancer
  - Carcinoid (bronchial)
  - ACTH levels higher than pituitary Cushing's
  - Causes more pronounced hyperpigmentation, muscle weakness and hypokalaemia
- ACTH independent:
  - Adrenal adenoma—ACTH suppressed by negative feedback
  - Adrenocortical carcinoma
  - Bilateral adrenal hyperplasia
  - Iatrogenic—long-term steroid use

How would you confirm the diagnosis in this patient?

- First confirm Cushing's syndrome
  - 24 hr urine cortisol
  - Raised midnight cortisol (loss of diurnal rhythm)
  - Low-dose dexamethasone test (should decrease the morning cortisol)
    - Exploits loss of negative feedback
- Then establish cause (i.e., is elevated cortisol ACTH dependent?)
  - ACTH
    - If raised, then ACTH dependent
    - High-dose dexamethasone suppression test (2 g, 6 hourly for 2 days)
      - Pituitary lesions retain some negative feedback and cortisol drops
      - Ectopic sources—cortisol remains high
    - If low or zero, then ACTH independent
- Follow blood tests with appropriate imaging studies
  - If high ACTH—CXR and MRI head to look for ectopic sources and pituitary adenomas
  - If low ACTH—CT and MRI abdomen to look for adrenal lesions
    - More than 3.5 cm suspicious for malignancy
    - Adenomas have higher water content on MR

The blood tests confirm the diagnosis, and a CT and MR show a left adrenal adenoma. How will you treat the patient?

- Perform laparoscopic adrenalectomy.
  - Prophylactic antibiotics are needed.
    - Patients are prone to postop infections.
  - Postoperative steroid cover is needed until normal adrenal function returns.
    - There is risk of fractures and hypoglycaemia.

If the CT was normal and a CXR showed a small-cell lung cancer, do you know how you could control the symptoms?

- Both metyrapone and mitotane will reduce circulating cortisol levels.

DAY-CASE SURGERY

How does day surgery differ from in-patient elective surgery?

- The former is planned admission of a surgical patient to hospital for a surgical procedure which, while recovering from a bed or trolley, allows the patient to return home the same day.

What procedures should be done as day cases?

- Day surgery strategy 2002—75% all elective surgery by 2005
- 1990—Audit Commission basket (20 cases)
- 1999—BADS (British Association of Day Surgery) trolley (20 cases)—
  50% as day cases
  - General surgical operations: laparoscopic hernia, hemithyroidectomy, WLE and ANC, haemorroidectomy, mastectomy, laparoscopic cholecystectomy
- 2001—Audit Commission updated the basket (25 cases—50% as day surgery)
  - General surgical operations: circumcision, orchidopexy, inguinal hernia repair, breast lump excision, anal fissure, haemorrhoidectomy, varicose veins, laparoscopic cholecystectomy

How would you set up a day-case unit?

- Dedicated day-case unit (theatre, ward staff, parking)
- Independent and separate from in-patient infrastructure
- Patient selection—no upper limits on age or BMI (unit guidelines range from 30 to 40), ASA I–III, home care for 24 hr, stop smoking 6 weeks or 12 hr before
- Preop assessment by trained triage nurses working on 'opt-in' basis
- Anaesthesia—regional blocks, GA (general anaesthesia) with LMA, IV propofol to reduce PONV, low use of pre-med, good analgesia
- Recovery—nurse initiated and criteria led based on strict guidelines (vital signs, patient activity, PONV, pain, bleeding)

Would you do a haemorrhoidectomy as a day case?

Say what YOU would do.

- Currently only 24% are done as day cases (BADS say 65% safe).
- Stapled and LigaSure™ procedures, with spinal anaesthesia, are less invasive and associated with less pain.
- It is vital to have good after-care of nonconstipatory analgesia, pre-emptive laxatives, GTN and metronidazole antibiotics to reduce incidence of pain and secondary haemorrhage.

Would you do a laparoscopic cholecystectomy as a day case?

Say what YOU would do.

- Day case rate varies from 0% to 60% (average is <10%).
- It is not done due to lack of availability of CBD exploration/C-arm in day surgery, and fears of reactionary haemorrhage, delayed haemorrhage and bile leak.
  - Reactionary occurs in 4–6 hr and can be addressed in a normal working day if patient is done in the morning.
  - Delayed occurs at 3–4 days, after most patients would have gone home.
  - Bile leak is rarely apparent until 48 hr after surgery—again, after most in-patients would have gone home.
- NHS Institute 2007 clinical pathway—70% could be safely performed as day cases; recommended as part of 18-week pathway.
- Patient selection needs to be rigorous: well-motivated and nonobese patients and attention to detailed surgical technique.

ELECTROSURGERY

How does diathermy work?

- Surgical diathermy involves the passage of high-frequency alternating current between two electrodes and through tissue.
- Where the local current density is the highest, a large amount of heat is produced in the tissue, resulting in tissue destruction.

What is the difference between monopolar and bipolar diathermy?

- Monopolar
  - High power (400 W)
  - A current is generated in the diathermy machine and passed to a hand-held electrode.
  - At the tip of this electrode, the current density is very high, resulting in very high local temperatures.
  - The current then dissipates over a large amount of tissue to the patient 'plate' electrode—with a large surface area of at least 70 cm^2, ensuring that the current density at the plate is low and thus causing minimal heating.
- Bipolar
  - Low power (50 W)
  - The current is passed from one electrode to another across a small amount of tissue.
  - The two electrodes are usually incorporated into a pair of forceps with which the surgeon can hold and coagulate tissue.
  - The power is much smaller and there is no need for a plate.
- This is commonly used in plastic surgery and neurosurgery for very precise coagulation.

Explain the different diathermy settings.

- Cutting:
  - Continuous output (AC generated is a pure, uninterrupted waveform of a few hundred volts) from the generator causes an arc to be struck between the active electrode and the tissue in monopolar diathermy.
  - Temperatures up to 1000°C are produced and cellular water is instantly vaporised, causing tissue disruption without much coagulation.
  - This setting is not available in bipolar diathermy.
- Coagulation:
  - Pulsed output from the diathermy generator (modulation) results in the sealing of blood vessels with the minimum of tissue disruption.
  - Modulation reduces the current flow and therefore the voltage has to increase to drive the current through the tissue.
  - Coagulation mode employs much higher voltages than cutting mode.
  - The highest voltage mode is fulguration or spray, which creates a rain of sparks that flash through the air to the tissue.
  - Any insulation under this condition would be minimal and therefore spray coagulation is regarded as inherently dangerous especially in laparoscopic surgery.
- Blend:
  - Used in monopolar diathermy
  - Continuous output with pulses to help coagulate as well as cut

What are the possible complications with using diathermy in theatre?

- Diathermy plate burns:
  - Due to incorrect placement of patient plate or poorly earthed/older diathermy machine
  - Plate needs good contact with dry, shaved skin
  - Contact surface area > 70 cm^2 (minimal heating)
  - Must be as far away as possible from bony prominences and tissue with poor blood supply (e.g., scar tissue)—poor heat distribution.
- Diathermy burns to skin/soft tissues or surgeon:
  - Careless technique (e.g., failure to replace electrode in insulated quiver after use)
  - Use of spirit-based skin prep with pooling, which can ignite if not left to dry prior to start of surgery
  - Surgeon pressing the cut or coag button when not actually operating
  - Active electrode not in view during laparoscopy
  - Use of metallic laparoscopic ports with plastic insulator cuffs—can create a capacitance in the port and local heating where the port meets the skin
- Risk of explosion in large bowel (methane and hydrogen)
- Gangrene of appendages (penis, digits, tissue pedicles) from monopolar diathermy:
  - Current concentrated along blood vessels and can cause tissue damage distant to the site of the electrode
  - In circumstances where coagulation is needed, bipolar should be used

- Local heating and tissue damage around metallic implants (e.g., hip prostheses)
  - Plate put on the opposite leg if possible

Why does diathermy induce very little neuromuscular stimulation?

- To produce profound neurostimulation, alternating current needs to be below 50 kHz. The mains electricity in the UK works at 50 Hz and a current of only 5–10 mA will cause painful muscle stimulation, whereas 80–100 mA across the heart will result in ventricular fibrillation.
- Surgical diathermy involves currents at 400 kHz–10 MHz and, with these frequencies; currents of up to 500 mA may be safely passed through the tissues.

You are a consultant vascular surgeon in outpatients and see a 75-year-old male who needs an elective open AAA repair. An EVAR is not an option here. You notice on physical examination that he has some sort of implantable device under his skin below his left clavicle. What are you going to do?

- Determine whether this is a pacemaker or implantable cardioverter defibrillator (ICD).
- Appreciate the difficulty with using diathermy in patients with these devices. There are two potential problems:
  - High frequency of the diathermy may result in induced currents in the logic circuits of the pacemaker, resulting in potentially fatal arrhythmias.
  - Diathermy close to the box itself may result in currents travelling down the pacemaker wires, leading to myocardial burns. This could either increase the threshold or at worst cause cardiac arrest.
- During preadmission screening, there should be close liaison with the anaesthetist and cardiologist. They will want to know the indication for the device, extent of any heart failure, degree of pacemaker dependency, implant complexity (bradycardia support, cardiac resynchronisation therapy), if the device is approaching replacement and if the device is part of a clinical investigation where restrictions apply.
- Consider additional perioperative support depending on how close the surgical procedure will be to the device. The more remote the device is from the operative site and the fact it has been checked and verified within the last months, risk of malfunction will be minimal.
- Cardiac pacing/ICD physiologist may need to be present before, during or after the operation (to confirm the correct functioning of the device, advise adjustments, programme an ICD prior to surgery to a monitor-only mode to prevent inappropriate shock delivery, etc.)
- During surgery, make sure of availability of CPR equipment, temporary external/transvenous pacing and appropriate cardiac personnel.
- Avoid diathermy completely if possible; if not, consider bipolar. If monopolar must be used, use only for short bursts and place the patient's plate so

that the current flows away from the pacemaker system. If any arrhythmias are noted, stop all diathermy immediately.

- If bipolar is not feasible, such as in an AAA repair, consider use of feedback—controlled bipolar (e.g., LigaSure), where the jaws of the instrument and therefore the area of coagulating tissue are larger. This is more effective than conventional bipolar electrosurgery. Also consider use of argon plasma where a stream of inert argon gas is passed over the tip of the electrosurgical instrument, confining the electrical current to an ionised stream and allowing precise directional control, whilst eliminating oxygen from the target area. This prevents tissue carbonisation.
- Where an ICD is deactivated and where access to the anterior chest wall will interfere with surgery (i.e., sterile field), consider connecting patient to an external defibrillator using remote pads. Also for patients with an ICD, consideration may be given to positioning a clinical magnet over the implant site to inhibit inappropriate shock delivery through noise detection.

GYNAECOMASTIA

What is gynaecomastia?

- Hyperplasia of stromal/ductal tissue of male breast
- Presents as a concentric painful swelling
- Due to altered oestrogen/androgen balance in favour of oestrogen, or increased breast sensitivity to a normal circulating oestrogen level
- Common, benign, unilateral or bilateral, usually reversible
- Pseudogynaecomastia is excess adipose tissue (no increase in breast tissue)

How do men produce oestrogen?

- Mainly through peripheral conversion of androgens to oestradiol and oestrone by aromatase
- Small amount from testicular secretion

What are the causes of gynaecomastia?

- Physiological—newborn infants, pubescent adolescents and elderly individuals
  - Elderly gynecomastia due to increased aromatisation of testosterone and gradual decrease of testosterone production in the aging testes.
- Pathological
  - Increase in production/action of oestrogen
    - Testicular tumours, lung cancer, liver disease
  - Decrease in production of testosterone
    - Klinefelter's syndrome, bilateral cyptorchidism, hyperprolactinaemia, renal failure
    - Testicular feminisation

- Increased aromatisation of testosterone
- Drug use
  - Antiandrogens (cyproterone acetate, finasteride)
  - Chemotherapy drugs (alkylating agents, methotrexate, vinca alkaloids)
  - Hormones (anabolic steroids, goserelin)
  - Recreational drugs (alcohol, cannabis, heroin, methadone)
  - Cardiovascular drugs (calcium channel blockers, ACE inhibitors, digoxin, spironolactone, amiodarone)
  - Antibiotics (metronidazole, minocycline, isoniazid, ketoconazole)
  - Psychoactive agents (diazepam, haloperidol, tricyclic antidepressants)
  - Others (omeprazole, metaclopramide, phenytoin, theophylline, methotrexate)

How would you investigate a patient with gynaecomastia?

- Take a history—age of onset and duration, recent changes in nipple size, nipple pain and discharge, history of testicular trauma, mumps, drug use, family history, sexual dysfunction, infertility, hypogonadism (impotence, decreased libido and strength).
- Examine the patient (breasts, abdomen, testes, signs of feminisation).
- If rapidly growing gynaecomastia/outside physiological age range:
  - Bloods (LFT, U+Es, prolactin, α-fetoprotein, βhCG, LH, oestradiol, total testosterone)
  - CXR
- Triple assessment of indeterminate lesions (exclude breast cancer)

How would you treat gynaecomastia?

- Physiological—reassurance only
  - Pubertal GM resolves within 3 years in 90% of patients
- Hypogonadism—testosterone replacement therapy
- Idiopathic gynecomastia or residual gynecomastia after treatment of the primary cause—weight loss, then consider medical therapy or surgery
  - Medication is unlikely to work if GM present > 1 year.
  - Tamoxifen is effective for recent-onset and tender gynecomastia. Up to 80% of patients report partial to complete resolution, but not currently licensed for use.
  - Danazol (synthetic derivative of testosterone) inhibits pituitary secretion of LH and FSH which decreases oestrogen synthesis from the testicles.
- Breast surgery—reduction mammoplasty or liposuction
  - Refer to oncoplastic surgical colleagues after GP has obtained funding.
  - Complications include contour irregularity, skin necrosis, haematoma, seroma and permanent nipple numbness.

HAEMORRHOIDS

A 27-year-old man presents to your clinic complaining of fresh rectal bleeding and constipation. How will you assess him?

- Take a history—change in bowel habit, quantity and quality of the rectal bleeding, pain on defecation, previous history of haemorrhoids, other 'red flag' symptoms (need to exclude coexisting rectal cancer and inflammatory bowel disease).
- Perform an examination—rectal examination and rigid sigmoidoscopy (if tolerated) to look for skin tags, anal fissures, haemorrhoids and other ano-rectal lesions.

What is the difference between an external and an internal haemorrhoid?

- External haemorrhoids are dilated vascular plexuses below the dentate line, covered by squamous epithelium. They present with severe thrombosis and pain (perianal haematoma) and develop into skin tags if left untreated.
- Internal haemorrhoids are engorged anal cushions above the dentate line, covered by transitional and columnar epithelium. They range in severity from first to fourth degree haemorrhoids.
- First degree haemorrhoids bleed but do not prolapse; fourth-degree haemorrhoids are irreducibly prolapsed.

The patient has been constipated for many years. On examination, there are second degree haemorrhoids. How will you treat him?

- I would try conservative measures, such as stool softeners, and changing his diet to treat the cause and prevent recurrence, with topical creams on a p.r.n. basis.
- If the patient wants formal treatment, I would perform a rubber band ligation in out-patients after counselling the patient about the risks of pain, bleeding and recurrence.

When would you consider operating on haemorrhoids? What surgery would you do?

Say what YOU would do (this depends on your chosen subspeciality and may involve referral) and then state the alternatives.

- I would operate on third and fourth degree haemorrhoids.
- There are three surgical options:
  - Conventional haemorrhoidectomy
  - Haemorrhoidal artery ligation (using a proctoscope with a Doppler probe to tie off the terminal branches of the superior rectal artery)
  - Stapled haemorrhoidopexy
  - A recent meta-analysis of stapled versus conventional surgery showed that the stapled procedure had a higher long-term risk of recurrence, prolapse and additional surgery.

What are the postoperative complications following haemorrhoidectomy?

- Pain, urinary retention, incontinence, primary and secondary haemorrhage, and a late anal stricture.
- Secondary bleeding is usually due to infection.
- Botox, topical GTN and metronidazole have all been shown to reduce postop pain.

HYDRADENITIS SUPPURATIVA

You see a 19-year-old girl in clinic with recurrent boils in her axillae. How would you manage her?

- The likely diagnosis is hydradenitis suppurativa.
- Take a history—pain, previous episodes, previous surgery, other sites affected, antibiotic history, smoker, diabetic, family history (40% have affected family members).
- Then, examine—check for other sites (groins, perianal to exclude Crohn's disease) looking for acute and chronic abscesses, sinuses and fistulae, fluctuance. Take a pus swab of any discharge.
- Treatment—start conservatively with lifestyle changes (e.g., stop smoking, control diabetes, regular hygiene and avoid deodorants).
- Refer initially to dermatologists to start medical treatment.
  - Undertake hormonal control with OCP (oral contraceptive pill) if associated with menses.
  - Prescribe low-dose, long-term antibiotics (clindamycin/minocycline).
  - Roaccutane
- Immunosuppressive therapy and radiotherapy can offer temporary relief, but these have potentially serious side effects and radiotherapy may make definitive surgery difficult.
- For acute inflammation, I would arrange incision + drainage and consider injecting intralesional steroids
- The definitive treatment is radical excision of the affected area, which may need either a VAC dressing or a skin graft. Liaise with plastic surgical colleagues to plan surgery.
- Ideally, there is a need for MDT management with a dermatologist, general and plastic surgeon, and GP.

What bacteria are commonly found?

- In the early stages—Staph/Strep/*E. coli*
- In later stages—anaerobes

What is the aetiology?

- Aetiology is not clearly understood; there is a genetic component.

- Follicular occlusion with secondary involvement of apocrine glands leads to inflammation and destruction of glands. Smoking may be a trigger.
- Shearing forces from obesity and tight clothing contribute to development.

What are the clinical stages?

- The classical three clinical stages as defined by Hurley are:
  - Stage 1: single or multiple abscesses formation, without sinus tracts and cicatrisation
  - Stage 2: recurrent abscesses, with tract formation and cicatrisation; single or multiple widely separated lesions
  - Stage 3: diffuse or near diffuse involvement or multiple interconnected tracts and abscesses across the entire area

HYDROCOELE

A 32-year-old man presents with a swelling in the right side of his scrotum. He first noticed it about a year ago and it has steadily increased in size since. It is not painful. What is the differential diagnosis?

- The differential here includes hydrocoele, hernia, epididymal cyst, varicocoele or testicular neoplasm.

What clinical signs would support the diagnosis of a hydrocoele?

- Hydrocoele is usually a slowly and uniformly enlarging painless swelling confined to the testes and usually inseparable from the testis.
- The swelling is normally firm (tense or lax), nontender and may transilluminate.
- One can easily get above it, and cannot separately feel the testicle.

What is the definition of a hydrocoele?

- A hydrocoele is an abnormal collection of serous fluid within the tunica vaginalis of the testis, which forms the outer covering of the testis.

How are hydrocoeles classified?

- Hydrocoele can be classified on the basis of aetiology and types.
  - Aetiology may be primary or secondary:
    - Primary: idiopathic; appears gradually and becomes large and tense—in children and the elderly.
    - Secondary: associated with an underlying testicular pathology. Usually occurs in males over 40. Appears rapidly in the presence of other symptoms—they are usually lax and often contain altered blood. The underlying pathology may include:

- Trauma
- Tumour
- Torsion—reactive hydrocoeles occur in up to 20% of cases
- Epididymo-orchitis
- Following inguinal hernia repair
- Lymphatic obstruction
- Types depend on which part of the processus vaginalis remains patent:
  - Vaginal hydrocoeles are the most common type whereby the processus vaginalis is obliterated and the fluid collects only around the testicle.
  - In congenital, the processus remains patent into the peritoneal cavity. This is seen in infants and usually resolves within the first 6–12 months of life but needs surgery if it persists after a year.
  - Infantile is rare. It involves the obliterated processus at or near the deep inguinal ring but remaining patent in the cord and scrotum. Thus, the fluid accumulates around the cord as well as around the testicle.
  - Hydrocoele of the cord is rarest. Fluid collection is restricted around the cord. Thus, unlike other hydrocoeles, the testicle can be felt separately.

Is ultrasound useful in the routine assessment of hydrocoeles?

- The diagnosis of a hydrocoele is usually clinical and rarely requires an ultrasound scan for diagnostic purposes.
- However, in suspicious cases and in cases of secondary hydrocoele, ultrasound scan can be performed to exclude testicular tumours and identify other underlying causes.

What are the treatment options?

- Nonsurgical:
  - Watchful waiting: if an underlying malignancy has been excluded clinically and with USS, it is reasonable to reassure the patient and not operate for asymptomatic, small hydrocoeles.
- Surgical:
  - Jaboulay's procedure: the sac is everted and approximated behind the cord via a longitudinal incision.
  - Lord's plication: the sac is plicated with a series of interrupted stitches to the junction of the testis and epididymis.
  - Aspiration is not advised as it potentially seeds infection and the recurrence rate is high.

What is the main complication following surgical repair?

- The main complication following surgical repair for hydrocoele is haematoma formation. Therefore, meticulous haemostasis is essential during the procedure.

HYPERTHYROIDISM

A 29-year-old woman presents in your clinic with a neck swelling and a history of weight loss and sweating. What do you do?

- This sounds like hyperthyroidism.
- I would first take a history—how long she has had the neck swelling, symptoms of hyperthyroidism (heat intolerance, weight loss, fatigue, sweating, palpitations, anxiety, diarrhoea).
- I would then examine her, confirm that the neck swelling is a goitre and feel for dominant nodules and listen for a bruit. Look for systemic signs of hyperthyroidism (tachycardia, brisk reflexes, tremor, acropachy, pretibial myxoedema). Look for thyroid eye signs seen in Graves' disease (exophthalmos, lid lag, lid retraction, red conjunctiva, squint and diplopia).
- The likely diagnosis given her age is Graves' disease, but I would want to exclude a toxic multinodular goitre, malignancy, subacute thyroiditis and an ovarian or pituitary tumour.

She has a diffuse goitre and bilateral exophthalmos. You suspect Graves' disease. How would you confirm this?

- Blood tests
  - TSH (low), free T3/T4 (raised)
  - IgG antibody to TSH receptor
- Neck ultrasound and radioisotope scan to look for a hot nodule or signs of malignancy

The blood tests confirm Graves' disease. How will you treat her?

- Because she has eye signs, radioiodine is not an option. I would discuss with her the pros and cons of medical treatment versus surgery, but surgery would be my treatment of choice.
- I would offer her a total thyroidectomy.

She does not want to have surgery because she is 12 weeks' pregnant. How will you treat her?

- I would give her propylthiouracil, since carbimazole is contraindicated in pregnancy.
  - It inhibits thyroid peroxidase and reduces T3/4 synthesis.
  - It works rapidly and there are no permanent side effects, but there is a risk of relapse.

She comes to see you in 1 year's time, having had a relapse, and is thyrotoxic. She wants to consider surgery. Are there any precautions you need to take prior to operating?

- She needs to be rendered euthyroid to prevent a postoperative thyroid storm.
- I would start her on propylthiouracil.
- I would also give her propranolol, which improves the symptoms of thyrotoxicosis and inhibits the peripheral conversion of T3 to T4. This must be continued for 5–10 days postoperatively because of the long half-life of circulating T4.
- I would ask her to take Lugol's iodine 7–10 days before surgery, to reduce the vascularity of the thyroid and make the gland firmer.
- I would tell her that she needs to take thyroxine for life postoperatively.

How would a thyroid storm present and how would you treat it?

- This is a life-threatening condition initiated by physiological stress such as surgery, but can also be induced by pregnancy, childbirth and infection. The mortality is 10%.
- Patients develop a fever, tachycardia, hyperthermia, diarrhoea, jaundice and a change in their mental state, ranging from agitation and delirium to a coma.
- They are treated on ITU, and given IV fluids, sedatives, cooling blankets, propylthiouracil, hydrocortisone and beta-blockers. They may need intubation.

IATROGENIC BILIARY INJURY

What do you tell your patients during the consent process for laparoscopic cholecstectomy?

- Overall, this is a safe procedure with a low incidence of complications.
- There is a 1 in 40 chance of conversion to open surgery.
- There is a 1 in 300 chance of bile duct injury.
- There is a small risk of postoperative bleeding, wound infection and port-site hernia formation.
- There is a 1 in 25 chance of common bile duct stones at cholangiogram, which would potentially require further treatment (*if you do a cholangiogram*).
- As with other operations, there is a small risk of chest infection, deep vein thrombosis and pulmonary embolism.

While on call at a district general hospital, your registrar calls you from theatre regarding a difficult emergency laparoscopic cholecystectomy. The patient is a 23-year-old female who was admitted yesterday with acute cholecystitis. During a difficult dissection, the ST7 says he can see bile, but cannot see where it is coming from. How would you manage this patient?

- Firstly, I would tell the ST7 to stop the dissection and then go to theatre myself, where I would read the notes, look at the preoperative imaging reports and assess the situation.

- I would not attempt to repair this laparoscopically; this is nearly always unsuccessful.
  - I would consider the possibility of unappreciated/missed injuries (e.g., resection of part of CBD, arterial injury, local diathermy injuries).
- If there was an obvious hole in the CBD, I would insert a T-tube.
- I would take photographs of the dissection and place a large Robinson drain in the subhepatic space.
- I would wash out the abdomen and start the patient on broad-spectrum antibiotics (e.g., IV Tazocin).
- I would then refer the patient to the local HPB specialist unit for definitive treatment (*unless you are an HPB surgeon, in which case you should describe your operative management*).
- Finally, I would have a debriefing with the SpR to go over the challenging points of the case and use it as a learning opportunity.

How could you establish the source of the leak?

- Conduct a postoperative MRCP, followed by ERCP if necessary to confirm the diagnosis and allow stent placement (to treat a small leak).
- If the CBD has been completely transected, I would proceed to a CT to delineate the anatomy.

How are biliary injuries classified?

- The two major classifications are Strasberg and Bismuth.
- However, both omit one of the most serious injuries—biliary leak with separation of the right and left ducts resulting from excision of the extrahepatic biliary tree.
- The most common is complete transection of the CBD, after mistakenly dividing the 'cystic' duct and/or further division of 'abnormal' extra ducts.

What are the common variations in bile duct anatomy?

- Right hemiliver
- Right anterior or right posterior sectoral duct insertion directly into the left hepatic duct
- Right posterior sectoral duct insertion below the right–left duct confluence
  - This is dangerous if it inserts into the cystic duct.

What is the risk of biliary injury during cholecystectomy?

- The risk for laparoscopic cholecystectomy is 0.3%–0.7%.
- The risk for open cholecystectomy is 0.13%.
- It occurs in elective straightforward cases as well as after pancreatitis/cholangitis and emergency cases.

- The main cause is misinterpretation of biliary anatomy—CBD confused with cystic duct.
- Associated injury to the right hepatic artery can occurs if it is mistaken for the cystic artery.
- Partial injury to the CBD can occur from a diathermy burn or after rigorous traction on the cystic duct, avulsing it from the CBD.

How can you avoid a biliary injury?

- Risk factors are inexperience, aberrant anatomy and inflammation. A recent study showed that a visual perceptual illusion is the most common cause.
  - 75% are missed intraoperatively.
- Dissect Hartmann's pouch at junction of gallbladder and cystic duct, and identify all structures in Calot's triangle prior to ligation (view of safety).
- Up to 25% of patients have drainage of a right sectoral duct directly into the common hepatic duct, and this can have a prolonged extrahepatic course, being mistaken for the cystic duct.
- There should be no blind clipping of arterial bleeding.
- Some surgeons advocate intraoperative cholangiography (IOC) or laparo-scopic USS in every case to avoid injury.
  - Routine IOC can reduce the risk of injury by twofold for inexperienced surgeons.
  - It can be interpreted incorrectly and injuries can still be missed.
  - If unclear anatomy, consider partial cholecystectomy/abandon surgery.

INFORMED CONSENT

What are the key components of informed consent?

- Consent is a partnership with the patient.
- It gives patients the information they need and want in terms they can understand.
- It explains options, including potential benefits, risks, burdens and side effects of each option, and the option to have no treatment.
- Patients must be given time to make the decision and should not be consented on the day of surgery.
- No one else can make a decision on behalf of an adult who has capacity.

Can you delegate consent to another member of the team?

- It is my responsibility to discuss consent with the patient if I will be performing the surgery.
- I can delegate if the junior doctor:
  - Is trained and qualified
  - Has sufficient knowledge of the proposed operation
  - Understands the risks involved
  - Acts in accordance GMC guidance

What level of risk would you mention?

- This depends on the individual patient and what he or she wants or needs to know.
- Adverse outcomes that may result from surgery, as well as those from not operating, must be identified.
- Risks include side effects, complications and failure of intervention.
- A patient must be told if surgery might result in a serious adverse outcome, even if the risk is very small (might affect their decision to consent).
- Patients also must be told about more common, less serious side effects, and what to do if they happen to the patient.

How can a patient give consent?

- In three ways:
  - Orally
  - In writing
  - Implied (rolling up sleeve for BP measurement)
- If there is not time to get written consent (ruptured AAA), oral consent can be relied upon, but the patient must still be given all the relevant information to make the decision. I would then record in the case notes the fact that the patient had given oral consent.

A child of 13 has acute appendicitis and her parents cannot be reached. Can you proceed with surgery?

- A child's capacity depends on the ability to weigh up options and make decisions, not on age.
- Children under 16 may have capacity to make decisions.
- It is the responsibility of the doctor to decide whether the child is Gillick competent.
- If the child is not competent, there is no need to delay an urgent operation if the parents cannot be contacted.

A 57-year-old man has been admitted with a stercoral perforation and is peritonitic. He thinks you are trying to kill him and refuses surgery. What would you do?

- Every patient has the right to refuse surgery, and his decision must be respected.
- You cannot force a patient with a mental illness to accept a treatment, even if this means that the outcome may be fatal. The patient still has the capacity to make decisions about his or her own care.
- The only treatment that could be forced on the patient is treatment of mental illness, after consulting with psychiatric colleagues.

What is the Mental Capacity Act?

- This is a legal framework from 2005 regarding treatment and care of patients who lack capacity. It presumes that every adult has mental capacity to make decisions about his or her care.
- If a patient lacks capacity, treatment options that provide overall clinical benefit for the patient must be considered. Previously expressed wishes, such as an advance directive, and the views of people close to the patient and whether those beliefs are in the patient's best interests must be taken into account.
- If there are no close relatives or caregivers, then an IMCA (independent mental capacity advocate) must be involved to decide whether elective treatment is in the patient's best interests.
- In an emergency setting, a patient can be treated without consent, provided the treatment is necessary to save his or her life.

IN-GROWING TOENAIL

A patient presents with an in-growing toenail. What is the cause?

- The cause is lateral projection of the nail growing into the periungual soft tissue.
- The vast majority occur on the great toe.
- Causes include extrinsic compression by footwear, nail cut too short laterally, infection, trauma, heredity.
  - The nail fold is penetrated; bacterial/fungal skin flora colonise.
  - Oedema, erythema and pain lead to abscess formation and hypertrophic granulation tissue.
- This can be the initiating pathway for osteomyelitis in patients with diabetes/ arterial insufficiency.

What is the anatomy of the nail?

- There is the nail plate—body (exposed portion) and root (proximal portion covered by skin fold—eponychium). It rests on a nail bed.
- The germinal matrix runs from the lunula to the eponychium.
- The cuticle is the most distal edge of the eponychium.

How would you treat this?

- Conservatively: dislodge lateral nail edge, then place sterile gauze under sharp corner of nail. Cut out shoe, replace gauze daily and order daily warm soaks until inflammation subsides. Educate the patient on proper nail care.
- Surgically: the preferred option is a wedge excision, but total removal of the nail plate can be performed.

Talk me through a wedge excision.

- Apply a local digital block with plain 1% bupivicaine without epinephrine.
- Place a rubber tourniquet around the proximal toe.
- Lift the lateral quarter of the nail using a haemostat.
- Divide the lateral nail down to and remove the underlying matrix with a scalpel.
- Grasp the nail fragment with the haemostat and roll medially to remove.
- Debride underlying tissue.
- Apply petroleum jelly to protect the skin.
- Apply 80% phenol to the exposed matrix with a cotton bud for 30–60 s.
- Irrigate with alcohol to remove excess phenol.
- Dress the toe and remove the tourniquet.

What are the postoperative complications?

- Ischaemia—excessive anaesthetic during digital nerve block or if adrenaline is used
- Recurrence or regrowth, and retained nail fragment
- Infection and bleeding

INGUINAL HERNIA

A 62-year-old male presents with a right inguinal hernia. The hernia has been present for 2 years and is asymptomatic. He is otherwise fit and well. What is your management plan?

- The plan is for elective mesh repair using a laparoscopic or an open approach; there is a 2% risk of developing complications. In addition, there is no increased incidence of chronic groin pain.
- Nonsurgical management such as a truss is used for symptomatic patients not fit for surgery.
- Do consider the feasibility of hernia repair under local anaesthesia.

What is a hernia?

- A hernia is an abnormal protrusion (sac) of a viscus through its normal covering or into an abnormal site.

What are the borders of the inguinal canal?

- Anterior—external oblique aponeuorsis with lateral third of internal oblique
- Posterior—transversalis fascia and conjoint tendon and reflected portion of inguinal ligament
- Inferior—inguinal ligament and medial third of lacunar ligament
- Superior—conjoint tendon

What are the types of inguinal hernia?

- There are two types of inguinal hernia:
  - Direct—slow increase in size with low risk of incarceration or strangulation (0.5% per annum)
  - Indirect—higher risk of acute events (2%–5% per annum)
  - Male-to-female ratio is 12:1, with the peak incidence in the sixth decade.
- The common presentation is a painless or painful groin lump and, in the elderly, an irreducible groin lump.
- Risk factors include advancing age, obesity, COPD, chronic constipation and connective tissue disorders.

What are the principles of inguinal hernia repair and what approaches are available?

- Definition of the anatomy, identification of the sac, assessment of the viability of its contents (in acute presentation) and repair using a synthetic material as a day-case procedure
- Modified Lichtenstein technique: widely used open technique and shown to have minimal long-term recurrence (<1% in 10 years)
- Laparoscopic repair—recommended for bilateral and recurrent hernias (NICE) and may be offered as an alternate approach to unilateral hernia. The two widely practiced approaches are total extra peritoneal mesh repair (TEP) and transabdominal preperitoneal mesh repair (TAPP).

What's the most favoured surgical approach and why?

- Laparoscopic approach is more widely used than open repair.
- The laparoscopic approach is preferred as it causes less postoperative pain and lowers the incidence of chronic groin pain, therefore facilitating early return to work (NICE).

Describe an ideal mesh.

- An ideal mesh should have the following characteristics:
  - Lightweight (<80 g/m^2)
  - Large pore (>1 mm) to avoid formation of solid fibrotic plate resulting in shrinkage of the mesh
  - Must be able to cope with transient increase in abdominal pressure during coughing, sneezing (>200 mmHg), etc.
  - Laparoscopic meshes should handle well and not cause bowel adhesions

How would you treat a patient with a recurrent inguinal hernia after a previous open repair?

- In addition to the laparoscopic approach, a transinguinal open and preperitoneal mesh repair/Rives or Stoppa procedure can be considered in selected cases. However, it has a higher risk of recurrence between 0.5% and 25% in 10 years and needs surgical expertise in performing this procedure.

You repair the inguinal hernia but he presents 3 months later with chronic groin pain (inguinodynia). How will you manage him?

- Inguinodynia affects up to 40% of patients.
- It can be due to neuropathic (local injury) or non-neuropathic (mesh-related) fibrosis of ilioinguinal, iliohypogastric and genital branch of genitofemoral nerves.
- Risk factors include young age, preoperative pain and pain at other sites.
- Management: lifestyle modification, NSAIDs and surgical or chemical neurectomy in selected cases offer a successful recovery, although there is no consensus in the treatment approach.
- A prophylactic neurectomy during hernia repair significantly decreases the incidence of inguinodynia.

IRON DEFICIENCY ANAEMIA

A 55-year-old man is referred to you with iron deficiency anaemia and weight loss. What are the likely causes of the anaemia?

- Gastrointestinal blood loss from gastric or colorectal cancer
- Coeliac disease
- Renal tract malignancy (present in 1% of patients)

How will you assess him in clinic?

- History:
  - 'Red flag symptoms'—rectal bleeding, change in bowel habit, dyspepsia, dysphagia, abdominal pain
  - Drug history (NSAIDs, PPIs, anticoagulants)
  - Family history of bleeding disorders
- Examination:
  - Abdominal masses, neck and groin lymph nodes
- Review blood tests from GP and repeat if necessary.
- Send a urine sample.

He has lost 1 stone in weight over the last couple of months. There is no history of rectal bleeding or change in bowel habit. How will you investigate the patient?

- In accordance with the British Society of Gastroenterology guidelines[4]:
- Screen for coeliac disease
  - Antitissue transglutaminase (tTG) antibodies
    - If negative, need D2 biopsies
- OGD (with D2 biopsies if tTG negative)
- Colonoscopy

What other options are available for visualising the large bowel?

- Colonoscopy is the preferred test.
  - The risk of perforation is 1:700, mortality following perforation is 10%.
- Flexible sigmoidoscopy is not good enough as it will not visualise the caecum and right colon.
- CT colonography is an option for patients who are not fit enough for a colonoscopy.
- Barium enema is the least preferred option.
  - There is a risk of perforation of 1:10,000, mortality 1:60,000.

He has an OGD. The tTG test was positive and the D2 biopsies confirm coeliac disease. Your ST6 asks if he can cancel the colonoscopy.

- No, the patient still needs the test.
- According to the guidelines, any patient >50 or with marked anaemia or a significant family history of colorectal carcinoma still needs a lower GI investigation, even if coeliac disease is confirmed.

What if the OGD and colonscopy were normal? Would you discharge the patient back to the GP?

- I would ask the GP to treat the anaemia with iron supplements.
- If the patient had persistent anaemia or was transfusion dependent, I would request a small bowel capsule endoscopy looking for telangiectasia.

A 46-year-old lady is referred to you with iron deficiency anaemia and abdominal pain. How will you investigate her?

- I would take a thorough history—and check whether she is pre- or postmenopausal.
- Only postmenopausal women need an OGD and colonoscopy, unless specific symptoms or strong family history warrant investigation.
- Premenopausal women should be screened for coeliac disease only.

LYMPHOEDEMA

A 30-year-old woman presents to your clinic with bilateral swollen lower legs that have got worse over the last couple of years. How will you assess her?

- This sounds like it could be lymphoedema.
- Take a history—how long have the legs been swollen? Does the swelling reduce with elevation? Is there a family history of leg swelling? Has she had a previous DVT?
- Perform an examination—look for evidence of pitting oedema, length of leg involved, skin changes (peau d'orange, waxy, thickened skin, ulceration).

What investigations would you request?

- Duplex scan—to exclude DVT
- Lymphangioscintigraphy

What are the causes of lymphoedema?

- Primary: due to developmental abnormality:
  - Congenital: <1 year
  - Praecox: <35 years
    - 70% unilateral, left leg > right
    - Milroy's disease: familial, sex-linked inheritance
  - Tarda: >35 years
- Secondary:
  - Cancer
  - Postop complication (e.g., axillary surgery)
  - Radiotherapy
  - Infection (filariasis)
  - After arterial–venous surgery

Why does lymphoedema develop?

- The lymphatic transport capacity is reduced.
- The normal volume of interstitial fluid production exceeds the rate of lymphatic return.
- This causes massive dilatation of the remaining outflow tracts and valvular incompetence.
- The lymphatic walls undergo fibrosis, and lymph nodes harden and shrink.
- The interstitial fluid accumulation initiates an inflammatory reaction, destroying elastic fibres and causing collagen deposition. This results in brawny nonpitting oedema.

Do you know the staging of lymphoedema?

- I—reduces with elevation
- II—pitting, no reduction with elevation
- III—elephantiasis

The duplex scan is normal, and you diagnose lymphoedema praecox. How will you treat her?

- Aims of treatment are to reduce limb swelling, improve limb function and reduce risk of infection.
- General advice is to exercise, lose weight, avoid infection/cellulitis; elevation may help.

- Medical therapy:
  - Manual lymphatic drainage—proximal to distal
  - Graduated compression stocking 50 mmHg once swelling is reduced
  - Intermittent pneumatic compression
  - Complex decongestive therapy
  - NO role for diuretics

When would you consider operating?

- Surgery is palliative, not curative.
- The goal of surgery is volume reduction to improve function, improve conservative therapy and help prevent complications.
- Patients still need medical therapy.
- There are two key approaches:
  - De-bulking procedures:
    - Homan's operation—elliptical excisions of skin and subcutaneous tissue with primary closure.
    - Charles' operation—radical excision of skin and subcutaneous tissue. Fascia is grafted using excised skin.
  - Bypass procedures (only for regional lymph blockade):
    - Enteromesenteric bridges
    - Lymphaticolymphatic or venous anastomosis

What are the complications of lymphoedema?

- Chronic lymphoedema for 10 years has a 10% risk of developing lymphangiosarcoma.
- It presents with a reddish purple discoloration/nodule that forms satellite lesions:
  - Highly aggressive
  - Requires radical amputation of the involved extremity
  - Very poor prognosis
- Most commonly seen in postmastectomy patients (Stewart–Treves syndrome)

MALIGNANT MELANOMA

A 45-year-old man presents with a lesion on his leg that has recently changed in size and colour. How would you investigate him?

- Take a history—change in size, shape, colour, bleeding, itching, ulceration?
- The risk factors for melanoma include sunburn, fair skin, family history, xeroderma pigmentosum, lentigo maligna.
- Perform an examination—lesion (site, size, margins, symmetry, pigmentation, ulceration), satellite lesions, complete skin survey including nail beds, regional nodal basins and hepatomegaly.

You suspect a melanoma. What are the different types?

- A melanoma is a malignant tumour of epidermal melanocytes, with radial and vertical growth phases. There are five types:
  - Superficial spreading (60%)—pre-existing mole, upper back and legs, often ulcerative
  - Nodular (30%)—most aggressive, more common in men, often bleeding
  - Lentigo maligna melanoma (7%)—arising from lentigo maligna, least aggressive type, in the elderly, strong link with sun exposure
  - Acral lentiginous (3% Caucasians; 35%–60% Asian/Hispanic/black populations), common on palms and soles, subungual
  - Amelanotic (1%)

How would you diagnose and treat him?

- I would photograph the lesion and perform a full thickness excision biopsy, aiming for a 2 mm margin of clearance.
  - Full-thickness biopsy is needed to measure Breslow's levels.
- Once the diagnosis is confirmed, I would perform further wide local excision to achieve clear margins:
  - In situ disease: 5 mm margin
  - <1 mm: 1 cm margin
  - 1.01–2 mm: 1–2 cm margin
  - 2.01–4 mm: 2–3 cm margin
  - >4 mm: 3 cm margin
- I would discuss at MDT and stage if stage III/IV disease—FBC, LFT, LDH (lactate dehydrogenase), CXR, FNA (fine needle aspiration) palpable nodes, USS liver, CT chest and abdomen/pelvis.
- No survival benefit for chemotherapy. No curative treatment for stage III/IV disease. Complete axillary dissection may offer local control. For limb recurrences, consider isolated limb perfusion with melphalan repetition, needs—risk of toxicity, lymphoedema and amputation.

How is melanoma classified?

- TNM:
  - I: <1.5 mm, no nodes
  - II: >1.5 mm, no nodes
  - III: regional nodes
  - IV: distant metastasis
- Breslow depth (from granular layer to deepest melanoma cell):
  - <1 mm: T1 (a—no ulcer; b—with ulcer)
  - 1–2 mm: T2 (a—no ulcer; b—with ulcer)
  - 2–4 mm: T3
  - >4 mm: T4

How would you investigate the lymph nodes?

- Sentinel lymph node biopsy for all melanomas > 1 mm in depth using radio-isotope and blue dye technique.
- MDT discussion regarding benefits of complete node dissection if the sentinel node is positive. Be cautious with deep groin dissection because it can cause severe lymphoedema and might not give a survival advantage.
- This is the only test that can upstage stage II to III disease and is a prognostic indicator.

MULTINODULAR GOITRE

A 56-year-old woman presents to your clinic with a large mass in the neck that she has had for several years. How would you assess her?

- This sounds like a multinodular goitre.
- I would take a history enquiring about the following symptoms:
  - Irritating cough, shortness of breath, stridor or hoarse voice
  - Pain—due to infarction or haemorrhage into a cyst
  - Dysphagia
  - Rapid growth—may indicate malignancy
  - Previous head and neck irradiation at a young age
  - Family history of MEN—may be relevant if dominant nodule
- I would examine her, assessing her thyroid status, the relevant features of the neck lump, whether there is a dominant nodule (risk of malignancy is the same as for a solitary nodule), cervical lymphadenopathy and retrosternal extension.
- Then, I would take blood for thyroid function tests (T4 and TSH) and arrange an initial USS ± FNA of any dominant nodules.
- If there was evidence of retrosternal extension and I was planning surgery, I would ask for a CT neck scan to assess the degree of extension.

What are the causes of a multinodular goitre?

- Most MNGs are due to enlargement of a simple goitre, which develops due to TSH stimulation secondary to low levels of thyroid hormones.
  - Iodine deficiency causes an endemic simple goitre, which appears in childhood and evolves into a colloid goitre at a later stage.
  - The increased demand for thyroid hormone in pregnancy and puberty causes enlargement of a goitre.
  - Dietary goitrous agents are in brassica vegetables; lithium and carbimazole also induce goitres.
  - Rare hereditary congenital defects in thyroid metabolism also cause goitres.
- Sporadic MNG can occur, commonly affecting middle-aged women.
- Previous radiotherapy to the neck (e.g., lymphoma) can also cause goitres.

You find a dominant nodule in the left-hand side of the goitre. How would you assess it?

- FNAC is mandatory, ideally under ultrasound guidance.
- Ultrasonography may also demonstrate enlarged cervical lymph nodes.
- If the FNAC is Thy 3, 4 or 5, then the nodule needs to be excised.

When would you offer surgery for a multinodular goitre?

- When there is a suspicion of malignancy
  - Rapid growth, FNA results
- Patients with pressure symptoms
  - Shortness of breath, dysphagia, stridor
- For cosmesis, in patients with a large neck swelling

What operation would you perform?

- For a dominant nodule, I would do a unilateral thyroid lobectomy.
- For a multinodular goitre, I would do a total thyroidectomy.
- Prior to surgery for an MNG, I would ask for an anaesthetic opinion, as this could be a difficult airway.
- Lung function tests with flow loop studies and a CT neck will evaluate the degree of airway compromise and the retrosternal extension and help plan surgery.
- The patient may need awake fibre-optic intubation.

MANAGEMENT OF DIABETES IN SURGICAL PATIENTS

How do you manage a diabetic patient having day-case surgery?

- The ASGBI guidelines regarding perioperative management of the adult patient with diabetes list six key points regarding surgical planning:
  - The patient should be carefully involved.
  - The patient should be prioritised on the operation list to allow for minimum starvation time.
  - Comorbidities should be optimised where possible.
  - Principles of enhanced recovery should be used to promote early mobilisation and return to normal diet.
  - Create a safe discharge plan for diabetes management.
  - The process and the outcomes should be audited regularly.
- Ideally, the blood glucose should be tightly controlled before surgery, since poor glycaemic control impairs the response to infection and slows wound healing. HbA1C should be checked during preadmission.

How do you manage a patient who will only miss one meal?

- If the patient is diet controlled, a patient should fast as normal, with qds BM measurements, and the diabetic team contacted if the BM > 10 for 24 hr.
- If the patient is tablet controlled, then these should be omitted on the morning and given postop with light meal.
- If the patient is insulin controlled:
  - Morning list: the patient should fast from midnight, be given a glucose drink at 06:00, and the insulin dose and breakfast should be given after the procedure.
  - Afternoon list: the patient should fast from 08:00, be given half the morning insulin dose with breakfast, a glucose drink at 10:30 and the midday insulin dose with lunch after the procedure.

How do you manage patients who will miss more than one meal?

- These patients need a variable rate intravenous insulin infusion (VRIII), which now replaces the historic sliding scale.
- The substrate solution is 0.45% NaCl/5% glucose and either 0.15% or 0.3% KCl. The dextrose is added to prevent proteolysis, lipolysis and ketogenesis.
- Capillary blood glucose should be monitored hourly during surgery and the immediate postop period.
- The WHO surgical safety checklist bundle should be implemented, with a target glucose of 6–10 mmol/l.
- S/C insulin should be given 30–60 min prior to stopping infusion.

How will you manage the daily fluid requirement for diabetic patients in the emergency setting?

- For all patients on a VRIII regimen, I would prescribe dextrose saline with KCl alongside the VRIII and adjust the KCl depending on the patient's electrolyte results. Diabetic patients need 180 g glucose/day and additional KCl to prevent hypokalaemia.
- If the patient is not on a VRIII regimen, I would prescribe Hartmann's solution to avoid hyperchloraemic metabolic acidosis.

What are the metabolic effects of starvation and surgery?

- Both induce a catabolic state, which is attenuated in diabetic patients on a glucose–insulin infusion. Hypoglycaemia also stimulates secretion of counter-regulatory hormones and exacerbates the catabolic response.
- Major surgery causes an increase in catabolic hormone secretion and inhibition of anabolic hormones, especially insulin.
- Type I diabetic patients have no insulin secretory capacity and therefore cannot respond to the increased demand for insulin.

- Type II diabetic patients have pre-existing insulin resistance with limited reserve, which reduces their ability to respond to the increased demand.

How will you manage patients taking metformin?

- If the patient is only missing one meal, he or she will take the metformin as normal, unless the patient takes it three times a day, in which case the lunchtime dose is omitted.
- If the patient has renal impairment, metformin should be stopped when the perioperative fast begins. Metformin is renally excreted, and there is a risk of lactic acidosis in renal failure in the emergency setting.

NECK LUMP

A 52-year-old man presents with a mass in the left-hand side of his neck. It has been there for about 4 months. He is a heavy smoker. How will you assess him?

- Take history—duration, drainage (? branchial cyst), pain, smoking and alcohol, hoarseness/change of voice, dysphagia, previous malignancy or HIV, systemic symptoms (malaise, weight loss, night sweats—TB/lymphoma).
- Conduct an examination—location, fixed to local structures, movement with swallowing, pulsatility, ears, nose and throat, neck nodal chains and axillae/groin nodes, skin, breasts, abdomen.
- Request tests—bloods (FBC, U+Es, Ca, LFTS, TFTs, smear,) FNA, CXR, USS neck, CT/MRI head and neck.

What is the differential diagnosis?

- Midline—thyroglossal cyst, dermoid cyst, pyramidal lobe of thyroid
- Lateral—lymph node, brachial cleft cyst
- Supraclavicular—lymph node
- Submandibular/preauricular—lymph node, salivary gland
- Infective causes of enlarged nodes—lymphadenitis, TB, toxoplasmosis, sarcoidosis, viral
- Remember the 'rule of 80s' after age 40:
  - 80% of nonthyroid neck masses in adults are neoplastic.
  - 80% of neoplastic masses are malignant.
  - 80% of malignant masses are metastatic.
  - 80% of metastases in adults are squamous cell carcinomas.
  - 80% of metastases are from primaries above level of clavicle.

How would you treat a thyroglossal cyst?

- USS neck to confirm presence of normal thyroid
- Sistrunk procedure—excision with middle portion of hyoid bone and follow any tissue to base of tongue

How would you treat a branchial cleft cyst?

- Make a careful surgical excision.
- The first cleft opens at the angle of the mandible and passes through branches of the facial nerve.
- The second cleft (most common) opens at the anterior border of sternoclei-domastoid (SCM) between carotid bifurcation.
- The third cleft opens at the lower border of SCM and passes behind the carotid artery.

How would you manage a solitary lymph node in the neck?

- Take a thorough history—eczema, rheumatoid arthritis, dental abscess, recent infective illness, previous malignancy.
- Examine the neck and all nodal chains, ear, nose and throat, including axil-lae and groins, and look for an obvious cause.
- Ask about recent infective illness or previous malignancy.
- Take an FNA for histology. Do not take a core; if the FNA shows a squa-mous cell carcinoma, then a biopsy will affect the subsequent resection margins; if FNA shows lymphoma, the patient needs an open biopsy.
- Remember that almost all nodes in the posterior triangle are next to the accessory nerve.

What would you do if an FNA of a node showed squamous cell carcinoma?

- Open excisional biopsy with panendoscopy of aerodigestive tract.

What would you do if an FNA of a node showed adenocarcinoma?

- Arrange for CT scan of neck/chest/abdomen/pelvis, bilateral mammograms in a female patient, OGD, barium enema and/or colonoscopy.
- If the primary tumour is found, this represents stage 4 disease and chemo-therapy may be offered.
- If no primary tumour is found, I would do an excisional biopsy to get formal histology, with ER/PR receptors and mucin stains to exclude breast cancer, melanoma and lymphoma.

What would you do if an FNA of a node showed lymphoma?

- I would perform an excisional biopsy of the node.
- I would request a CT scan of neck/chest/abdomen/pelvis, and consider a bone marrow biopsy (stage 4 disease).
- I would determine the disease stage (number of nodal groups, which side of diaphragm is involved).
- I would refer to the haematology MDT.

What are the boundaries and contents of the anterior triangle in the neck?

- Boundaries—midline, anterior border of SCM, lower border of the mandible
  - Subdivided into submental, submandibular, muscular and carotid triangles
- Contents—internal jugular vein, facial vein, retromandibular and external jugular vein, lymph nodes, hyoid bone, larynx, thyroid, parathyroid, carotid sheath, branches of external carotid artery, ansa cervicalis, oesophagus

What are the boundaries and contents of the posterior triangle of the neck?

- Boundaries—SCM, trapezius and middle third of the clavicle
  - Subdivided into occipital and supraclavicular triangles
- Contents—XI nerve, nodes, occipital artery, inferior belly omohyoid, external jugular vein, suprascapular vessels, cutaneous branches of cervical plexus
- Beneath prevertebral fascia—brachial plexus, subclavian artery, cervical plexus and phrenic nerve

PAEDIATRIC UMBILICAL HERNIA

A 6-month-old male infant presents with a painless swelling in the umbilical region, which increases in size when he cries and disappears when he is asleep. What is the most likely diagnosis, and what is the natural history of this condition?

- This is most likely an umbilical hernia.
- This is a common surgical problem of newborn infants and is present in 10% of Caucasian babies.
- The umbilical ring closes over a period of time after birth, and the fascia of the umbilical defect strengthens.
- Most (95%) will spontaneously resolve by 3 years of age.

The parents are anxious and are very keen to get the hernia repaired as quickly as possible. Will you offer them surgery?

- No—I would explain to them the natural history of umbilical hernias and that it is not standard practice to repair these until the child is at least 3 years old.
- It is incredibly rare for umbilical hernias to become incarcerated, because they are wide necked.
- I would discharge them back to their GP and ask them to refer the child back if the hernia persists after 3 years of age.
- It is safe to wait to see if the hernia resolves spontaneously. If the hernia is still present at 4 years of age, it is unlikely to close on its own.

What are the surgical principles of repair of paediatric umbilical hernia?

- Secure closure of the fascia
  - Transverse fashion using nonabsorbable sutures
- Preservation of the appearance of the umbilicus (avoid button-holing the skin)

What conditions are commonly associated with umbilical hernia?

- Prematurity and low birth weight
- Down syndrome
- Trisomy 18
- Trisomy 13
- Mucopolysaccharidoses
- Congenital hypothyroidism
- Beckwith–Wiedemann syndrome.

PHAEOCHROMOCYTOMA

A 40-year-old man is referred to your clinic with hypertension, headaches, palpitations and sweating. How will you investigate him?

- This sounds like it could be a phaemochromocytoma.
- I would take a history, looking for other specific symptoms (headaches, visual problems, dizziness) and ask about a family history. The symptoms are classically paroxysmal. Direct trauma and stress can precipitate symptoms.
- Phaeochromocytoma is seen with MEN 2A and 2B syndromes, neurofibromatosis and von Hippel Lindau syndrome (cerebellar haemangiomas and renal tumours).
- I would perform a full examination and then confirm the diagnosis with blood and urinalysis.

How is this diagnosed?

- Hyperglycaemia and hypercalcaemia
- Raised plasma metanephrine
- 24 hr urine collection for creatinine, total catecholamines, vanillylmandelic acid, and metanephrines (urine container should be acidified and kept cold and dark to prevent degradation of catecholamines)
- If these tests confirm the diagnosis, the patient needs to be alpha-blocked before staging tests are performed, as uncontrollable hypertension can be fatal.

What radiological tests confirm the diagnosis?

- MRI is preferred over CT, with a sensitivity of up to 100%, and it is better at detecting extra-adrenal tumours. They appear hyperintense on T2-weighted images (light-bulb sign) because of the high water content.

- A I^{123} MIBG scan is 95% sensitive and specific, as it resembles norepineph-rine and concentrates within the tumour, and is good for detecting meta-static deposits.

Why do patients get symptoms?

- The adrenal medullary tumour produces excessive amounts of catechol-amines and their derivatives.
- Alpha and beta receptors' stimulation causes hypertension, increased heart rate and contractility, and hyperglycaemia.
- 10% are bilateral, 10% are extra-adrenal and 10% are malignant.

What preoperative steps must be taken prior to surgery?

- Alpha-blockade with phenoxybenzamine or doxazosin, escalating the dose until postural hypotension occurs and the patient is maximally vasodilated
- The alpha-blockade should start 7–10 days preop to allow for expansion of blood volume
- Beta-blockade only given once the alpha-blockade is adequate (if given too soon, the patient has a hypertensive crisis), together with IV fluids to coun-ter the tachycardia

What is the surgical approach for removing a phaeochromocytoma?

- A laparoscopic approach is recommended.
- If the tumour is large or malignant, then open surgery is required.
- There should be minimal tumour handling to avoid the catecholamine secretion and an unstable blood pressure.
- Once the tumour is devascularised, there is a sudden drop in catecholamine levels and the patient may become hypotensive, needing significant volume replacement, so regular communication with the anaesthetist is vital during the procedure.
- If a phaeochromocytoma is found incidentally during surgery (unusual rises in blood pressure/pulse and arrhythmias during induction), it should be left alone.
- Postoperatively, blood glucose should be monitored. Severe hypoglycae-mia is common due to the sudden removal of the glycolytic effects of the secreted catecholamines.

PILONIDAL SINUS

A 25-year-old man comes in via A+E with a painful swelling on his left buttock, which he has had for 3 days. On examination, you see an abscess just to the left of the natal cleft. What is it and how will you treat him?

- This sounds like an acute pilonidal abscess.
- I would treat him with incision and drainage of the abscess and would leave the wound to heal by secondary intention.

In theatre, you see several midline pits and evidence of recurrent abscesses. Will you remove those as well?

- No—there is a high risk of recurrence if excisional surgery is performed at the same time (up to 60%).
- Incision and drainage will lead to a definitive cure in up to 50% of patients.

How do pilonidal sinuses develop?

- In-growing hairs in the natal cleft become a focus of infection.
- They are also seen in finger web spaces of hairdressers.
- They can discharge, often in the midline, leaving a sinus tract and a visible pit.

What are the risk factors for developing pilonidal disease?

- Male gender
- Hirsute individuals
- Sitting occupations (e.g., lorry drivers)
- Deep natal cleft and hair in natal cleft
- Family history
- Obesity—risk factor for recurrence

What bacteria are typically found?

- Mixed aerobic and anaerobic cocci are found.
- *Staphylococcus aureus* is the most common skin commensal.

The patient comes back to see you in clinic a couple of months later, after another abscess that drained spontaneously. He wants surgery to stop it from happening again. How will you advise him?

- Inform him of all the treatment options.
- Conservative—the patient should lose weight, consider regular hair removal, keep the area clean, avoid sitting for long periods of time
- Surgical—the patient must be aware of the risks of recurrence and problems with healing and wound breakdown.
- Surgical options—scrape out the tract and close with fibrin glue, Bascom's procedure, Karydakis flap, Limberg rhomboid flap.

Describe the operation you are most familiar with; Karydakis flap is easiest to understand.

- Karydakis flap
  - Prone position
  - Ellipse of skin and fat lateral to midline containing all pits and tracts

- Medial skin flap undermined and mobilised laterally to close wound
- Flattens natal cleft

PNEUMOPERITONEUM

Why is a pneumoperitoneum necessary for laparoscopic surgery?

- Safe laparoscopic surgery requires visual clarity, space in which to operate and manoeuvre instruments and the maintenance of a normal physiological state.

What gases can be used to induce pneumoperitoneum?

- Carbon dioxide, air, oxygen, nitrous oxide, argon and helium

What factors govern selection of the gas for pneumoperitoneum?

- Physiologic compatibility
- Type of anaesthesia
- Ease of use
- Safety profile
- Toxicity
- Delivery methods
- Cost
- Combustibility

Why is carbon dioxide generally preferred?

- It is a normal end-product of metabolism which is rapidly cleared by the body.
- It is highly soluble in tissue (avoids risk of embolisation).
- It is noncombustible.
- It has a high diffusion coefficient.
- It has the lowest risk of gas embolism.

What are the disadvantages of CO_2?

- In patients with cardiac disease it may trigger arrhythmias (nitrous oxide may be preferred).
- It may also cause hypercarbia in these patients.

What are the potential complications that may occur when establishing a pneumoperitoneum?

- Visceral or vascular injury
- Bleeding or gas dissection within the abdominal wall

What maximum pressure do you set?

- A maximum intra-abdominal pressure of 15 mmHg is usually set.

What happens at higher pressures?

- Undesirable physiological effects start to manifest as pressure rises, especially above 25 mmHg.
- Airway pressure rises.
- Intrathoracic pressure rises.
- Central venous pressure rises.
- Signs of cardiovascular stimulation (i.e., tachycardia and hypertension) occur.

Why do the gas delivery systems include a filter?

- The gas cylinders store gas as liquid under pressure.
- As time passes, organic and inorganic contamination accumulates in the cylinder, requiring the gas to be filtered before insufflation into the patient.

Why does fogging of the lens occur?

- This is due to the dry cold lens being introduced into the warm moist environment of the peritoneal cavity, which causes the dew point on the lens to be reached.
- The result is condensation on the inner surface of the lens.
- It can be prevented by heating and hydrating the gas and applying a surface wetting agent.

Why else should the gas be hydrated?

- It prevents dessication of the peritoneal surfaces, which in turn reduces adhesion formation and preserves peritoneal surface integrity.

Why is the gas warmed?

- It is warmed to prevent hypothermia.
- CO_2 is stored at about 20°C.
- In addition, gas flow causes evaporation from tissue surfaces, leading to further temperature loss.
- Patients lose about 0.3° for every 60 L of CO_2 insufflated.

PROSTATE CANCER

On your post-take ward round you see a 69-year-old man who was admitted by the new FY1 overnight with retention (2l residual urine volume). You notice that he is finding it difficult to get out of bed. What is your immediate management?

- This is potentially a missed emergency.
- The suspicion is of retention secondary to spinal cord compression. I would ask him to stay in bed and perform a neurological exam to confirm a neurological deficit and ascertain the level.
- I would perform a digital rectal examination to look for prostate cancer/pelvic malignancy as a cause for this and assess reduced anal sphincter tone. It is not uncommon for metastatic prostate cancer to present in this manner.

What are your next steps?

- If a neurological deficit is confirmed and a level found, I would organise:
  - An urgent MRI of the spinal cord
  - Serum PSA and U+Es
  - Review by an orthopaedic and/or neurosurgical and oncology team

The MRI shows multiple metastases causing spinal cord compression at T12 to L3 levels. Meanwhile, his PSA returns as 3000 ng/ml. What is the immediate management?

- If there is an isolated metastasis, a decompression laminectomy can be performed. However, depending on the local infrastructure or availability of emergency spinal surgery, surgery may not be recommended.
- In such cases and for patients with multiple metastases, dexamethasone (8 mg bd) and radiotherapy are an alternative treatment.
- Additionally, urgent referral to the urology MDT should be made to plan treatment of the prostate cancer.

What are the treatment options for the prostate cancer? Do you need a biopsy to confirm the diagnosis?

- A biopsy is not necessary unless the diagnosis is in doubt or the patient is suitable for a clinical trial.
- The treatment options are surgical (immediate subcapsular orchidectomy) or medical (LHRH antagonist, e.g., degaralix) to drop testosterone levels immediately.
- If the patient has spinal metastases and needs radiotherapy, then an LHRH analogue is started, with antiandrogen cover (e.g., cyproterone acetate 100 mg tds or bicalutamide 150 mg for 2 weeks before and after).
- If there is hydronephrosis, the patient may need nephrostomies and stents.

Can you discuss the mechanisms of action of the various antiandrogens used in prostate cancer treatment and the rationale for use?

- Testosterone is produced by the testicles in response to the pulsatile release of LH from the anterior pituitary, which in turn is produced by pulsatile release of LHRH from the hypothalamus.

- For patients with metastatic disease:
  - LHRH agonists cause a surge of testosterone release, followed by a castrate effect as there is no pulsatile/release of LH
  - Due to the testosterone surge, the initial dose is covered by an antiandrogen to prevent the testosterone flare (can make spinal cord compression worse).
  - LHRH antagonists exert a similar effect by blocking LHRH and do not need antiandrogen cover.
  - Oestrogen preparations (e.g., stilboesterol) suppress androgen release and also have direct antitumour properties.

PYLORIC STENOSIS

A 6-week-old male infant is brought to A+E with a 1-week history of projectile vomiting. You have been asked to see him. How will you manage him?

- I would take a history—was the child feeding normally up to now? Is the vomit milky or bilious? Is he hungry after feeding? Weight loss? Family history of similar problems?
- I would perform an examination. Dehydration? Abdominal distension? Palpable lump (olive) in RUQ (easier to feel when feeding)?

He has lost 10% body weight, is always hungry and you think you can feel a mass in the RUQ. His father had a similar problem when he was a baby. What is the differential diagnosis?

- Given the classical history of nonbilious projectile vomiting, positive family history and examination findings, the most likely diagnosis is hypertrophic pyloric stenosis.
- Other differentials include gastro-oesophageal reflux, overfeeding, congenital adrenal hyperplasia, pylorospasm and raised intracranial pressure.

What is the epidemiology of pyloric stenosis?

- Incidence is one to four per 1000 live births.
- It is more common in first-born, male infants.
- A positive family history is a significant risk factor.

How will you confirm the diagnosis?

- Clinically, this can be done in 80% of cases by palpating the pyloric mass.
- Ultrasound is the gold standard of investigation.
  - Muscle thickness is greater than 4 mm and length is greater than 16 mm.
  - There is obstruction in the progress of feeds across the pylorus.

How will you manage the condition?

- Firstly, resuscitate the baby and correct the electrolyte imbalance:
  - Hypochloremic, hypokalemic metabolic alkalosis due to vomiting
  - If not corrected, can proceed to 'paradoxical aciduria'
- I would refer the baby to my paediatric surgical colleagues to have a Ramstedt pyloromyotomy.
  - This can be performed by either an open or a laparoscopic approach.
  - Incise longitudinally (2–3 cm) along the anterior, avascular surface of the pyloric 'olive'.
  - Split the hypertrophic muscle with a spreader down to the intact submucosa.

RADIATION-INDUCED BOWEL INJURY

How does radiation-induced bowel injury present?

- It can present early—anorexia, nausea, vomiting, cramps, diarrhoea, tenesmus, mucoid discharge and rectal bleeding.
  - Most symptoms resolve in 2–6 months.
  - There is poor correlation between severity of mucosal damage and symptoms.
- It can present late—several months to years after radiotherapy.
  - Colicky abdominal pain, vomiting and nausea are due to small bowel obstruction.
  - Watery diarrhoea and/or steatorrhoea are due to malabsorption, bile acid-mediated diarrhoea, bacterial overgrowth, impaired motility.
  - There can be faeculent vaginal discharge or pneumaturia, tenesmus, mucoid rectal discharge, rectal bleeding, constipation, and decrease in stool calibre (if rectal involvement).

What are the clinical signs?

- Weight loss and malnutrition (malabsobrtion)
- Abdominal tenderness/peritonism (perforation)
- Abdominal mass (inflammatory response)
- Distended abdomen, tinkling bowel sounds (bowel obstruction)
- Rectal tenderness and bleeding (rectal involvement)

What are the risk factors for radiation-induced bowel injury?

- Previous surgery causing adhesions that fix the intestines in the radiation field.
- Hypertension, diabetes mellitus, and atherosclerosis offer an increased risk for vascular injury.
- Thin, elderly and female individuals may have more small intestine lying in the pelvis—subject to more radiation exposure.

- Certain chemotherapeutic agents (adriamycin, methotrexate, 5-fluorouracil, bleomycin) increase sensitivity to radiation.

How would you diagnose it?

- Plain AXR may show ileus, air–fluid levels (obstruction) and thumb printing (mucosal oedema).
- Barium contrast studies provide better mucosal detail and document the presence of fistulae. Fixed loops with poor distension, absent haustral markings, diffuse mucosal ulceration, or a single ulcer may be seen.
  - When this is not in an emergency setting, use gastrograffin.
- A CT scan will confirm bowel obstruction and location, rule out abscesses and further delineate fistula.
- Colonoscopy ± endoscopic therapy—ability to take biopsies. Perform cautiously in acute setting—friable, oedematous mucosa, ulceration and inflammation. Chronic changes include fibrosis, smooth strictures and pale, granular mucosa and submucosal telangiectasia.

How would you treat it?

- For acute symptom control, consider antidiarrhoeal agents, bile-sequestering agents, antiemetics, and 5-aminosalicylic acid compounds.
- Consider topical steroids and sucralfate enemas if symptoms are related to rectal involvement.
- Consider rectal 4% formalin installation for intractable radiation proctitis.
- Surgery is a last resort or in the presence of complications (perforation, obstruction, abscess drainage, fistulae). It should be as conservative as possible.
  - Resection causes a higher incidence of leakage and mortality than bypass, but the diseased bowel left behind can cause more bleeding, perforation and fistulisation.
- Rectovaginal fistulae may close spontaneously, or after a diversion colostomy; other fistulae require surgical repair.

RADIOTHERAPY

What is radiotherapy?

- The use of ionising radiation to treat malignancy.
  - It is measured in grays (Gy)—measure of the amount of energy deposited in the tissue.
- A linear accelerator produces an electron stream, releasing free radicals which cause oxygen-dependent DNA damage.
- Normal cells trigger apoptosis when they divide, whilst tumour cells die.
- Radiation dose is given in fractions.
  - It improves the therapeutic ratio.
  - It allows normal cells to recover.

- The degree of tumour destruction depends on:
  - Radiosensitivity of tumour
  - Repopulation (potential proliferation rate of tumour)
  - Rate of cell loss (radioresponsiveness)
  - Tolerance of surrounding healthy tissue.

How would you classify radiotherapy?

- Primary: main treatment of tumour (head and neck, bladder, cervical, lung)
- Neoadjuvant: before surgery to downsize (rectal cancer)
- Adjuvant: after surgery (breast cancer)
- Palliation: bone pain, spinal cord compression, SVC obstruction, brain metastases.

How is radiotherapy given?

- External beam radiotherapy using a linear accelerator
- Locally (brachytherapy—radioactive implants)
- Systemically—radioactive isotopes (iodine^{131} in thyroid cancer)
- Intraoperatively: breast cancer

What are the side effects of radiotherapy?

- Usually localised to irradiated site
- Acute:
  - Skin thinning, desquamation, diarrhoea, rectal bleeding, mucositis, oesophagitis, dysuria
- Delayed:
  - Infertility (stem cell damage)
  - Endarteritis obliterans
  - Lymphoedema
  - Malignancy (breast cancer after mantle cell radiotherapy, angiosarcoma of the breast after breast radiotherapy)

ROLE OF THE CORONER

What is a coroner?

- The coroner is an independent judicial office holder, appointed and paid for by the local health authority.
- The coroner must be a lawyer or a doctor of at least 5 years' standing.

What do coroners do?

- They inquire into violent or unnatural deaths, sudden deaths of unknown cause and deaths that occurred in prison.

- They issue death certificates and maintain death records.
- Purposes of coroner service:
  - Establish whether an inquest is required.
  - Establish identity of person who died, and how/when/where that person came to die.
  - Assist in prevention of future deaths.
  - Provide public reassurance.

When is a death reported to the coroner?

- No doctor attended the deceased during the last illness.
- Deceased was not seen within 14 days of death or after death.
- Cause of death is unknown.
- Death occurred during an operation/before recovery from anaesthetic.
- Death was due to industrial disease.
- Death was sudden/unexpected/unnatural.

What can the coroner do when a death has been reported?

- Issue a death certificate if the cause is evident and natural.
- Ask for a postmortem (does not need permission from relatives).
- Order an inquest.

What is an inquest?

- It is a limited, fact-finding enquiry to establish who died, how, when and where.
- It does not establish liability or blame.
- The coroner's court is a court of law; the coroner may summon witnesses, and people found to be lying are guilty of perjury.

Who can certify a death?

- Any GMC-registered medical practitioner can certify death.
- Any doctor can issue an immediate death certificate if he or she attended the patient within 14 days of death.

When should you as a doctor disclose relevant information about a patient who has died?

- To help a coroner with an inquest
- When disclosure is required by law or justified in the public interest (education and research)
- For national confidential inquiries for local clinical audit
- On death certificates
- For public health surveillance

- When a person has right of access to records—*Access to Health Records Act 1990*

SCREENING

What criteria should apply to implement a screening program?

- In 1968, Wilson and Jungner (WHO) identified 10 key points:
  - The condition should be an important health problem.
  - The natural history should be well understood.
  - It should be recognisable at an early stage.
  - The treatment is better at an early stage.
  - A suitable test exists.
  - An acceptable test exists.
  - Adequate facilities exist to cope with abnormalities detected.
  - Screening is done at repeated intervals when the onset is insidious.
  - The chance of harm is less than the chance of benefit.
  - The cost should be balanced against the benefit.

What is the difference between screening and surveillance?

- Screening is designed to detect unsuspected disease in a population of apparently healthy people.
- Surveillance is designed to detect disease in an already diseased population.

What biases exist in a screening programme?

- Lead-time bias—survival is measured from detection to death, and this will be longer because the disease is detected earlier.
- Selection bias—individuals who present for screening are more likely to be health conscious and may not represent a true sample of the population.
- Length bias—slow growing tumours are more likely to be detected by screening than rapidly growing tumours, which would present between screening intervals.

What are the problems with screening programmes?

- Increased morbidity without affecting prognosis (i.e., overtreatment of cancers that may never have led to death)
- Excessive treatment of benign or indeterminate lesions
- Anxiety in the target population
- Costs

What do you understand by the sensitivity and specificity of a screening test?

- A positive or negative test does not mean that a patient has or does not have the disease, as there are false negatives and false positives in every programme.

- Sensitivity is the ability of the test to identify the disease in patients with the disease.
- Specificity is the ability of the test to exclude the disease in the absence of the disease.

What surgical screening programmes are there?

- Breast, cervical, colon and AAA

Tell be briefly about the NHS Cervical Screening Programme.

- It was set up in 1988 to prevent cancer by detecting and treating early abnormalities that would progress to cancer if left alone. It is not based on a test for cancer. A cervical cell sample is taken and sent for analysis.
- All women between 25 and 64 years are eligible for a screening every 3–5 years. Women are first invited at 25 years, then 3 yearly from 25 to 49, and 5 yearly from 50 to 64 years of age.
- A single smear has been shown to reduce the incidence of cancer by 40%–70%, depending on the age group.

Tell me briefly about the NHS Abdominal Aortic Aneurysm Screening Programme.

- The 10-year Multicentre Aneurysm Screening Study (*BMJ* 2009) showed that the NHS screening programme could prevent a significant number of AAA ruptures and deaths, and that the number of lives saved would outweigh the number of elective postop surgical deaths (assumes 80% attendance and 5% elective postop mortality).
- The screening programme aims to reduce AAA-related mortality by screening the male population during their 65th year, and men over 65 can arrange to be scanned. It aims to reduce rupture-related deaths by 50%.

Tell me briefly about the NHS Breast Screening Programme.

- It was introduced in 1988, following the Forest Report.
- It screens every woman from the age of 50, every 3 years, with a phased extension of the age range from 47 to 73 years, which should have been completed in 2012. Digital mammography is used, and two views are taken at every screen.
- The NHSBSP has reduced mortality in the screening age group, and 2.5 lives are saved for every overdiagnosed case. One-third of breast cancers are now detected through screening.

SCROTAL SWELLING

A GP refers a 35-year-old man to your clinic with a scrotal swelling. How will you assess him?

- Take a history:
  - How long has the lump been there?
- Perform an examination—gentle palpation of testes, epididymii and cord.
  - Is it possible to get above it?
  - Is the whole testis enlarged, or is the swelling attached to the testis/epididymis/cord?
  - Is there a hydrocoele or varicocoele?

What is the differential diagnosis of a scrotal lump?

- Cutaneous causes:
  - Sebaceous cysts, haemangioma (rare)
- Arising from the scrotal sac:
  - Hydrocele (transilluminates)
  - Testicular—tumours, epididymo-orchitis, cysts
  - Epididymal—cysts, tumours
  - Cord—cysts
- Arising from the abdomen:
  - Inguinoscrotal hernia
  - Varicocele

What is the differential diagnosis of a scrotal ultrasound?

- In ambiguous cases (adenomatoid tumours, non-resolving epididynmo-orchitis can mimic a tumour that has bled)
- When there is a suspicion of malignancy
  - New irregular lump
  - Rapidly growing hydrocoele in man < 55 years

You find a varicocoele. What is a varicocoele?

- An abnormal enlargement of the pampiniform venous plexus in the scrotum, which drains the testes.
- Idiopathic varicocoele occurs when the valves in the veins are defective
- Secondary varicocoele is due to external compression of the venous plexus. Right varicocoeles should raise suspicion of a retroperitoneal tumour, and a sudden left varicocele should raise suspicion of a renal tumour, especially when newly diagnosed in a man older than 40 years of age.

How are varicocoeles graded?

- Subclinical—identified incidentally on USS, not clinically palpable
- Grade I—palpable with Valsalva manoeuvre only
- Grade II—palpable at rest
- Grade III—visible all the time

How would you manage the patient?

- I would refer him to a urological colleague to discuss the options.
- Surgery is offered for symptom control.
- A recent Cochrane database review showed insufficient evidence that surgery will improve fertility.
- The varicocoele can be excised through an inguinal, retroperitoneal (high ligation) and subinguinal approach. It has also been done laparoscopically. Alternatively, radiological embolisation can be done.

SKIN CANCERS

A 75-year-old man presents with a pearly nodule at the angle of his eye. How would you assess him?

- The likely diagnosis is a basal cell carcinoma (BCC).
- Take a history—risk factors (sunburn, arsenic exposure, immunosuppression, xeroderma pigmentosum).
- Examine the lesion (BCC—pearly nodule with a raised, rolled edge, central ulceration and scabbing), perform a full skin survey and check nodal basins.

How do these lesions spread?

- They spread slowly by local infiltration, destroying surrounding tissues— hence, 'rodent ulcer'.

What is a BCC?

- It is a slow growing, locally invasive malignant epidermal skin tumour.
- It occurs in any part of the body including the anal canal.
- Most (90%) occur above the line from the angle of the mouth to the ear.
- It occurs in twice as many men as women.

How would you treat him?

- Refer to a dermatologist, if clinical diagnosis is uncertain, for a diagnostic shave biopsy.[5]
- Excise the lesion with a 4–6 mm margin. As it is close to the eye, I would liaise with my plastic surgical colleagues; he is likely to need an advancement flap for primary closure.
- If the lesion is advanced, then primary radiotherapy is an option.
- Generally, these have a good prognosis.

A 70-year-old woman presents with an ulcer on her scalp. How would you assess her?

- The likely diagnosis is a squamous cell carcinoma (SCC).
- Take a history—pre-existing lesion (actinic keratosis), sun exposure, previous burns (Marjolin's ulcer), immunosuppression (e.g., organ transplant, lupus).
- Examine the lesion (ulcer with a raised, everted edge and a central scab, may be hyperkeratotic and crusty), perform a full skin survey, examine nodal basins.

How do these lesions spread?

- Locally and by lymphatic invasion (5%–10% metastasise)
- Face and backs of hands exposed to sun
- Men more than women

How would you treat it?

- Request a full thickness punch biopsy for diagnosis[6] (shave would miss a deep cancer in the skin).
- Make a wide local excision with minimum margin of 4 mm—wider for poorly differentiated lesions. Lymph node dissection and radiotherapy are considered for metastatic nodal spread.

SKIN GRAFTS AND FLAPS

What is a skin graft?

- A skin graft is a section of skin including epidermis and dermis that has been completely separated from its blood supply and transplanted to a recipient bed.
- Skin grafts should not be used on exposed bone/tendon/cartilage/implants and radiation-damaged tissue, as these offer a poor vascular bed.
  - Partial or split thickness—epidermis and portion of dermis. It is harvested with dermatome (Humby knife, air-driven or electric—adjust for width and depth of cut).
  - Full thickness includes epidermis and all the dermis. These are less prone to contracture and are often used on the face.

How do skin grafts develop a blood supply?

- Imbibition—the first 24–48 hr nutrients diffuse from wound to extracellular fluid and graft capillaries. Graft begins to fix with fibrin bonds.
- Inosculation—there is alignment of donor capillary buds with graft capillaries and establishment of circulation.
- In revascularisation, connecting vessels differentiate into arterioles and venules.

How do skin graft donor sites heal?

- Split sites heal by epithelialisation from epidermal appendages (hair follicles, sweat glands, sebaceous glands). This can take up to 21 days.
- Full sites heal by primary closure or granulation and contraction.

What are the causes of graft failure?

- Loss of contact with the recipient bed—haematoma, seroma, pus, shearing.
- Meshing the graft helps overcome this.

What is a flap and when would you use it?

- A flap is a section of tissue that comes with its original blood supply. The tissues used are skin, fascia, muscle, bone, nerve and omentum. They can be characterised as follows:
  - Blood supply (random/axial)
  - Method of transfer (advancement, rotation, transposition, free)
  - Tissue composition (musculocutaneous, fasciocutaneous etc)
- I would use a flap to cover exposed bone/vessels/implanted devices, open joints and wounds that are too large for primary closure.

What is the difference in blood supply between random and axial flaps?

- Random—derived from the dermal and subdermal plexus. Most local flaps on the face rely on the dermal and subdermal plexus.
- Axial—derived from cutaneous arteries and veins, oriented longitudinally in the flap.

What is the difference between a transposition and an interpolation flap?

- Transposition is a triangular, square or rectangular flap that moves laterally about a pivot point into an adjacent defect (e.g., a Z-plasty).
  - It leaves a defect which may be closed directly or by a skin graft.
- Interpolation is a flap that moves laterally about a pivot point into a defect that is not immediately adjacent (e.g., nasolabial island flap to nasal tip, deltopectoral flap to head and neck).
  - The pedicle is passed over or under an intervening skin bridge.

What is a Z-plasty?

- It is the transposition of two triangular flaps.
- It is used to increase the area of tissue or length of a scar, break up a straight scar and realign a scar.

- The gain in length depends on local tissue elasticity and tension.
- At completion, the Z has rotated by 90°.

What muscular flaps do you know?

- Pedicled flaps—latissimus dorsi and TRAM flaps are used for breast reconstruction.
- Free flaps—DIEP (deep inferior epigastric perforator), SGAP (superior gluteal artery perforator), TUG (transverse upper gracilis) and ALT (anterolateral thigh) flaps are used in breast and other soft tissue reconstruction.
- The perforator flaps are based on an innominate vessel going through subcutaneous tissue to the skin.

SURGICAL SITE INFECTION

What is a surgical site infection?

- This is a wound infection occurring after an invasive or surgical procedure.
- This accounts for 20% of all healthcare-associated infections.
- Five percent of patients having a surgical procedure develop an SSI.
- Most are caused by contamination of an incision with bacteria from the patient's own body during surgery.
- The majority are preventable.

What are the risk factors for developing an SSI?

- Patient related:
  - Extremes of age
  - Malnutrition and obesity
  - Diabetes
  - Smoking
  - Immunosuppression
  - MRSA colonisation
- Surgery related:
  - Length of scrub and skin antisepsis
  - Shaving
  - Length of surgery, theatre ventilation
  - Inappropriate antibiotic prophylaxis
  - Foreign material in situ, use of surgical drains
  - Poor haemostasis and tissue trauma
  - Postoperative hypothermia

How would you categorise SSIs?

- Superficial:
  - Within 30 days of surgery

- At least one of pain/swelling/erythema/heat
- *S. aureus,* β-haemolytic strep isolated from the wound
- Deep visceral:
  - Purulent drainage (not from abdomen)
  - Fever > 38°C/pain/tenderness
  - Abscess in deep incision
- Organ/space:
  - Within 30 days
  - Purulent discharge from drain
  - Abscess or collection diagnosed
  - Anaerobes, *E. coli* or enterobacteria isolated from pus

What are the preoperative preventative measures?

- Patient—preop shower with soap, theatre clothing, no hair removal prior to surgery, no routine bowel prep or nasal decontamination
- Hair removal—electronic clippers in theatre
- Antibiotic prophylaxis—clean (if using prosthesis/implant), clean/ contaminated, contaminated or dirty surgery, single IV dose at induction
  - NOT for inguinal hernia repair or laparoscopic cholecystectomy
- Staff—theatre clothes, remove hand jewellery and nail polish

What are the intraoperative measures?

- Operating team—first, scrub using aqueous antiseptic surgical solution and nail pick; further scrubs with alcoholic hand rub or antiseptic surgical solution, sterile gowns.
- Patient—prep skin using antiseptic (aqueous or alcohol-based) povidone-iodine or chlorhexidine; allow to dry by evaporation.
- Diathermy should not be used for the surgical incision.
- Patient homeostasis should be maintained during surgery (avoid hypothermia and hypoxia [sats > 95%] during surgery and recovery).
- Cover incisions with an interactive dressing at the end of surgery.

What are the postoperative measures?

- Use an aseptic nontouch technique for changing or removing surgical wound dressings.
- Use sterile saline for wound cleansing in the first 48 hr after surgery and tap water for further cleaning.
- Use an appropriate interactive dressing to manage surgical wounds that are healing by secondary intention and refer to a tissue viability nurse for dressing advice.
- When an SSI is suspected, treat with an antibiotic that covers the likely causative organisms.

Explain clean, contaminated and dirty operations.

- Clean—elective, no infection or transection of GI, GU or biliary tract
- Clean-contaminated—urgent clean case, controlled opening of GI, GU or biliary tract with minimal spillage
- Contaminated—gross soiling of operative field, surgery on open traumatic wounds
- Dirty—abscess, preoperative perforation of GI, GU or biliary tract, penetrating trauma > 4 hr old

What antibiotics would you use to treat an SSI?

- This depends on site of infection, likely organisms and local protocols:
  - Skin—*S. aureus, S. epidermidis*
  - GU tract—*E. coli, Proteus, Klebsiella, Enterobacter*
  - Colon—*E. coli, Klebsiella, Enterobacter, Bacteroides, Clostridia*
  - Biliary tract—*E. coli, Klebsiella, Proteus, Clostridia*
- Gram-positive aerobes (*S. aureus, S. pneumonia, Enterococcus*)
  - Co-Amoxiclav, gentamicin, teicoplanin, vancomycin
- Gram-positive anaerobes (*C. difficle*)
  - Metronidazole, vancomycin
- Gram-negative aerobes (*Bacteroides*)
  - Co-Amoxiclav, metronidazole
- Gram-negative anaerobes (*E. Coli, Klebsiella, Pseudomonas*)
  - Co-Amoxiclav, gentamicin

TESTICULAR CANCER

As the surgeon on call, you admit a 25-year-old man with confusion, shortness of breath and an abdominal mass. Your keen junior mentions that on examination, his right testis is hard. A chest x-ray shows multiple lung metastases. You confirm that there is a suspicious hard testis on examination. What are the key points in the history?

- Symptoms and duration (10% present with metastatic symptoms)
- Risk factors (undescended testis, family history, HIV, history of intratesticular germ cell neoplasia [ITGCN] which could be secondary to cryptorchidism, extragonadal germ cell tumour, previous or contralateral testicular cancer, atrophic contralateral testis, infertility or 45XO karyotype)
- Does the patient have children and has he completed his family?

What investigations would you order?

- After confirming clinical findings and suspicion of testicular cancer, and examining the state of the contralateral testis, investigations other than routine blood tests and CXR would include serum tumour markers and CT scans of head, chest, abdomen and pelvis.

What tumour markers are used to diagnose testicular cancer?

- AFP—expressed by trophoblastic and yolk sac elements
  - Raised in 50%–70% of nonseminomatous germ cell tumours (NSGCT)
  - Not raised in pure seminomas
  - Other causes of positive results: carcinomas of pancreas, biliary tree, gastric and duodenal malignancy.
- HCG—expressed by syncytiotrophoblastic elements
  - Raised in 100% of choriocarcinomas, 40% of teratomas and 30% of seminomas
  - Also raised in other tumours (e.g., breast, kidney, bladder, liver, stomach, biliary tree, hydatidiform mole)
- LDH—marker of tumour burden
  - Also part of the staging of testicular tumours—depends on the degree of elevation

What would your management plan be if the CT showed retroperitoneal metastases and raised tumour markers?

- Most low to intermediate staged tumours can be managed by orchidectomy followed by staging and then chemotherapy.
- However, in stage 4 disease presenting with distant symptomatic metastases, initial treatment is with neoadjuvant chemotherapy followed by surgery.

UNDESCENDED TESTIS

You are called to see a full-term, 1-day-old baby boy with an absent right testis. What do you do?

- Take a history from the mum. Were there any problems during pregnancy? Has the right testis ever been seen or was it absent since birth?
- Examine the baby. Check that the left testicle is present in the scrotum, check the penis (look for hypospadias), examine the right hemiscrotum (hydrocele/hernia), gently palpate from the inguinal region down toward the scrotum, feeling for an undescended testicle or a retractile testicle.

The left testicle is in the scrotum. You feel a testis-like lump in the right groin that can be brought down to the top of the scrotum. What advice will you give the parents?

- This is an undescended testis that can be brought down into the groin.
- If there is no other anomaly, I would review the baby in 6 months.
- If the testis had not reached the base of the scrotum by that time, I would recommend surgery.

Is there a role for ultrasonography in undescended testes?

- No—ultrasound is not required for a palpable undescended testis.
- USS findings do not change the management plan in a nonpalpable case.
- Diagnostic laparoscopy is the gold standard for diagnosis and management of nonpalpable undescended testis.

When would you operate?

- The current consensus for operative repair is at 1 year of age.
- There is a debate about operating earlier to preserve the spermatogenesis.
- Timing of surgery is based on experimental studies that suggest that damage to the undescended testis may begin occurring as early as 6 months of age.

What is a retractile testis?

- The testis is pulled back into the inguinal canal because of a strong cremasteric reflex.
- It can be milked down into the scrotum and will stay there.
- The cremasteric reflex is more pronounced in the first 3 months of life and after puberty.

If this boy's testis was impalpable on examination, where could it lie?

- In the inguinal canal—10%
- Intra-abdominal—40%
  - High, undescended testis
  - Ectopic testis (beyond the normal path of descent)
- Absent—50%
- The possibility of disorder of sexual differentiation should be kept in mind in cases with bilateral nonpalpable, undescended testes and those with ambiguous genitalia.

What is the most important restricting factor in the mobilisation of an intra-abdominal testis and what are the various options?

- The testicular vessels are the most important restricting factor.
- Surgical options (laparoscopic or open):
  - Generous mobilisation and single-stage pull-down of the testis
  - Division of the testicular vessels and pull-down of the testis in a single stage (single-stage Fowler–Stephens)
- Division of the testicular vessels at first surgery, delay of 6 months for collaterals to develop and subsequent pull-down of the testis in a second surgery (two-stage Fowler–Stephens)

What are the long-term chances of malignancy in undescended testes?

- The undescended testes are 5–10 times more likely to develop a malignancy.
- Testicular self-examination should be promoted for early diagnosis.

What is the effect on fertility?

- Unilateral—paternity rates of 80%–90%:
  - 55%–95% of men have normal semen analysis
- Bilateral—paternity rates of 45%–65%
  - 25%–30% of men have normal semen analysis

VASECTOMY

A 35-year-old man attends your outpatient clinic requesting a vasectomy. What specific assessments do you make?

- Assess the patient's contraceptive needs and discuss alternative methods of contraception (i.e., whether he has completed his family, number of children, likelihood of wanting more children, age of partner, previous urological history which may influence surgery [e.g., if he had undescended testis and was brought down in a two-stage procedure, then ligation of vas may compromise blood supply to testis]).
- Perform a clinical examination to assess ease of palpability of vas; this determines a recommendation of LA or GA procedure.
- Undertake a general discussion of the surgical technique, tailored to the individual (LA vs. GA).
- Undertake a frank and honest discussion of the risks and specific complications associated with vasectomy.

How would you consent this patient?

- Inform him of the success of the procedure compared to alternatives.
- It is more effective than withdrawal (19% first year failure), condoms (3%–14% first year failure), reversible female methods (0.1%–3% first year failure), female tubal ligation (1/500 failure).
- Risks/complications:
  - Acute complications:
    - Bleeding, haematoma and infection (5% overall), unilateral absent vas (0.25%)
  - Chronic complications:
    - Early failure (0.43%), related to experience
    - Late failure (rare: <0.001%)
    - Chronic pain (reports vary from 5% to 15%)
- Irreversibility and the need to continue to use an alternative form of contraception until given the all clear

How would you perform a vasectomy?

- There are various techniques (e.g., scalpel vs. no-touch/no scalpel technique).
- There is evidence that fascial interposition and intraluminal diathermy and surgical experience are superior in reducing failure rates.

How would you follow up the patient?

- Ideally, two semen analyses are done at 12 and 16 weeks.
- Patients are more likely to fail to provide the single sample at 16 weeks as compared to at 12 weeks (66% vs. 79% submission rates). Of the patients who submit a sample at 12 weeks, submission rates can be as low as 42%.
- Failure to provide two specimens occurs in 4.5%–40% of patients.

What would you do if his semen analysis at 12 weeks showed the following: a volume of 2 ml, 1,000 nonmotile sperm per high-power field?

- I would ask if the patient has been ejaculating and repeat the analysis after 4–6 weeks, after encouraging the patient to ejaculate more.
- It is likely that the patient is sterilised, but this would be worth confirming on further analyses for 'special clearance'.

What if the semen analysis showed a volume of 3 ml, five motile sperm per high-power field?

- This could be a case of failure or due to a low number of ejaculations to clear the reproductive tract.
- I would warn the patient of failure and the possible need for a repeat vasectomy if a subsequent sample confirms motile sperm (1:17000 men could have a double vas).

REFERENCES

1. Darouiche, Rabih O, Matthew J Wall, Kamal M F Itani, Mary F Otterson, Alexandra L Webb, Matthew M Carrick, Harold J Miller, et al. 2010. Chlorhexidine-alcohol versus povidone-iodine for surgical-site antisepsis. *New England Journal of Medicine* 362 (1): 18–26. doi:10.1056/NEJMoa0810988.
2. Noorani, A, N Rabey, S R Walsh and R J Davies. 2010. Systematic review and meta-analysis of preoperative antisepsis with chlorhexidine versus povidone-iodine in clean-contaminated surgery. *British Journal of Surgery* 97 (11): 1614–1620. doi:10.1002/bjs.7214.
3. DOH website. 2012. Updates: Guidance on the diagnosis and reporting of *Clostridium difficile*. http://www.dh.gov.uk/prod_consum_dh/groups/dh_digitalassets/@dh/@en/documents/digitalasset/dh_133016.pdf.
4. Goddard, Andrew F, Martin W James, Alistair S McIntyre and Brian B Scott. British Society of Gastroenterology. 2011. Guidelines for the management of iron deficiency anaemia. *Gut* doi:10.1136/gut.2010.228874.

5. Telfer, N R, G B Colver and C A Morton, British Association of Dermatologists. 2008. Guidelines for the management of basal cell carcinoma. *British Journal of Dermatology* doi:10.1111/j.1365-2133.2008.08666.x.

6. Multiprofessional guidelines for the management of the patient with primary cutaneous squamous cell carcinoma 2009 (update of original article *British Journal of Dermatology* 2004 146(1): 18–25). http://www.bad.org.uk/portals/_bad/guidelines/clinical%20guide-lines/scc%20guidelines%20final%20aug%2009.pdf.

BIBLIOGRAPHY

ASGBI issues in professional practice: The perioperative management of the adult patient with diabetes. May 2012. http://www.asgbi.org.uk/en/publications/issues_in_professional_practice.cfm.

Clayton, E S J, S Connor, N Alexakis and E Leandros. 2006. Meta-analysis of endoscopy and surgery versus surgery alone for common bile duct stones with the gallbladder in situ. *British Journal of Surgery* 93 (10): 1185–1191.

Department of Health website. Day surgery: Operational guide. http://webarchive.nationalarchives.gov.uk/+/www.dh.gov.uk/en/Publicationsandstatistics/Publications/PublicationsPolicyAndGuidance/DH_4005487?IdcService = GET_FILE&dID = 17206&Rendition = Web.

Marsden, J R, J A Newton-Bishop, L Burrows, M Cook, P G Corrie, N H Cox, M E Gore, et al. 2010. Revised UK guidelines for the management of cutaneous melanoma 2010. *Journal of Plastic, Reconstructive & Aesthetic Surgery* 63 (9): 1401–1419. doi:10.1016/j.bjps.2010.07.006.

Martin, D J, D R Vernon and J Toouli. 2006. Surgical versus endoscopic treatment of bile duct stones. *Cochrane Database Systems Review* 2:CD003327.

Tranter, S E and M H Thompson. 2002. Comparison of endoscopic sphincterotomy and laparoscopic exploration of the common bile duct. *British Journal of Surgery* 89 (12): 1495–1504.

5 Breast Surgery

Elizabeth Ball, Amy E E Burger and Sue K Down

CONTENTS

ADVANCED BREAST CANCER

A 48-year-old premenopausal woman who underwent WLE and axillary sampling 8 years previously presents with a new lump deep to the scar and palpable axillary nodes. Describe your initial management.

- Take a history—duration of new symptoms, associated symptoms (e.g., weight loss, bone pain, jaundice), details about previous breast cancer treatment and pathology.
- Complete a triple assessment.
- Perform an examination—including supraclavicular fossae, liver
- Request imaging—mammograms, US of breast and axilla with core biopsy of lump and FNA of nodes.
- Request details of previous breast cancer treatment, previous imaging and pathology slides for review in MDT.

Core biopsies confirm recurrent invasive lobular cancer, grade 2, ER Aldred score 8/8, HER2 positive on FISH. Imaging shows a 25 mm mass, with several suspicious axillary lymph nodes. She previously underwent radiotherapy and took tamoxifen for 5 years. What further investigations would you recommend?

- Blood tests—FBC, U&Es, Ca, LFTs, CEA, CA15-3
- Staging CT (chest, abdomen, pelvis)

- Isotope bone scan—to look for metastatic deposits in long bones and skull
- If recurrence not visible on mammography, MRI may be of value in assessing the contralateral breast

Staging CT shows metastatic nodules in both lungs and involved internal mammary nodes. What systemic treatments would you suggest?

- I would suggest ovarian suppression (surgical oophorectomy or LH-RH agonist, e.g., Goserelin)
- Chemotherapy consists initially of anthracyclines (risk of cardiomyopathy; cannot be repeated). If disease progression on anthracyclines, offer first line docetaxel, second line vinorelbine or capecitabine.
- Trastuzumab is given in combination with a taxane. Because of the associated cardiac toxicity, avoid use with anthracyclines; monitor cardiac function (MUGA/echo). Continue as single agent whilst disease is responsive. If brain metastasis develops, continue Trastuzumab and treat mets with surgery/radiotherapy.
- If relapse occurs with trastuzumab, I would consider lapatinib in combination with capecitabine.
- For endocrine adjuvant therapy, I would consider tamoxifen as >1 year since therapy ceased.
- Otherwise, I would use an aromatase inhibitor in combination with LH-RH agonist.

Is there a role for primary surgery?

- It is used for local control (e.g., fungating tumours).
- Discuss the role of axillary clearance at MDT; give only further prognostic information because patient is already being offered chemotherapy; this would prevent axillary recurrence in the future.
- There is a possible survival advantage in removing primary disease.
- Postoperative complications can delay systemic treatment, resulting in a worse prognosis.

Five months later, she develops severe lower back pain. A repeat isotope bone scan confirms an isolated vertebral body metastasis. What treatment can you offer?

- Bisphosphonates (*you should know the oral and intravenous preparations*)
  - Inhibit osteoclast activity
  - Decrease bone resorption
  - Reduce the risk of further skeletal morbidity (metastases, fractures, etc.)
  - Reduce bone pain
  - Side effects—renal impairment and osteonecrosis of the jaw, possible increased risk of oesophageal cancer with oral bisphosphonates—should

be taken with water on an empty stomach, then patient needs to remain upright for 60 min with no further oral intake
- Pain control with simple NSAID analgesia (e.g., diclofenac) or external beam radiotherapy (single fraction, 8 Gy)
- Systemic therapy regime changed due to disease progression (i.e., switch from tamoxifen to AI, from AI to exemestane)

AXILLARY MANAGEMENT IN BREAST SURGERY

How do you manage the axilla in a woman with invasive breast cancer?

- Axillary status remains of vital importance for providing prognostic information and guiding adjuvant treatment.
- I would complete a preoperative triple assessment if identified through screening—clinical examination, mammograms and ultrasound of the axilla.
- Prominent/suspicious nodes should have FNA or core biopsy (FNA in most centres).
  - Features of suspicious nodes include round rather than elliptical shape, thickened/irregular/eccentric cortex.
- Positive FNA/core for lymph node metastasis/high level of suspicion on USS/patient request calls for primary axillary clearance.
- Clinically/radiologically node negative calls for sentinel lymph node biopsy.
- Overall 10-year survival is 75% for node-negative patients versus 25%–30% for multiple node-positive patients.

What is the evidence that supports the use of sentinel node biopsy?

- ALMANAC trial[1]
  - Level 1 evidence for use of sentinel node biopsy
  - Compared SLNB with standard axillary clearance
  - Improved quality of life outcomes and arm morbidity for SLNB group

How would you perform sentinel node biopsy?

- I would use a dual technique (blue dye and radio-labelled technetium), as described in the ALMANAC trial.
- The consensus at ABS is that a single-agent isotope technique, which provides a good axillary signal, is also acceptable.
- Single-agent blue dye is not acceptable and should be used as part of a four-node axillary sample.

Are you aware of any intraoperative methods of assessment of the SLN and how will this affect the patient management?

- Broadly, there are three methods of intraoperative analysis—frozen section, touch imprint cytology (TIC) and OSNA.

- Frozen section—half of bisected node snap frozen and assessed by pathologist
  - Pros—sensitive and specific, tissue retained for future reference
  - Cons—requires dedicated pathologist for immediate assessment, does not assess the whole node
- TIC—bisected node imprinted on slides and assessed
  - Pros—high specificity, lower sensitivity, entire node available for further assessment, cheap
  - Cons—cytologist availability, low sensitivity
- OSNA—node homogenised and PCR performed for epithelial cytokeratins (cytokeratin 19); can quantify between macro- and micromets and ITCs
  - Pros—very sensitive and specific, almost eliminates false negatives and therefore need for second operation
  - Cons—expensive equipment, no tissue remaining for future assessment; some false positives due to contamination, therefore unnecessary axillary clearance
- These assessments let me perform a completion axillary clearance at the time of initial operation, avoiding return for second operation after the SLN histology is assessed. However, there is an increase in patient anxiety and uncertainty prior to surgery.

What is your opinion on the management of the axilla on discovery of a positive SLN?

- There are three degrees of positivity—macromet (>2 mm), micromet (<2 mm) and isolated tumour cells.

State whether you would clear an axilla for macromets, micromets or ITC. Some units now do not perform ANC for a micromet.

- Current guidelines state that a completion clearance should be performed for macromets (>2 mm) and micromets (0.2 mm), but not for isolated tumour cells
- This, however, may be dependent on the tumour factors, patient preferences and the number of SLNs retrieved. If four SLNs are retrieved with a micromet in only one, the MDT decision may be that completion ANC is unnecessary, in contrast to a micrometastasis in a single retrieved SLN.
- In patients with a positive SLN, in 47%–68% of cases this will be the only positive SLN. Therefore, the majority of patients with preoperatively, clinically and radiologically node-negative axillae and a positive SLN are being overtreated by axillary clearance and have the long-term potential morbidity of lymphoedema.
- NSABP B-04 trial[2]—4008 SLN procedures were randomised to four groups.
  - Positive SLN ± ANC, and negative SLN ± ANC
  - After FU of 31 months, axillary recurrence rate low (0.25%)

- Axillary relapse more common in the +ve SLN, no ANC group; overall axillary relapse rate very low

What study has aimed to examine whether completion ANC is required? Do you have any criticisms of it?

- The ACOSOG Z0011 study[3] randomised patients with a positive SLN to either completion clearance or no further treatment. It aimed to recruit 1,900 patients, but recruited 891.
  - The primary end point was overall survival.
  - It involved T1/2 tumours, only patients undergoing WLE and radiotherapy and only patients with less than three positive SLNs.
  - Of the ANC group, 27% had additional positive nodes (therefore, a similar number should be present in the no-further-treatment group).
  - End points—at 6 years, no difference in overall survival; SLN was the only group that had slightly fewer local recurrences than the ANC group.
  - Concerns:
    - Early stage tumours
    - Older average age
    - High ER positivity
    - All WLE; therefore, having tangential field radiotherapy may include some lower axillary nodes
    - High rates of chemotherapy use
    - Micromets only—37.5%
    - Short length of follow-up—just after completion of adjuvant hormones

Are you aware of any studies that are further investigating management of the axilla?

- POSNOC trial (positive sentinel node: observation versus clearance)
  - Primary objective—to assess whether axillary recurrence rate in patients not having completion axillary clearance is inferior to those who do undergo clearance
  - Secondary objectives—assessment of arm morbidity, quality of life, locoregional and distant recurrence, overall survival
    - Involved T1/T2 tumours, with less than three macromets, clinically and radiologically negative axilla
    - Exclusion criteria—extranodal extension in a positive SLN, neoadjuvant chemo
- AMAROS trial (after mapping of the axilla: radiotherapy or surgery?)
  - Compares completion axillary clearance and axillary radiotherapy after positive sentinel node
  - No difference in the choice of adjuvant chemotherapy/hormonal manipulation

- Aims to show noninferiority of radiotherapy compared with surgery in terms of axillary recurrence (and other secondary outcome measures such as distant mets, overall survival)

BRCA/FAMILY HISTORY OF BREAST CANCER

How do we assess breast cancer risk associated with family history?

- An initial assessment is made in primary care according to NICE guidelines, followed by referral to secondary or tertiary unit.
- Overall, 4%–5% of breast cancers are currently thought to have a genetic cause.
- In women under 30 years old, this rises to approximately 25%.
- Obtain full and accurate history of affected relatives, gender, age, bilaterality (ask patients to fill out a family history proforma).
- Refer to geneticist to confirm details and degree of risk.
- Discuss the patient in family history MDT.
- Computer prediction models include BOADICEA, Tyrer—Cuzick.
- Calculate the likelihood of a genetic defect or risk above the average.

Broadly, how would you classify the groups of risk levels?

- Population risk:
  - <17% lifetime risk; 10-year risk: <3% aged 40–49
    - Managed in primary care
- Moderate risk:
  - Lifetime risk of 17%–30%, 10 year risk: 3%–8% aged 40–49
    - Managed in secondary care
- High risk:
  - Lifetime risk: >30%, 10 year risk: >8% aged 40–49
  - More than 20% chance of a faulty BRCA1, 2 or TP53 gene
    - Managed in tertiary care

What are the cancer risks associated with BRCA1 and 2?

- BRCA1: breast cancer lifetime risk: 60%–80%
  - Ovarian cancer: 40%–50%
  - Male breast cancer: 1%–2%
  - Prostate cancer (men): ~ two times background risk
  - Pancreatic cancer: two to three times the background risk
- BRCA2: Breast cancer: 40-85%
  - Ovarian cancer: 10-25%
  - Male breast cancer: 6%
  - Prostate cancer: ~33% by age 65
  - Pancreatic cancer: three to four times the background risk
- Also, increased risk of melanoma, colon and haematological malignancies

What are the pathological characteristics of BRCA breast cancers?

- BRCA1:
  - High grade, less ER/PR positivity, increased expression of basal cyto-keratins—CK5/6, CK14, CK17—less in situ disease, 'pushing' margins on ultrasound, less likely to be sensitively detected on mammograms
- BRCA2:
  - More similar to nonfamilial tumours, lower grade, more ER/PR positivity, more in situ disease, mammograms more sensitive

What are the NICE guidelines for screening patients with gene defects and family history?

- BRCA1/2—annual MRI (30–49 yrs), annual mammography (30–69 yrs)
- TP53—annual MRI (20–69 yrs), no mammography (RT-induced cancer risk)
- High risk family history (>30% lifetime risk):
  - <30% BRCA gene
    - annual mammography (40–59 yrs)
  - >30% BRCA gene
    - annual mammography (40–59 yrs)
    - annual MRI (40–69 yrs)
    - offer MRI 30–49 yrs – BRCA positive/>30% BRCA gene
  - Uncertainty about value of mammographic screening in younger women
- Moderate risk family history (8–17% lifetime risk):
  - Annual mammography (40–49 yrs)
  - Enter NHS Breast Screening Programme if over 50 years

What are the benefits of screening these women?

- Identifying cancer at an earlier stage, not reducing risk
- Reducing morbidity associated with breast cancer treatment
- No mortality benefit

How else can these patients be managed?

- Chemoprevention:
  - Offer Tamoxifen/Raloxifene (depending on presence/absence of uterus) for 5 years to high risk, and consider offering to moderate risk women.
    - Risk of endometrial cancer, DVT, PE
    - Will only prevent ER +ve cancers
- Risk reduction surgery for breast cancer:
  - Discuss at risk reduction MDT (geneticist, psychologist, breast care nurse, surgeon). It takes 6–12 months to complete the process.
    - Risk reduction for breast cancer is ~95% (i.e. not elimination of risk).[4]
- Risk reduction for ovarian cancer:
  - There is a proven mortality benefit in BRCA1 mutation carriers.[5]

- Do not begin before the age of 35.
- Oophorectomy reduces ovarian and breast cancer risk independently of any surgery to the breast.
- Give lifestyle advice to reduce breast cancer risk.
  - Advise stopping OCP/HRT/smoking, reducing alcohol intake and losing weight to achieve healthy BMI.

How would you approach a patient with a known breast cancer who is a BRCA1 carrier?

- Index cancer is the primary concern.
- Mortality is linked to the index cancer rather than possible future risk to the contralateral breast.
- Surgical and oncological treatment of the index cancer.
- Risk-reducing surgery may be offered contemporaneously; however, bear in mind the risk of delay to adjuvant treatment if complications arise.
- The patient must be aware that contralateral surgery will not prevent her dying from breast cancer.
- If the patient is premenopausal, counsel and advise regarding completion of family and possible oophorectomy.

Do you know of another group of patients at increased risk of breast cancer?

- Li Fraumeni syndrome
- TP53 mutation
  - MRI screening approved from age 20 (NICE guidelines, CA 164)

How does the outcome of family history analysis affect the patient?

- If family history suggests a genetic defect, there is a need to discuss genetic testing and implications.
  - Ask how the patient would deal with a result confirming mutation.
  - Ask about the effect on job, family, children.
  - The patient should consider financial implications—insurance, mortgage.
- The patient should meet with a trained genetic counsellor for pretest counselling—ideally, two sessions.
- If a genetic defect is not suggested but the patient is at increased risk (moderate risk), early screening (mammography or MRI depending on level of risk) can be offered.

What are the problems with screening these patients?

- Screening does not prevent breast cancer.
- Anxiety occurs, especially after recall for indeterminate lesions.

Do you know of any family history studies?

- FH01 study[6]:
  - Mammographic screening for young women (40–49) with intermediate risk family history (not known gene carriers).
  - Yearly mammograms resulted in predicted lower mortality compared with external comparison groups.
- MRISC trial[7]:
  - MRI is more sensitive than mammograms for detecting invasive cancer.
  - However, screening is limited in mutation carriers and no evidence yet has indicated that screening improves survival.

BREAST CANCER IN PREGNANCY

How would you assess a breast lump in a pregnant woman?

- The differential diagnosis should be cancer until proven otherwise.
- A full history should be taken and both breasts examined, axillae and SCF examined.
- Mammogram can be performed, if required, with foetal shielding.
- All solid masses should be assessed with core biopsy rather than FNA.

What are the factors to consider with a woman with confirmed breast cancer in the various trimesters of pregnancy?

- First trimester:
  - Ensure correct dates.
  - Choriovillous sampling may be performed at 10–12 weeks and amniocentesis at 15 weeks.
  - This is the most risky period for the foetus. There are increased miscarriage rates even without treatment.
  - Bearing in mind the mother's outcomes, the option of termination of the pregnancy must be discussed.
  - The foetus is most vulnerable to the effects of radiation: Avoid bone scans; CXR with foetal shielding is acceptable.
  - Chemotherapy is associated with a 20%–30% risk of miscarriage in this trimester and a 10%–25% risk of malformations.
    - It is essentially contraindicated.
- Second trimester:
  - Termination is still an option, but the foetus is now less vulnerable.
  - Foetal parts USS can be conducted at 16 weeks.
  - Surgery may be performed more safely in this trimester.
  - Chemotherapy is associated with intrauterine growth retardation and decreased birth weight, but is overall considered safe if oncologically required.
- Third trimester:
  - Decisions are less difficult.
  - Surgery is safer.

- Chemotherapy may be administered as appropriate.
- Treatment may, in some cases, be delayed until after birth.
- Consider expediting delivery to around 34 weeks, with betamethasone given for lung maturation.

What are the issues surrounding surgery in the pregnant woman?

- The anaesthetic risk to the foetus reduces throughout the duration of pregnancy, but may induce early labour in the third trimester.
- This requires close collaboration with the obstetrician throughout management:
- Breast conserving surgery versus mastectomy:
  - This is the same decision-making process as for any other breast cancer.
  - It is necessary to factor in the delay in giving radiotherapy until after delivery (therefore less effective treatment).
- Sentinel node biopsy
  - Blue dye not recommended
  - Tc99 foetal dose very small (<4 mGy) but full effect unknown
- Consider four-node sample

What are the outcomes with pregnancy-associated breast cancer?

- Patient:
  - The 5- to 10-year survival and recurrence rates are the same as age-matched controls, if full treatment is completed.
  - There is increased frequency of BRCA-related tumours due to the skewed age distribution.
  - Histology is the same as for age-matched controls, and HER-2 status is the same.
  - There is some evidence of increased lymph node involvement, possibly due to later presentation.
  - There is an increased presentation at a later stage.
  - There is no adverse effect on any future pregnancies after breast cancer, but if patient is >40 years old, she may often be amenorrhoeic after chemotherapy.
- Foetus:
  - First trimester termination rates increase.
  - Congenital abnormalities and reduced birth weight are associated with chemotherapy use.
  - There is a possible risk of future malignancy with use of alklyating agents.
  - There are few long-term data on the late effects of chemotherapy on the foetus (i.e., reduced fertility themselves in adult life).
- Options for future pregnancy:
  - Ovarian function can be preserved with Zoladex, which puts ovaries 'to sleep' before chemotherapy and can protect ovarian function, especially if the patient is <40 years old.

- Uncertainties about the effect on tumour response to chemotherapy should be discussed on an individualised basis.
- Embryo cryopreservation may be considered—egg harvest, IVF and cryopreservation.
  - These strategies may delay the start of chemo.
  - There are funding issues.

What are the issues surrounding systemic treatment and radiotherapy in pregnancy-associated breast cancer?

- Timing of chemotherapy due to foetal toxicity means that neoadjuvant chemotherapy may be used less than in age- and tumour-matched controls.
- Chemotherapy drugs that transfer to the foetus are of low molecular weight, lipid soluble and have low plasma protein binding.
  - 5-FU—teratogenic
  - Methotrexate—maternal and foetal toxicity due to third space distribution
  - Doxorubicin—maternal and foetal cardiotoxicity
  - Cyclophosphamide—decreased maternal efficacy, gonadal toxicity
  - Herceptin—anecdotal reports only; can use in metastatic setting; if to be used in adjuvant setting, delay until after birth
  - Avastin—avoid
  - Taxanes—unknown risk of malformation and miscarriage; avoid unless high risk/metastatic disease
  - Tamoxifen—avoid
- After birth, chemotherapeutic drugs may be used as standard. However, due to the transfer of drugs into breast milk, the infant cannot be breastfed.
- Radiotherapy should be avoided in pregnancy unless it is life saving. If it is essential, foetal shielding may be used.

BREAST CANCER SCREENING

On what principles are screening programmes based?

- The condition being screened for should be an important health problem.
- The natural history of the condition should be well understood.
- There should be a detectable early stage.
- Treatment at an early stage should be of more benefit than at a later stage.
- A suitable test should be devised for the early stage.
- The test should be acceptable.
- Intervals for repeating the test should be determined.
- Adequate health service provision should be made for the extra clinical workload resulting from screening.
- The risks, both physical and psychological, should be less than the benefits.
- The costs should be balanced against the benefits.
- Wilson–Jungner criteria (WHO) should be followed.[8]

TABLE 5.1
Summary of Breast Screening Trials

RCT	Year started	Age group	Approx. no. of subjects (total)	Mortality reduction (%)	Ref.
HIP, New York	1963	40 to 64	62,000	25	9
Two-county, Sweden	1977	40 to 74	133,000	30	10
Malmo, Sweden	1976	45 to 69	42,000	4	11
Edinburgh, Scotland	1979	45 to 64	45,000	17	12
Stockholm, Sweden	1981	40 to 64	60,000	29	13
NBSS 1, Canada	1980	40 to 49	50,000	−36	14
NBSS 2, Canada	1980	50 to 59	39,000	3	15
Gothenburg 1993	1982	40 to 59	50,000	14	16
UK age trial 2006	1991	39 to 48	161,000	17	17

What is the evidence for breast screening?
See Table 5.1.

Describe the history of the NHSBSP.

- It was introduced in 1988 following the Forrest report.[18]
- An interval of 3 years was chosen to emulate the Swedish two-county trial and confirmed by UKCCCR trial.[19]
- Two-view digital mammography is currently being extended to the 47–73 age range.
- Can also provide annual MRI surveillance for women at high risk of developing familial breast cancer (NICE guideline 41).
- It costs £96 million per year.

What types of bias may influence the apparent improvements in breast cancer survival?

- Lead-time bias:
  - Screening advances the date of diagnosis but does not affect the date of death, thereby falsely increasing the survival period.
- Length bias:
  - More slow growing tumours or noninvasive diseases, which have an intrinsically better prognosis, are detected.
- Selection bias:
  - Only health-conscious individuals will attend a screening programme and they are likely to have a better prognosis anyway.

What quality assurance processes are in place in the NHSBSP?

- Regional Quality Assurance Reference Centres (QARCs) monitor standards in all disciplines (radiology, surgery, pathology, etc.).

- Screening units have regular QA visits to ensure they meet minimum standards and to identify outlying units.

What surgical quality assurance guidelines exist for breast screening?

- NHSBSP 20 QA guidelines for surgeons in breast cancer screening, March 2009[20]
- ABS surgical guidelines for the management of breast cancer, 2009[21]

Describe current controversies in breast cancer screening.

- Gotzsche and Nielson reviewed seven randomised trials in 2011[22]:
  - Reduction in breast cancer mortality by 15%, but 30% overdiagnosis and overtreatment
- Review of NHSBSP and Swedish two-county study suggests 2–2.5 lives saved per case overdiagnosed.[23]
- Possibility of radiation-induced breast cancer from mammography was estimated at 1 per 35 lives saved.[24]
- An independent review of breast screening in October 2012, chaired by Professor Sir Michael Marmot, concluded that for every 10,000 women invited to screening for 20 years, 43 deaths from breast cancer will be prevented and 129 cases will be overdiagnosed. The review panel concluded that breast screening should continue but women should receive more information to allow them to make an informed decision.[25]

DCIS

A 48-year-old patient is recalled from her first-round screening with a mammogram showing 4 cm of suspicious pleomorphic calcification. Biopsy shows high-grade DCIS. How would you manage this patient?

- Explain the diagnosis—what DCIS is, its implications if left untreated, and the management options.
- Take a history—including general fitness, family history and other risk factors, any previous breast operations.
- Examine both breasts, axillae and SCF. Assess breast size and ptosis, proximity of calcification to nipple.
- Review imaging including USS at MDT and review extent of microcalcifications.
- Enter data into the Sloane project (completing its collection of DCIS data and in phase 2 will be gathering information on lobular in situ neoplasia and ADH).

Would you offer breast-conserving surgery?

- This is a possible option in a large breast with peripherally placed calcifications.

- There is risk of inadequate clearance/poor cosmetic outcome in a small breast, or with centrally placed calcification, although a central WLE may be possible.
- Discuss the risks with the patient:
  - Risk of positive margins—need for further surgery, may lead to mastectomy
  - Defect in breast shape if >20% volume removed
  - Long-term recurrence risk with BCS versus mastectomy (recurrences after DCIS tend to be invasive cancer)
  - Risk of not treating the DCIS—progression to invasive cancer with metastatic spread
- Therapeutic mammoplasty (TM) is an option in large breasts—need to ensure adequate clearance the first time, excision of margins is difficult to do after TM.

What should the local recurrence rate be after BCS for DCIS?

- <10% at 5 years (according to ABS guidelines)
- However, higher than expected recurrence rates after BCS for DCIS
- Trial of observation versus surgery for low-grade DCIS due to commence 2013/2014

Would you perform sentinel lymph node biopsy in a patient with DCIS?

- Generally, it is not performed if breast conserving surgery is performed.
- If occult microinvasive or invasive focus is detected after surgery, then SLNB would be offered.
- Always perform SLNB in these circumstances:
  - Mastectomy for DCIS—cannot do SLNB afterward if occult invasive disease on histology
  - Mass-forming DCIS (suspicious of occult invasion)
  - Documented microinvasion in core biopsy
  - More than 4 cm calcification and undergoing breast conserving surgery
    - There is a 20%–40% chance of occult invasion; mammograms often underestimate the final size.

Is there evidence for use of adjuvant radiotherapy in DCIS?

- Trials have shown a 50% reduction in local recurrence rates with radiotherapy after BCS for DCIS.
- There is no effect on overall survival (however, the trials were not powered to show a survival difference).
- NSABP–B17[26]:
  - This included 818 women; 80% were detected by mammogram.
  - There was a 12-year follow-up.
  - Overall recurrence was reduced from 31.7% to 15.7% with radiotherapy.

- Invasive recurrence was reduced from 16.8% to 7.7%.
- DCIS recurrence was reduced from 14.6% to 8.0%.
- Comedo necrosis was the only significant risk factor for recurrence.
- EORTC–10853[27]:
  - This included 1,010 women; 71% were detected by mammogram.
  - There was a 10.5-year follow-up.
  - Overall recurrence was reduced from 26% to 15%.
  - Invasive recurrence was reduced from 13% to 8%.
  - DCIS recurrence was reduced from 14% to 7%.
  - Risk factors for recurrence included:
    - Age < 40, mass-forming disease, intermediate-/high-grade DCIS, cribriform/solid growth pattern, indeterminate margins
- NICE[28] and ABS[29] guidelines for radiotherapy in DCIS suggest that it should be offered to patients following adequate breast-conserving surgery after discussion of risks and benefits.
- Patients who have had mastectomy for DCIS do not require radiotherapy.

Is there any evidence for use of hormonal manipulation in DCIS?

- Currently, NICE does not recommend the use of tamoxifen in patients with DCIS.
- There is conflicting evidence to support its use, especially if surgery is adequate (i.e., margins well clear). The result of the IBIS 2 DCIS trial is awaited.
- NSABP–B24[30]:
  - There were 1,804 women.
  - BCS + RT versus BCS + RT + tamoxifen for 5 years was studied (positive or unknown margins in 23% patients).
  - At 5 years, breast cancer events reduced from 13.4% to 8.2% in the tamoxifen group.
  - Invasive recurrence was reduced by 50% in the tamoxifen group.
  - Contralateral cancers were reduced by 50%.

ENDOCRINE MANIPULATION

You see a woman in the postop results clinic. She is 60 years old and has had surgery for a T2N0M0 tumour with WLE and SLNB. It was ER/PR positive and HER2 negative. She is going to have radiotherapy. What other adjuvant treatment would you recommend?

- Any decision should be based on a discussion of the benefits and side effects of treatment. All patients with ER + tumours can potentially benefit from hormonal manipulation.
- Options for this patient, assuming that at 60 years old she is postmenopausal, would be adjuvant oestrogen suppression either with tamoxifen or an aromatase inhibitor.

- As her tumour is T2, she should ideally be offered an AI (anastrozole or letrozole) according to the NICE guidelines for early breast cancer.[31]

Would any benefit be derived if she were ER–ve (Allred score 1)?

- The Early Breast Cancer Triallists Collaborative Group Oxford Overview[32] concluded that ER–ve women do not benefit from hormonal manipulation (but, of course, are still at risk from the side effects).

Which aromatase inhibitor would you give in this immediate postop situation and why?
You need to say which drug you would prescribe as a consultant, not what is currently offered in your unit. According to NICE guidelines, either anastrozole or letrozole may be offered in the immediate adjuvant setting.

- ATAC trial (arimidex, tamoxifen, alone or combination)[33]:
  - The trial included 9,366 postmenopausal women with early breast cancer postoperatively randomised per the study name. The combination arm was discontinued, as the results were equivocal to the tamoxifen-only arm.
  - After 5 years, arimidex significantly improved disease-free survival (HR 0.87, p = 0.01), time to recurrence (0.79, p = 0.0005), distant metastases and contralateral breast cancers.
  - Benefits in terms of recurrence and distant mets were also detectable at 10 years.
  - There was no difference in overall survival.
- BIG 1-98 (letrozole vs. tamoxifen, monotherapy or sequential)[34]:
  - This included 8,010 postmenopausal women with ER+ve disease, postoperatively randomised to letrozole, tamoxifen or a switch (Let-Tam/Tam-Let).
  - A 2.9% DFS benefit for the letrozole monotherapy group was found at 5 years over tamoxifen.
  - There was no advantage to a switch over to letrozole alone and no difference in overall survival.

How long would you give this?

- The standard treatment duration is 5 years; however, a number of studies have shown improved outcomes with extended treatment in some high-risk patient groups.
- When using tamoxifen, endometrial cancer risk continues to increase; hence, use is often limited to 5 years.
- Currently, NICE recommends that patients with lymph node positive, ER+ve early breast cancer who have been previously treated with tamoxifen can be offered extended treatment with letrozole for a further 2–3 years.

Are you aware of any trials that looked at extended endocrine therapy?

- ATLAS trial[35] looked at longer term tamoxifen; there was small further reduction in recurrence rate and, as yet, no difference in overall survival.
- NSABP B-14[35] showed no advantage with 10 versus 5 years of tamoxifen for node-negative patients. The possibility was raised that prolonged treatment may in fact be detrimental.
- MA-17 trial[36] extended adjuvant letrozole given to women with ER+ve tumours after discontinuation of tamoxifen. It improved disease-free survival (HR 0.58, $p < 0.001$), improved distant DFS (HR 0.60, $p = 0.002$) and also overall survival (HR 0.61, $p = 0.04$). In addition, patients who switched to letrozole after unblinding also showed benefit in terms of DFS and OS.
  - Criticism was that patients were unblinded at 2.4 years, and most switched from placebo to the active agent.
- NSABP B-42[37] involved 5 years of letrozole versus placebo in patients who had completed 5 years of hormonal therapy with either Tamoxifen or an AI. This trial is ongoing and there has been no early unblinding.

What do you know about endocrine therapy 'switching'?

- The NICE guidelines give advice about postmenopausal women who have been treated with tamoxifen up front.
- Women who have been treated with tamoxifen for 2–3 years and are not 'low risk' may be offered a switch to either exemestane or anastrozole.
- The IES trial[38] involved 2–3 years tamoxifen and then a switch to exemestane. There was a DFS benefit in the switch group (HR 0.68, $p < 0.001$) and an absolute DFS benefit of 4.7%. No significant difference in overall survival was found.

What other factors should be considered when starting a patient on endocrine manipulation?

- Patients commencing on an AI should have a baseline DEXA scan.
- Advise patients about the side effect profile of these agents:
  - Tamoxifen: menopausal symptoms
    - Endometrial hyperplasia/risk of cancer
    - Risk of deep venous thromboembolism
    - Reduced cognition, reduced libido
    - Benefit: increased bone density due to agonist action
  - AIs: menopausal symptoms
    - Bone density loss
    - Joint symptoms
    - Rarely, liver and renal dysfunction, adrenal insufficiency

Can you tell me anything about neoadjuvant hormonal manipulation and any evidence emerging about this?

- POETIC—perioperative endocrine therapy individualising care:
  - AI for 2 weeks before and standard duration after surgery is hypothesised to improve outcomes.
  - Measurement of Ki-67 proliferative marker in the excised cancer after 2 weeks of endocrine treatment may predict DFS better than pretreatment measurements.
  - Inclusion criteria are early breast cancer, postmenopausal, ER+, palpable and/or >1.5 cm.
- NEO-EXCEL—16-week preoperative treatment with an AI (exemestane or letrozole) ± COX-2 inhibitor:
  - Inclusion criteria are early breast cancer, postmenopausal, ER+ve and >2 cm on clinical examination.

HERCEPTIN/TRASTUZUMAB

What is HER2?

- Human epidermal growth factor receptor 2 (also known as HER2, ErbB2, HER2-neu and CD340) is a tyrosine kinase protein present on all epidermal cells.
- Dimerisation of the HER2 protein results in activation of cell signalling pathways, which stimulate cell proliferation.
- HER2 is overexpressed in approximately 30% of breast cancers and is associated with more aggressive disease and a poorer prognosis.
- HER2 overexpression is associated with tamoxifen resistance in ER-positive tumours.[39]
- HER2 expression confers sensitivity to anthracycline-based chemotherapy agents, although this combination is associated with increased cardiac toxicity.[40]

How is HER2 measured?

- Immunohistochemistry—antibodies directed against the HER2 protein are visualised with chromogenic detection. This is a widely available method. Score is 0, 1+, 2+ or 3+. There is a 10% false negative rate. Equivocal results (2+) are retested by FISH.
- FISH is fluorescence in situ hybridisation and is a quantitative measurement of gene amplification. It requires specialist equipment and is relatively expensive.
- CISH (chromogenic in situ hybridisation) and SISH (silver in situ hybridisation) are quantitative measurements using immunohistochemical techniques to visualise HER2 expression directly; CISH is lower cost than FISH, with similar sensitivity and specificity to the FISH technique.[41]

Describe the mechanism of action and current indications for the use of trastuzumab.

- Trastuzumab (Herceptin) is a recombinant humanised IgG1 monoclonal antibody directed against the extracellular domain of HER2 which prevents the activation of cell signalling pathways and therefore inhibits cell proliferation.
- The most significant side effect is cardiac toxicity; patients require pretreatment echo with LVEF > 55%. Echo should be repeated every 3 months during treatment and trastuzumab suspended if LVEF drops by 10% or to below 50%. Treatment can be reinstigated on recovery of cardiac function.
- It is unable to cross the blood–brain barrier.
- Early-stage HER2-positive breast cancer—used following surgery, chemotherapy and radiotherapy at 3-week intervals for 1 year.[42]
- Advanced HER2-positive breast cancer—used in combination with paclitaxel in patients who have not had chemotherapy and for whom anthracycline treatment is inappropriate. It is used as a single agent therapy in patients who have already undergone treatment with antracycline/taxane and hormones.[42]

Are you aware of any trials involving trastuzumab in early breast cancer?

- HERA (Herceptin adjuvant trial):
  - Trastuzumab was taken for 1–2 years following early HER2 positive breast cancer and adjuvant chemotherapy.
  - There was a 46% reduction in disease recurrence.[43]
  - An 8-year follow-up has shown no advantage of 2 years over 1 year.
- NSABP-B-31:
  - This was a phase III randomised study of doxorubicin and cyclophosphamide followed by paclitaxel with or without trastuzumab in women with node-positive breast cancer that overexpresses HER2.
- NCCTG-N9831:
  - This was a phase III randomised study of doxorubicin plus cyclophosphamide followed by paclitaxel with or without trastuzumab in women with HER-2 overexpressing node-positive or high-risk node-negative breast cancer.
- In a combined analysis of US trials, there was a 52% reduction in disease recurrence and 33% decrease in morbidity.[44]
- Current trials:
  - EPHOSB:
    - Neoadjuvant short course of trastuzumab/lapatinib
  - SOLD:
    - Additional 12 months of trastuzumab following standard adjuvant treatment with FEC and taxane/trastuzumab
  - PERSEPHONE:
    - Six months versus 12 months of trastuzumab

- APHINITY:
  - Comparing trastuzumab and pertuzumab versus trastuzumab alone as adjuvant therapy

Describe the mechanism of action and current indications for the use of lapatinib.

- Lapatinib (Tyverb) is a protein kinase inhibitor that targets the intracellular components of HER2, preventing activation of the tyrosine kinase and inhibiting cell division.
- It is licensed for use in advanced breast cancer and administered orally with capecitabine or an aromatase inhibitor.
- Side effects include gastrointestinal effects.
- It can cross the blood–brain barrier.
- Lapatinib is not recommended for routine use by NICE, except within a clinical trial.
- Lapatinib in combination with an aromatase inhibitor is not recommended as first-line treatment for metastatic breast cancer.[45]
- The ALTTO trial (adjuvant lapatinib and/or trastuzumab treatment optimisation) compared trastuzumab and lapatinib alone or in combination for early breast cancer.
- The lapatinib-only arm of the trial was discontinued following a high rate of disease recurrence, and final study results are awaited.

What other drugs are being developed to treat breast cancer?

- Bevacizumab (Avastin):
  - This antiangiogenic monoclonal antibody inhibits vascular endothelial growth factor A (VEGF-A).
  - It slows progression of metastatic disease but has no effect on overall survival or quality of life, and has significant side effects including hypertension.
  - It is not recommended by NICE for metastatic breast cancer.
  - It can be prescribed off licence via the Cancer Drugs Fund for triple negative recurrent tumours and cancers which have progressed despite prior taxane treatment.
- Pertuzumab:
  - This is a HER2 dimerisation inhibitor effective in combination with trastuzumab and docetaxel for metastatic disease (CLEOPATRA phase III trial).
  - Further trials are ongoing to assess effectiveness in early breast cancer.
  - NICE guidance is expected in November 2013.
- Neuvax:
  - This is a combination of a synthetic derivative of HER2 peptide and GMCSF which targets CD4 T cells to HER2 overexpressing cells.
  - Phase 3 clinical trials are ongoing.
- Serum HER2 levels can be used to monitor response to treatment.[46]

LIPOMODELLING AND ONCOPLASTIC BREAST CONSERVING TECHNIQUES

A 56-year-old woman presents with a significant defect in the upper inner quadrant of her left breast following WLE and completion of radiotherapy 9 months previously. She is otherwise fit and well. What are the options for symmetrisation?

- Volume replacement
  - Lipomodelling, miniflap
- Volume displacement
  - Contralateral reduction/mastopexy (to reduce breast parenchyma, skin or both)

Describe the classification of deformities following breast-conserving surgery.

- Type I—symmetrical breast with reduced volume but no deformity
- Type II—deformity of the breast amenable to partial reconstruction
- Type III deformity—major deformity requiring mastectomy and reconstruction[47]

The woman expresses an interest in lipomodelling. Please detail the factors you would discuss with her, including potential risks.

- At least 12 months should be allowed to elapse following radiotherapy before performing lipomodelling to ensure that acute reaction has subsided.
- There is a lack of evidence regarding long-term oncological safety and aesthetic outcomes.
- Initial postoperative breast imaging is performed prior to surgery according to local protocol. Further imaging should not be performed for at least 6 months following surgery.
- Risks include fat necrosis (10%), calcification (5%), wound infection (1%), donor site morbidity and bowel perforation (from lipoharvesting techniques).
- A proportion of graft volume will be lost (up to 30%), so there may be a need for further staged operations.
- This is contraindicated in smokers due to increased risk of fat necrosis and wound complications.
- The patient should not be actively dieting at the time of surgery or immediately postoperatively.[48]

Describe the various techniques for lipomodelling.

- Fat harvesting can be performed freehand following infiltration with local anaesthetic/adrenaline or a commercial water-assisted liposuction device can be used.

- In the Coleman technique, fat is harvested under low pressure and centrifuged at 3000 rpm for 1–3 min to separate the fat graft from an upper lipid layer and a lower tumescent serosanguinous layer.
- Graft preparation uses a commercially available closed system to purify the graft prior to use.
- In cell-assisted fat transfer, adipose-derived regenerative stem cells (ADRCs) are harvested from the fat sample and used to enrich the graft.
  - It may improve graft survival, but has only been used in the context of clinical trials or prospective audits at present.[49]

What are the main indications for lipomodelling?

- Following breast cancer surgery
  - To correct WLE defects, improve coverage of implant-based reconstructions, stimulate neovascularisation following radiotherapy, augment autologous tissue reconstruction
- For congenital abnormalities
  - To correct volume asymmetry, chest wall abnormalities
- For aesthetic enhancement
  - To correct contour problems following reduction/mastopexy, camouflage implant rippling, breast enhancement, disguise capsular contracture

If the patient had no suitable donor sites for lipomodelling, what other volume replacement techniques could you consider?

- Latissimus dorsi myocutaneous or miniflap (myosubcutaneous flap based on thoracodorsal pedicle) or ICAP (intercostal artery perforator) flap
  - Donor site morbidity
- Pedicled TRAM flap (transverse rectus abdominis myocutaneous)
  - Increased risk of fat necrosis, abdominal wall hernia
- Implant reconstruction
  - Risk of capsular contracture; may limit subsequent mammographic surveillance

What are the initial oncoplastic options to avoid cosmetic deformity for primary tumours in the UIQ of the breast?

- Level I technique (for <20% excision volume):
  - Periareolar or radial incision
  - Excise tumour and approximate local glandular flaps, recentre NAC if required[48]
- Level II technique (20%–50% excision volume)[49,50]:
  - Depends on position of cancer in breast
  - May require contralateral symmetrisation
  - Scar choice independent of pedicle

- Lower pole—superior pedicle mammoplasty (Wise pattern or vertical scar)
- Lower inner quadrant—superior pedicle mammoplasty (Wise pattern or vertical scar)
- Upper inner quadrant—round block mammoplasty, inferior pedicle mammoplasty, batwing excision
- Upper pole—round block mammoplasty, inferior pedicle mammoplasty
- Upper outer quadrant—inferior pedicle mammoplasty, racquet mammoplasty
- Lower outer quadrant—superior pedicle mammoplasty, J-mammoplasty
- Retroareolar—Grisotti excision

NIPPLE DISCHARGE

A 45-year-old woman presents to your clinic with unilateral blood-stained nipple discharge. How will you manage her?

- Take a history and examine the patient. Is the discharge spontaneous? Is it from single or multiple ducts? What colour is it? Is there a family history of breast cancer, OCP use, smoking history, previous breast surgery?
- Investigate (to complete triple assessment):
  - Digital mammogram
  - USS useful if palpable lump behind nipple
  - Haemoccult test (only 50% sensitivity)
- Pathology:
  - Nipple discharge cytology (poor sensitivity)—may be increased by duct lavage
  - US-guided core or vacuum-assisted biopsy

What are the indications for surgery for single-duct discharge?

- Blood-stained or haemoccult positive test
- Persistent discharge
- Associated mass
- Postmenopausal status
- U3 or M3 lesion on imaging

What are the most common causes of nipple discharge?

- Duct ectasia—may also cause duct shortening and nipple retraction. It is not usually blood stained, may be bilateral and is rarely spontaneous.
- Papillomas are discrete/multiple/juvenile. They are most common in the 30- to 50-year age group. Blood-stained discharge may be present 50% of the time. It may be associated with in situ carcinoma.

- In DCIS, 30% of symptomatic noninvasive breast cancers present with nipple discharge. It is associated with Paget's disease.
- In pregnancy, it could be benign, due to hypervascularity of breast tissue.
- In adenoma, papillary growth on a nipple can cause erosion and bleeding. It is most common in the 40- to 50-year age group.
- With granular cell tumours, neurological neoplasm arising from Schwann cells. They are usually benign but treated by WLE to prevent recurrence.

What are the surgical options?

- Ductoscopy allows for visualisation/targeted biopsy of lesions.
- Microdochectomy can be performed if a single duct discharge can be identified on the day of surgery.
  - Cannulate the duct and isolate with either a probe or methylene blue dye.
  - Access via the periarolar incision.
  - This allows for subsequent breastfeeding.
- Total duct excision (Hadfield's procedure) is used for single or multiple duct discharge in patients who have completed their family.
  - This has greater sensitivity and lower false-negative rates than for microdochectomy.
  - Risks include nipple necrosis, reduced sensation and nipple inversion, and recurrence.
  - Cover with broad-spectrum antibiotic.

The patient undergoes total duct excision. Pathology shows multiple intraductal papillomas. How would you counsel her?

- The definition is more than five separate papillomas, usually peripheral from the nipple (>3 cm).
- There is an associated risk of in situ malignancy and bilateral disease.
- It requires regular surveillance with digital mammography or MRI (discuss in MDT).
- Further lesions warrant excision with VAB to ensure no malignancy and minimise cosmetic deformity.
- Patients may opt for prophylactic mastectomy.

REFERENCES

1. Mansel, Robert E, Lesley Fallowfield, Mark Kissin, Amit Goyal, Robert G Newcombe, J Michael Dixon, Constantinos Yiangou, et al. 2006. Randomized multicenter trial of sentinel node biopsy versus standard axillary treatment in operable breast cancer: the ALMANAC Trial. *Journal of the National Cancer Institute* 98 (9): 599–609.
2. Fisher, B, C Redmond, E R Fisher, M Bauer, N Wolmark, D L Wickerham, M Deutsch, E Montague, R Margolese and R Foster. 1985. Ten-year results of a randomized clinical trial comparing radical mastectomy and total mastectomy with or without radiation. *New England Journal of Medicine* 312 (11): 674–681.

3. Giuliano, Armando E, Kelly K Hunt, Karla V Ballman, Peter D Beitsch, Pat W Whitworth, Peter W Blumencranz, A Marilyn Leitch, Sukamal Saha, Linda M McCall and Monica Morrow. 2011. Axillary dissection vs. no axillary dissection in women with invasive breast cancer and sentinel node metastasis: A randomized clinical trial. *Journal of the American Medical Association* 305 (6): 569–575.

4. Meijers-Heijboer, H, B van Geel, W L van Putten, S C Henzen-Logmans, C Seynaeve, M B Menke-Pluymers, C C Bartels, et al. 2001. Breast cancer after prophylactic bilateral mastectomy in women with a BRCA1 or BRCA2 mutation. *New England Journal of Medicine* 345 (3): 159–164.

5. Domchek, Susan M, Tara M Friebel, Susan L Neuhausen, Theresa Wagner, Gareth Evans, Claudine Isaacs, Judy E Garber, et al. 2006. Mortality after bilateral salpingo-oophorectomy in BRCA1 and BRCA2 mutation carriers: A prospective cohort study. *Lancet Oncology* 7 (3): 223–229.

6. FH01 collaborative teams. 2010. Mammographic surveillance in women younger than 50 years who have a family history of breast cancer: Tumour characteristics and projected effect on mortality in the prospective, single-arm, FH01 study. *Lancet Oncology* 11 (12): 1127–1134.

7. Rijnsburger, Adriana J, Inge-Marie Obdeijn, Reinoutje Kaas, Madeleine M A Tilanus-Linthorst, Carla Boetes, Claudette E Loo, Martin N J M Wasser, et al. 2010. BRCA1-associated breast cancers present differently from BRCA2-associated and familial cases: Long-term follow-up of the Dutch MRISC screening study. *Journal of Clinical Oncology: Official Journal of the American Society of Clinical Oncology* 28 (36): 5265–5273.

8. Wilson, J M and Y G Jungner. 1968. [Principles and practice of mass screening for disease.] *Boletín de la Oficina Sanitaria Panamericana.* Pan American Sanitary Bureau 65 (4): 281–393.

9. Shapiro, S. 1997. Periodic screening for breast cancer: The hip randomized controlled trial. Health insurance plan. *Journal of the National Cancer Institute.* Monograph no. 22: 27–30.

10. Tabar, L, B Vitak, H H Chen, S W Duffy, M F Yen, C F Chiang, U B Krusemo, T Tot and R A Smith. 2000. The Swedish two-county trial twenty years later. Updated mortality results and new insights from long-term follow-up. *Radiologic Clinics of North America* 38 4 (4): 625–651.

11. Andersson, I, K Aspegren, L Janzon, T Landberg, K Lindholm, F Linell, O Ljungberg, J Ranstam and B Sigfússon. 1988. Mammographic screening and mortality from breast cancer: The Malmö mammographic screening trial. *British Medical Journal* (clinical research ed.) 297 (6654): 943–948.

12. Alexander, F E, T J Anderson, H K Brown, A P Forrest, W Hepburn, A E Kirkpatrick, B B Muir, R J Prescott and A Smith. 1999. 14 Years of follow-up from the Edinburgh randomised trial of breast-cancer screening. *Lancet* 353 (9168): 1903–1908.

13. Frisell, J and E Lidbrink. 1997. The Stockholm mammographic screening trial: Risks and benefits in age group 40–49 years. *Journal of the National Cancer Institute.* Monograph no. 22: 49–51.

14. Miller, A B, C J Baines, T To and C Wall. 1992. Canadian national breast screening study: 1. Breast cancer detection and death rates among women aged 40 to 49 years. *Canadian Medical Association Journal* [*Journal de l'Association Medicale Canadienne*] 147 (10): 1459–1476.

15. Miller, A B, C J Baines, T To and C Wall. 1992. Canadian national breast screening study: 2. Breast cancer detection and death rates among women aged 50 to 59 years. *Canadian Medical Association Journal* [*Journal de l'Association Medicale Canadienne*] 147 (10): 1477–1488.

16. Bjurstam, Nils, Lena Björneld, Jane Warwick, Evis Sala, Stephen W Duffy, Lennarth Nyström, Neil Walker, et al. 2003. The Gothenburg breast screening trial. *Cancer* 97 (10): 2387–2396.

17. Moss, Sue M, Howard Cuckle, Andy Evans, Louise Johns, Michael Waller and Lynda Bobrow, Trial Management Group. 2006. Effect of mammographic screening from age 40 years on breast cancer mortality at 10 years' follow-up: A randomised controlled trial. *Lancet* 368 (9552): 2053–2060.

18. Forrest, A P M. 1987. Breast cancer screening. Report to the Health Ministers of England, Wales, Scotland and Northern Ireland by a working group chaired by Sir Patrick Forrest. London: HMSO (http://www.cancerscreening.nhs.uk/breastscreen/publications/forrest-report.pdf).

19. Breast Screening Frequency Trial Group. 2002. The frequency of breast cancer screening: Results from the UKCCCR randomised trial. United Kingdom Co-Ordinating Committee on Cancer Research. *European Journal of Cancer* 38 (11): 1458–1464.

20. NHSBSP. 2009. 20 QA guidelines for surgeons in breast cancer screening (http://www.cancerscreening.nhs.uk/breastscreen/publications/nhsbsp20.pdf).

21. Association of Breast Surgery. 2009. Surgical guidelines for the management of breast cancer. *European Journal of Surgical Oncology* 35:1–22.

22. Gøtzsche, Peter C and Margrethe Nielsen. 2011. Screening for breast cancer with mammography. *Cochrane Database Systems Review* 1:CD001877.

23. Duffy, Stephen W, Laszlo Tabar, Anne Helene Olsen, Bedrich Vitak, Prue C Allgood, Tony H H Chen, Amy M F Yen and Robert A Smith. 2010. Absolute numbers of lives saved and overdiagnosis in breast cancer screening, from a randomized trial and from the breast screening programme in England. *Journal of Medical Screening* 17 (1): 25–30.

24. Screening for Breast Cancer in England: Past and future. 2006. Advisory Committee on Breast Cancer Screening. NHSBSP publication no. 61.

25. Independent UK Panel on Breast Cancer Screening. 2012. The benefits and harms of breast cancer screening: An independent review. *Lancet* 380 (9855): 1778–1786.

26. Antoniades, K. 1995. Pathologic Findings from the National Surgical Adjuvant Breast Project (NSABP) Protocol B-17: Intraductal carcinoma (ductal carcinoma in situ). *Cancer* 76 (11): 2385–2387.

27. Bijker, Nina, Philip Meijnen, Johannes L Peterse, Jan Bogaerts, Irène Van Hoorebeeck, et al. 2006. Breast-conserving treatment with or without radiotherapy in ductal carcinoma-in-situ: Ten-year results of European Organisation for Research and Treatment of Cancer Randomized Phase III Trial 10853—A study by the EORTC Breast Cancer Cooperative Group and EORTC Radiotherapy Group. *Journal of Clinical Oncology* 24 21 (21): 3381–3387.

28. NICE guidelines for early breast cancer (CG80). February 2009.

29. Association of Breast Surgery. 2009. Surgical guidelines for the management of breast cancer. *European Journal of Surgical Oncology* 35:1–22.

30. Fisher, B, J Dignam, N Wolmark, D L Wickerham, E R Fisher, E Mamounas, R Smith, et al. 1999. Tamoxifen in treatment of intraductal breast cancer: National Surgical Adjuvant Breast and Bowel Project B-24 randomised controlled trial. *Lancet* 353 (9169): 1993–2000.

31. NICE guidelines for early breast cancer (CG80) (February 2009).

32. Early Breast Cancer Trialists' Collaborative Group (EBCTCG). 2012. Effects of chemotherapy and hormonal therapy for early breast cancer on recurrence and 15-year survival: An overview of the randomised trials. *Lancet* 365 (9472): 1687–1717.

33. Cuzick, Jack, Ivana Sestak, Michael Baum, Aman Buzdar, Anthony Howell, Mitch Dowsett and John F Forbes, ATAC/LATTE investigators. 2010. Effect of Anastrozole and Tamoxifen as adjuvant treatment for early-stage breast cancer: 10-Year analysis of the ATAC trial. *Lancet Oncology* 11 (12): 1135–1141.

34. Regan, Meredith M, Patrick Neven, Anita Giobbie-Hurder, Aron Goldhirsch, Bent Ejlertsen, Louis Mauriac, John F Forbes, et al. 2011. Assessment of Letrozole and Tamoxifen alone and in sequence for postmenopausal women with steroid hormone receptor-positive breast cancer: The BIG 1-98 randomised clinical trial at 8·1 years median follow-up. *Lancet Oncology* 12 (12): 1101–1108.

35. Davies, Christina, Hongchao Pan, Jon Godwin, Richard Gray, Rodrigo Arriagada, Vinod Raina, Mirta Abraham, et al. 2013. Long-term effects of continuing adjuvant Tamoxifen to 10 years versus stopping at 5 years after diagnosis of oestrogen receptor-positive breast cancer: ATLAS, a randomised trial. *Lancet* 381 (9869): 805–816.

36. Goss, Paul E, James N Ingle, Silvana Martino, Nicholas J Robert, Hyman B Muss, Martine J Piccart, Monica Castiglione, et al. 2005. Randomized trial of Letrozole following Tamoxifen as extended adjuvant therapy in receptor-positive breast cancer: Updated findings from NCIC CTG MA.17. *Journal of the National Cancer Institute* 97 (17): 1262–1271.

37. Mamounas, Eleftherios P, Barry Lembersky, Jong-Hyeon Jeong, Walter Cronin, Barbara Harkins, Charles Geyer, Donald Lawrence Wickerham, Soonmyung Paik, Joseph Costantino and Norman Wolmark. 2006. NSABP B-42: A clinical trial to determine the efficacy of five years of letrozole compared with placebo in patients completing five years of hormonal therapy consisting of an aromatase inhibitor (AI) or tamoxifen followed by an AI in prolonging disease-free survival in postmenopausal women with hormone receptor-positive breast cancer. *Clinical Breast Cancer* 7 (5): 416–421.

38. Coombes, R Charles, Emma Hall, Lorna J Gibson, Robert Paridaens, Jacek Jassem, Thierry Delozier, Stephen E Jones, et al. 2004. A randomized trial of exemestane after two to three years of Tamoxifen therapy in postmenopausal women with primary breast cancer. *New England Journal of Medicine* 350 (11): 1081–1092.

39. Hurtado, Antoni, Kelly A Holmes, Timothy R Geistlinger, Iain R Hutcheson, Robert I Nicholson, Myles Brown, Jie Jiang, William J Howat, Simak Ali and Jason S Carroll. 2008. Regulation of ERBB2 by oestrogen receptor-PAX2 determines response to tamoxifen. *Nature* 456 (7222): 663–666.

40. Gennari, Alessandra, Maria Pia Sormani, Paolo Pronzato, Matteo Puntoni, Mariantonietta Colozza, Ulrich Pfeffer and Paolo Bruzzi. 2008. HER2 status and efficacy of adjuvant anthracyclines in early breast cancer: A pooled analysis of randomized trials. *Journal of the National Cancer Institute* 100 (1): 14–20.

41. Ross, Jeffrey S, W Fraser Symmans, Lajos Pusztai and Gabriel N Hortobagyi. 2007. Standardizing slide-based assays in breast cancer: Hormone receptors, HER2, and sentinel lymph nodes. *Clinical Cancer Research: An Official Journal of the American Association for Cancer Research* 13 (10): 2831–2835.

42. NICE guidelines for early breast cancer (CG80) (February 2009).

43. Piccart-Gebhart, Martine J, Marion Procter, Brian Leyland-Jones, Aron Goldhirsch, Michael Untch, Ian Smith, Luca Gianni, et al. 2005. Trastuzumab after adjuvant chemotherapy in HER2-positive breast cancer. *New England Journal of Medicine* 353 (16): 1659–1672.

44. Romond, Edward H, Edith A Perez, John Bryant, Vera J Suman, Charles E Geyer, Nancy E Davidson, Elizabeth Tan-Chiu, et al. 2005. Trastuzumab plus adjuvant chemotherapy for operable HER2-positive breast cancer. *New England Journal of Medicine* 353 (16): 1673–1684.

45. NICE technology appraisal guidance 257: Lapatinib or trastuzumab in combination with an aromatase inhibitor for the first-line treatment of metastatic hormone receptor-positive breast cancer that overexpresses HER2 (June 2012).

46. Ali, Suhail M, Walter P Carney, Francisco J Esteva, Monica Fornier, Lyndsay Harris, Wolfgang J Köstler, Jean-Pierre Lotz, et al. 2008. Serum HER-2/Neu and relative resistance to Trastuzumab-based therapy in patients with metastatic breast cancer. *Cancer* 113 (6): 1294–1301.

47. Clough, K B, J Cuminet, A Fitoussi, C Nos and V Mosseri. 1998. Cosmetic sequelae after conservative treatment for breast cancer: Classification and results of surgical correction. *Annals of Plastic Surgery* 41 (5): 471–481.
48. Lipomodelling guidelines for breast surgery (August 28, 2012). Joint guidelines from the Association of Breast Surgery, the British Association of Plastic, Reconstructive and Aesthetic Surgeons and the British Association of Aesthetic Plastic Surgeons.
49. Dixon, J M, ed. 2009. *Breast surgery: A companion to specialist surgical practice.* Philadelphia: Saunders Elsevier.
50. Clough, Krishna B, Gabriel J Kaufman, Claude Nos, Ines Buccimazza and Isabelle M Sarfati. 2010. Improving breast cancer surgery: A classification and quadrant per quadrant atlas for oncoplastic surgery. *Annals of Surgical Oncology* 17 (5): 1375–1391.

BIBLIOGRAPHY

Anon. 2009. NICE—Advanced breast cancer—Full guidance (February 20): 1–122.
Blamey, R W. 1999. British Association of Surgical Oncology Guidelines in the management of metastatic bone disease in the United Kingdom. *European Journal of Surgical Oncology* (February 10): 1–21.
Debnath, Debasish, Dhafir Al-Okati, and Wael Ismail. 2010. Multiple papillomatosis of breast and patient's choice of treatment. *Pathology Research International* 2010:540590.
Green, Jane, Gabriela Czanner, Gillian Reeves, Joanna Watson, Lesley Wise and Valerie Beral. 2010. Oral bisphosphonates and risk of cancer of oesophagus, stomach, and colorectum: Case-control analysis within a UK primary care cohort. *British Medical Journal* (clinical research ed.) 341:c4444.
Pavlakis, N, R L Schmidt and M Stockler. 2005. Bisphosphonates for breast cancer. *Cochrane Database Systems Review* (3): CD003474.
Rapiti, Elisabetta, Helena M Verkooijen, Georges Vlastos, Gerald Fioretta, Isabelle Neyroud-Caspar, André Pascal Sappino, Pierre O Chappuis and Christine Bouchardy. 2006. Complete excision of primary breast tumor improves survival of patients with metastatic breast cancer at diagnosis. *Journal of Clinical Oncology: Official Journal of the American Society of Clinical Oncology* 24 (18): 2743–2749.
Ross, J R, Y Saunders, P M Edmonds, S Patel, K E Broadley and S R D Johnston. 2003. Systematic review of role of bisphosphonates on skeletal morbidity in metastatic cancer. *British Medical Journal* (clinical research ed.) 327 (7413): 469.
Royal College of Obstetricians and Gynaecologist guidelines for treatment of breast cancer in pregnancy (http://www.rcog.org.uk/files/rcog-corp/GTG12PregBreastCancer.pdf).

6 Colorectal Surgery

Edward Courtney, Gillian Tierney and Samson Tou

CONTENTS

ANAL CARCINOMA

A 70-year-old man presents to your clinic with a painful ulcerated anal lesion. The appearances are suspicious for an anal carcinoma. There are some enlarged inguinal lymph nodes in the right groin clinically. How would manage the patient?

- I would take a complete medical history with performance status assessment, asking about anal pain, bleeding and discharge, history of anal intercourse, genital warts (HPV infection) and HIV.
- I would examine the patient, feeling for regional lymphadenopathy and hepatomegaly, and inspect the anal lesion. It is important to differentiate between tumours arising in the anal canal versus those arising from the anal margin. Small lesions at the margin may be treated by surgery alone, unlike true canal tumours.
- Anal margin lesions look like malignant ulcers with a raised, everted, indurated edge. Anal canal lesions may not be visible, may be painful on PR examination and may have rectal extension. Perirectal nodes may be palpable.
- I would list the patient for an urgent EUA, rigid sigmoidoscopy and biopsy. At EUA I will assess the tumour size and involvement of local structures. I will also arrange an FNA/biopsy of the inguinal nodes (50% of enlarged inguinal nodes will show evidence of metastases, whilst the rest are enlarged due to secondary infection).
- Finally, I would request an MRI to assess the extent of local disease, and a CT to look for distant metastases.

Biopsies confirm a squamous cell carcinoma, which on EUA is extending into the anal canal and is 3 cm in maximum diameter. What would your management be?

- I would have a network cancer MDT discussion with surgeons, pathologists, radiologists and medical and radiotherapy oncologists.
- I would request chemoradiotherapy:
  - High-dose radiotherapy in 2 courses
  - IV 5-FU and Mitomycin C
  - Superior local control from combined therapy over radiotherapy alone
  - Complications of chemotherapy: diarrhoea, mucositis, myelosuppression, skin erythema and desquamation, anal stenosis and fistula formation.

How do anal cancers spread?

- Locally—cephalad, so they can appear to originate from the rectum
- Outward invasion into local structures (rectovaginal septum, perineal body, scrotum or vagina)
- To lymph nodes—perirectal nodes followed by inguinal, haemorrhoidal and lateral pelvic nodes
- Late haematogenous spread (liver, lung, bone) associated advanced local disease

The patient has a complete response initially, but at a 12-month check-up he has an ulcerated lesion at the site of the previous ulcer, suspicious for recurrence. What would your management be?

- Repeat EUA and biopsy to confirm recurrence.
- Biopsies need to be of sufficient size/depth to differentiate from postradiotherapy change.
- If there is no metastatic disease on restaging, the patient may be considered for a salvage abdominoperineal resection of the rectum and anus. In fit patients with extensive disease extending around the vagina or bladder, a pelvic exenteration may need to be considered (high morbidity and impaired wound healing after RT).

BOWEL SCREENING

What is the definition of screening?

- Screening is a process of identifying apparently healthy people who may be at increased risk of a disease/condition.
- A screening test should have a high sensitivity and specificity and be acceptable to the screening population, cost effective and safe to perform.

Why do we screen for bowel cancer?

- About 1 in 20 people in the UK will develop bowel cancer during their lifetime.
- It is the third most common cancer in the UK, and second leading cause of cancer deaths, with over 16,000 people dying from it each year.
- The natural history is known, with a premalignant lesion which, when treated, reduces the risk of developing cancer.
- The prognosis after treatment is much better in early-stage disease.

What is the evidence for NHS bowel screening?

- A meta-analysis of four trials from a Cochrane review reported a 16% reduction in bowel cancer specific mortality with FOB screening.

- The bowel cancer FOB screening pilot, finished in 2007, invited 500,000 men and women aged 50–59 years for screening. The FOB test was completed by 50% of them. The PPV was 10.9% for cancer and 35% for adenoma.
- A recent once-only flexible sigmoidoscopy multicentre trial for the 55- to 64-year age group resulted in the reduction of colorectal cancer incidence (23%) and mortality (31%). This will soon be rolled out across the UK, in conjunction with FOB screening.

How does the FOB test work?

- FOB is a guaiac-based test which detects the peroxidase-like activity of haematin in faeces. The activity decreases as it passes through the GI tract, so it is much more likely to detect lower over upper GI bleeding.
- False positives are due to ingestion of vegetables that contain peroxidase and animal haemoglobin.
- The sensitivity is 70%–80%, so it is more of a risk-reduction programme because the sensitivity is low.
- Screening is currently offered biannually to everyone aged 60–69 years.
- People over 70 can request a screening kit.

What is the detection rate of the NHS screening programme?

- For every 1,000 people screened 20, will have a positive FOB test.
- The offered colonoscopy is accepted by 16 of the 20.
- Eight have a normal colonoscopy. Six have polyps. Two have bowel cancer.

How do you follow up people with colonic adenomas?

- They are divided into three risk groups, depending on the number and size of the adenomas, and are screened until 75 years of age:
  - Low risk (one or two small adenomas)—no surveillance or every 5 years, stopping after a negative exam
  - Intermediate risk (three or four small adenomas, or one adenoma > 1 cm)—every 3 years screenings until two negative exams
  - High risk (more than five adenomas, three or more with at least one larger than 1 cm)—colonoscopy at 1 year. If negative or low risk adenomas, repeat in 3 years. If further high risk adenoma, repeat in 1 year.

FAECAL INCONTINENCE

A 60-year-old woman has been referred to you with faecal incontinence. How will you assess her in clinic?

- I would take a history—frequency, stool type (Bristol stool chart), urgency, use of pads, type of leakage (flatus, mucus, liquid stool, solid stool), obstetric history (significant tears/use of forceps), previous bowel surgery (IBD, anal surgery, fissures/fistulas).

- I would calculate the faecal incontinence score (e.g., Cleveland Clinic, Wexner).
- I would perform an examination—abdominal examination, inspection of perineum for scars/deformity, soiling, anal gape (previous obstetric injury/pelvic neuropathy), perineal descent, digital examination (resting and squeeze tone), anorectal angle, length of sphincter, palpable sphincter defects, rectocoele, enterocoele.
- I would perform proctoscopy/rigid sigmoidoscopy.
- Depending on the findings, I would request anal manometry and physiology and proceed to endoanal USS (2D/3D) and defecating proctogram if required.

What are the most likely causes of faecal incontinence in a woman of this age?

- Obstetric:
  - Sphincter injury (forceps damage to external sphincter),
  - Pudendal neuropathy (long second stage delivery, abnormal perineal descent causing nerve traction/damage) causing low anal squeeze pressures and reducing anal canal sensation
  - Increasing risk of incontinence with number of vaginal deliveries and the delivery of large babies
- Internal rectal prolapse/intussusception
- Iatrogenic (previous anal surgery, e.g., Lord's procedure)

She had natural vaginal deliveries of large babies, and her anorectal physiology shows low maximum squeeze pressures, with no evidence of a sphincter defect on endoanal USS and no rectoanal intussception on defaecating proctogram. How will you treat her?

- I would start with conservative management, using a combination of loperamide and bulking agents to produce a solid stool. I would also suggest a trial of a low-fibre diet to see if this improves symptoms.
- Glycerin suppositories might help to ensure compete rectal evacuation.
- If this did not work, I would arrange pelvic floor physiotherapy, which improves symptoms in a proportion of patients.

If all these conservative treatment options fail, what other management options are there?

- Because her problem is mainly neurological and there is no evidence of sphincter damage, I would recommend that a trial period of sacral neuromodulation could be offered.
- A percutaneous wire is inserted under either local or general anaesthesia into the second, third or fourth sacral foramina. Correct positioning is indicated by a 'bellows' contraction (anal contraction and lifting up of the perineum) and flexion of the ipsilateral big toe. If successful after a 2- to 3-week stimulation period, a permanent implant can be inserted.

- Approximately 75%–80% of patients experience an improvement of 50%, with 50% having normal continence. Posterior tibial nerve stimulation is also an evolving treatment being used for the treatment of faecal incontinence, with several small, published series showing improvement of symptoms in the short term.

How would your management change if the endoanal USS showed a large sphincter defect?

- If the patient had a posterior defect, I would repair this directly.
- If it was an anterior defect, I would do an anterior sphincter repair with a levatorplasty.
- If there was insufficient residual sphincter, a previous failed repair or a major neurological deficit, I would consider sphincter augmentation (gracilis muscle transposition, electrically stimulated gracilis neosphincter).

FAMILIAL ADENOMATOUS POLYPOSIS

An 18-year-old male presents with fresh painless rectal bleeding for 3 months, without a change in bowel habit. How will you assess him in clinic?

- I would take a history—timing and nature of bleeding, straining at stools, history of haemorrhoids, family history of bowel cancer and inherited syndromes, weight loss and abdominal pain.
- I would perform general and rectal examinations including proctoscopy and rigid sigmoidoscopy.

There are no other red-flag symptoms. He was adopted, so does not know his family history. You see over 20 polyps in the rectum during rigid sigmoidoscopy. What do you do next?

- I will biopsy one of the polyps and arrange a colonoscopy, as he could have FAP.

How would you classify colonic polyps?

- Adenomatous—sporadic, familial adenomatous polyposis (FAP) including attenuated FAP, hereditary nonpolyposis colorectal cancer (HNPCC), MYH-associated polyposis
- Hyperplastic
- Inflammatory (ulcerative colitis/Crohn's disease)
- Hamartoma (juvenile polyposis, Peutz–Jeghers syndrome)

What clinical features characterise patients with FAP?

- Usually have family history
- More than 100 adenomatous polyps from second decade (less in attenuated FAP)

- Duodenal adenomatous polyps
- Extraintestinal manifestations
- Mutation in APC gene chromosome 5q (80% of individuals) on testing

What are the extracolonic features of FAP?

- Adenomas and carcinomas of the duodenum, stomach, small bowel, biliary tract, thyroid, adrenal cortex
- Epidermoid cysts, pilomatrixoma, osteomas
- Fundic gland polyps
- Desmoid tumours
- Hepatoblastoma
- Tumours of the central nervous system
- Congenital hypertrophy of the retinal pigment

The colonoscopy showed over 100 polyps, confirmed as FAP with genetic testing. How will you follow up this patient and when would you offer surgery?

- He needs an annual colonoscopy with chromoendoscopy because adenomas have been detected. Asymptomatic mutation carriers should have biannual flexible sigmoidoscopy as teenagers, converting to annual colonoscopy when adenomas are seen.
- Upper GI endoscopy (with side-viewing scope to examine ampulla of Vater) should be performed every 1–3 years, generally starting at 20–25 years of age.
- There should be regular physical examinations for extraintestinal features of FAP.
  - Any desmoid tumours need US/CT to evaluate them prior to abdominal surgery.
- As the risk of cancer for patients with FAP is nearly 100% and it is very difficult to remove all the precancerous polyps endoscopically, surgery should be offered as soon as it is practical, often during summer holidays or gap years.

What are the surgical options?

- Restorative proctocolectomy with ileal pouch anal anastomosis (two-stage procedure, with covering ileostomy)
  - No risk of polyps or cancer in retained rectum, although cancers have been reported in retained cuff of mucosa at the stapled anastomotosis
  - Risk of pelvic nerve damage during proctectomy and postop pouch complications
  - Adverse fertility effects in women
  - Needs annual surveillance with PR and flexible sigmoidoscopy
- Colectomy and ileorectal anastomosis (one-stage procedure with lower morbidity and mortality compared with pouch)
  - Lower morbidity and mortality

- Function (stool frequency and leakage) that is better than a pouch.
- Increased risk of rectal cancer (especially if numerous rectal polyps, mutations at codon 1309 on genetic testing, over age 30)
- Cumulative rectal cancer risk of up to 30% by 60 years of age
- Needs annual surveillance with PR and flexible sigmoidoscopy
- Total proctocolectomy and end ileostomy (mainly for those with low rectal cancer)
  - No postop surveillance needed

FISTULA-IN-ANO

What is a fistula-in-ano?

- A fistula-in-ano is a hollow tract lined with granulation tissue, connecting a primary opening inside the anal canal to a secondary opening in the perianal skin.
- Secondary tracts may be multiple and can extend from the same primary opening.

What are the causes of anal fistulas?

- Chronic cryptoglandular disease
- Crohn's disease, TB
- Pilonidal disease, hidradenitis suppuritiva, trauma, foreign bodies
- Malignancy

How do you classify them?
I use Park's classification (you might be asked to draw a diagram):

- Intersphincteric fistula (70%)—the tract passes within the intersphincteric space.
- Trans-sphincteric fistula (25%)—the tract passes through the external sphincter into the ischiorectal fossa.
- Suprasphincteric fistula (5%)—the tract passes above the puborectalis and then curls down through the levators and ischiorectal fossa.
- Extrasphincteric (<1%)—the tract runs without relation to the sphincters, often passing from the rectum above the levators.

How do you manage a trans-sphincteric fistula?

- EUA—assess location of internal and external opening, course of the primary track, presence of secondary extensions and other diseases that might complicate the fistula (e.g., Crohn's disease).
- Drain the infection and if the tract can be easily probed, insert a loose draining Seton.
- If the fistula does not heal, I would request an MRI to evaluate the fistula.

- Subsequent surgical options include fibrin glue, collagen plugs, advancement flap and LIFT procedure (ligation of the intersphincteric fistula tract).

How do you classify perianal disease in Crohn's disease?
Hughes' classification of perianal lesions:

- Primary lesions—anal fissure, ulcerated oedematous pile, cavitating ulcer, aggressive ulceration
- Secondary lesions—skin tags, anal/rectal strictures, perianal abscess/fistula, carcinoma
- Incidental lesions—haemorrhoids, perianal abscess/fistula, skin tags, cryptitis, hidradenitis suppuritiva

What are the treatment options for a Crohn's perianal fistula?

- Drain sepsis, be conservative, find the tract, place a loose draining Seton and subsequently open if superficial.
- If the fistula is high, then an advancement flap or plug is called for.
- Consider a defunctioning stoma.
- A loose Seton can be used as a long-term treatment.
- Protracted cases may need proctectomy.

HOT TOPICS IN COLORECTAL SURGERY

THE MALIGNANT POLYP

- The incidence is 2% and is likely to increase due to screening.
- Size is the most important factor when determining risk of malignant transformation within a polyp.
- There are two classification systems: Haggit (pedunculated malignant polyps) and Kikuchi (sessile malignant polyps).
- In practice, the classification is difficult to apply as many pedunculated polyps have short stalks that are destroyed during mechanical snaring or diathermy.
- Haggitt classification:
  - Level 0: carcinoma in situ or intramucosal carcinoma, not invasive
  - Level 1: carcinoma invading through muscularis mucosa into submucosa, but limited to the head of the polyp
  - Level 2: carcinoma invading the level of the neck of the adenoma
  - Level 3: carcinoma invading any part of the stalk
  - Level 4: carcinoma invading into the submucosa of the bowel wall below the stalk of the polyp, but above the muscularis propria
- Kikuchi classification (depth of invasion into submucosa):
  - SM1: superficial 1/3 submucosa (risk of nodal metastasis = 2%)
  - SM2: middle 1/3 submucosa (risk of nodal metastasis = 8%)
  - SM3: deep 1/3 submucosa (risk of nodal metastasis = 23%)

- Polyps are treated by endoscopy (loop snare or submucosal dissection) or TEMS/TEO for rectal polyps. The resection margin should be > 2 mm.

TREC Trial

- From ACPGBI guidelines, local excision for cure in rectal cancer should be restricted to T1 and <3 cm lesions with good or moderate differentiation. With recent advances in chemoradiation, local excision can be used selectively for T2 lesions with neoadjuvant or adjuvant therapy.
- TREC (transanal endoscopic microsurgery and radiotherapy in early rectal cancer) is a feasibility study comparing radical total mesorectal excision (TME) surgery versus short-course preoperative radiotherapy with delayed local excision at 8–10 weeks.
- Patients with T1–T2 with negative lymph nodes are considered for the study.

Extralevator APE

- Abdominoperineal excision (APE) is associated with higher rates of intraoperative perforation and circumferential margin (CRM) involvement compared to anterior resection.
- Cylindrical extralevator dissection (extralevator APE) has been suggested to avoid 'coning down' or 'surgical wasting' as dissection approaches the anal canal from above and below.
- Multicentre study has shown extralevator APE is associated with less CRM involvement and intraoperative perforation than standard APE.

ILEOANAL POUCH

A 24-year-old female with ulcerative colitis had a subtotal colectomy and ileostomy performed as an emergency 6 months ago and comes to your clinic asking what happens next? What do you tell her?

- The surgical options are:
  - No further surgery—would need annual rectal surveillance
  - Ileorectal anastomosis—only if minimal inflammation in the rectum and no dysplasia, and also needs annual surveillance (cancer risk in rectal stump, 5% at 20 years)
  - Restorative proctocolectomy and ileoanal pouch anastomosis
  - Proctocolectomy and permanent ileostomy—no surveillance needed

When offering pouch surgery, what other aspects do you need to consider?

- Good anal sphincter function
- Exclude Crohn's disease (high failure rate)

- Should not be performed in patients with active anal lesions (fissure, anorectal sepsis or ulceration)
- Exclude sclerosing cholangitis (relatively contraindicated due to high incidence of pouchitis)
- Fecundity—decrease in female infertility after pouch surgery (likely due to the rectal dissection), so either delay surgery or accept the risk of reduced fertility

When consenting patients for pouch surgery, what complications do you mention?

- Pouch failure (10%)—up to 30% in Crohn's disease due to pelvic sepsis, poor function and mucosal inflammation
- Anastomotic leak (5%)
- Stricture and small bowel obstruction (10%)
- Pelvic sepsis (15%; may lead to pouch excision and poor function or fistulas if late presentation)
- Pouchitis (30%; in FAP, 10%), chronic pouchitis (5%–10%)
- Reduced fertility in women and sexual dysfunction (up to 30% in women, 25% in men); however, generally improved sexual satisfaction after pouch formation, probable overall improvement of health
- Stool frequency—mean of six per day, two per night
- Incontinence to flatus and/or stool—5% during the day and 10% during night
- Operative mortality rate of 0.4%, morbidity rate of 30%, reoperation rate of 16%

What is pouch failure?

- Failure is defined as the need to remove the pouch and establish a permanent ileostomy.
- The learning curve in pouch surgery is related to pouch failure.

KEY COLORECTAL TRIALS

QUASAR STUDY (QUICK AND SIMPLE AND RELIABLE)[1]

- Stage 2 patients with colon or rectal cancer were randomised to receive either 5FU-based chemotherapy or observation. A small absolute survival benefit at 5 years (3.6%) was seen in the chemotherapy group.

SWEDISH RECTAL CANCER TRIAL[2]

- There was an improved survival and reduced local recurrence (11% vs. 27%, 5-year follow-up) with short course preop radiotherapy compared to surgery alone.

Dutch TME Trial[3]

- Local recurrence with short-course preop radiotherapy and surgery (2.4%) was compared with surgery alone (8.2%; 2-year follow-up). The 5-year recurrence rate was 5.6% versus 10.9% with no survival difference.

MRC-CR07 Trial[4]

- Preop short-course radiotherapy was tested against selective postop chemo-radiotherapy in patients with rectal cancer (multicenter RCT); there were 80 centres in four countries. Results were reduction of local recurrence (6.2% in 3 years) in the preop radiotherapy group and improvement of disease-free survival (6% in 3 years) in the preop radiotherapy group compared to selective postop chemotherapy group.

German CAO/ARO/A10 94 Trial[5]

- The trial compared preop versus postop CRT (standard TME). The preop approach had lower recurrence (6% vs. 12%) and lower complications (acute and late), but overall survival unaffected.

Mercury Trial[6]

- MRI predicted CRM has strong correlation of pathological findings (involvement of the CRM is a strong predictor of local recurrence).

Laparoscopic Colorectal Surgery Trials

- COST (comparison of laparoscopic-assisted and open colectomy for colon cancer)[7]
- Spanish (Lacey)[8]
- CLASSIC (conventional versus laparoscopic-assisted surgery in colorectal cancer; only trial to include rectal cancer)[9]
- COLOR (colon cancer laparoscopic or open resection)[10]
- Overall, it was shown that laparoscopic surgery has a longer operating time, reduced wound infection rate, less postop pain, less narcotic use, less over-all morbidity, a shorter hospital stay and comparable oncological outcomes (short to medium term).

Current Trials

CREST Trial (Colorectal Stenting Trial)

- This multicentre randomised trial assessed the effects (morbidities, stoma formation, QoL) of stenting in obstructing colonic/upper rectal tumours versus surgery. It was open to recruitment in 2009; currently, 48 centres are participating.

DREAM Trial (Dexamethasone Reduces Emesis after Major Gastrointestinal Surgery)

- This double blind, phase 4, multicentre RCT has been designed to determine if preop dexamethasone reduces postoperative nausea and vomiting in patients undergoing elective colorectal resections.

ROLARR Trial (Robotic versus Laparoscopic Resection for Rectal Cancer)

- This is an international, multicentre, prospective RCT of robotic-assisted versus laparoscopic surgery for the curative treatment of rectal cancer.

FIAT Trial (the Fistula-in-Ano Trial)

- This compared Surgisis anal fistula plug versus surgeon's preference for transphinteric fistula-in-ano (advancement flap, fistulotomy or cutting Seton).

FOxTROT Trial (Fluoropyrimidine, Oxaliplatin and Targeted Receptor Preoperative Therapy for Colon Cancer)

- This randomised trial assessed whether preoperative chemotherapy and/or an anti-EGFR monoclonal antibody improve outcomes in high-risk operable colon cancer.

HubBLe Trial (Haemorrhoidal Artery Ligation (HAL) versus Rubber Band Ligation (RBL) for Haemorrhoids)

- This multicentre RCT compared rubber band ligation with haemorrhoidal artery ligation in the management of symptomatic second- and third-degree haemorrhoids.

eTHoS Trial (Either Traditional Haemorrhoidectomy or Stapled Haemorrhoidopexy for Haemorrhoidal Disease)

- A pragmatic multicentre RCT compares stapled haemorrhoidopexy to traditional excisional surgery for haemorrhoidal disease.

The Ladies Trial: Laparoscopic Peritoneal Lavage or Resection for Purulent Peritonitis and Hartmann's Procedure or Resection with Primary Anastomosis for Purulent or Faecal Peritonitis in Perforated Diverticulitis

- This is a two-armed RCT. One arm compares laparoscopic lavage with either a Hartmann's procedure or resection and primary anastomosis. The second arm compares a Hartmann's procedure with primary anastomosis in Hinchey 4 diverticulitis.

OBSTRUCTIVE DEFAECATION

A 40-year-old lady referred by the GP is having problems with defaecation and sometimes digitation per vagina is required to help to evacuate. How will you assess her in clinic?

- Take a history, asking whether she strains at stool, whether there is a feeling of incomplete evacuation, and how often she digitates to help remove the stool. I would also ask about her obstetric history and whether she has had previous gynaecological surgery (e.g., colposuspension).
- This is probably a rectocoele, which is not usually painful.
- A rectocoele is a hernia of the anterior rectal wall through the rectovaginal septum.
- I would perform a rectal exam, looking for perineal descent/prolapse and feeling for sphincter tone and the position of the rectocoele (anterior or posterior).

How would you investigate this lady?

- I would perform an endoscopic examination (flexible sigmoidoscopy/colonoscopy), if indicated, to exclude an underlying neoplastic lesion.
- I would perform a colonic transit study to exclude slow transit constipation.
- Defaecography (MR) is useful to exclude other causes of obstructive defaecation (internal intussusception).

You find an anterior rectocele. What are the treatment options?

- Initially, I would treat with conservative measures, such as laxatives, suppositories, dietary manipulation and biofeedback.
- If that fails, surgery is an option, performed by either a gynaecologist or a colorectal surgeon, and there are several routes (transvaginal, perineal, transanal, transabdominal) which use suture plication, mesh reinforcement, excision of redundant tissue and fixation of the rectum/vagina/perineal body and reinforcement of the pelvic floor to repair the rectocoele.

Describe one surgical technique that you might use in your practice.

- One is the transanal approach—STARR (stapled transanal rectal resection).
- It is similar to stapled haemorrhoidopexy but the purse string suture is full thickness anteriorly and only mucosal posteriorly.
- It is necessary to exclude an enterocoele prior to surgery; if one is found, it should be repaired preop by a gynaecologist or laparoscopically in conjunction with the STARR procedure.
- Put the patient in a Lloyd–Davies or prone jackknife position and insert an anal retractor.
- Purse-string sutures are placed in the anterior wall (1 cm apart and 4 cm above the dentate line).
- The staple gun is inserted, the purse-string is tightened and the gun is closed, ensuring the vaginal wall is clear before firing by performing vaginal examination (PPH-03 device).

What are the complications of this technique?

- Sphincter damage, incontinence, stenosis, bleeding, urinary retention, perineal pain and recurrence

How would your management change if she had a high-grade internal rectal prolapse?

- I would recommend a laparoscopic ventral mesh rectopexy to eliminate the intussception by fixation of the lower anterior rectal wall to the sacral promontory, as well as correcting the associated rectocoele.
- The Oxford pelvic floor group reported success rates of 75%–80% in patients with obstructive defecation. Avoiding posterior mobilisation of the rectum preserves the autonomic nerve supply to the rectum, thus avoiding the postoperative constipation traditionally seen with posterior sutured rectopexy.

POUCHITIS

A 25-year-old female patient who had ileoanal pouch surgery previously attends follow-up clinic and complains of bloody diarrhoea and urgency. What is the likely cause and how would you manage it?

- This is pouchitis (acute inflammation of pouch), characterised by stool frequency and urgency, liquid stool, abdominal pain and fever. It is more common in smokers
- The incidence is 30% in UC patients and 10% in FAP patients with 5%–10% of patients complaining of chronic pouchitis.
- The diagnosis is based on the history and findings at rigid sigmoidoscopy, but endoscopic examination and histology may be needed to confirm the diagnosis.
- I would treat it in the first instance with a 2-week course of oral antibiotics (metronidazole, ciprofloxacin or augmentin) and probiotics (e.g., VSL3).
- A majority (80%) of patients will respond.

What are the side effects of long-term metronidazole?

- Metronidazole should not be taken for more than 6 weeks because of the risk of peripheral neuropathy.

If antibiotics did not control her symptoms, what would you do?

- Arrange a flexible sigmoidoscopy and obtain tissue for histology and microbiology, to confirm the diagnosis and exclude infective causes (e.g., *C. difficile* and CMV).

- Start a 1-month course of ciprofloxacin and metronidazole.
- If there was still no response, I would resend stool cultures and alter the antibiotic accordingly, for another month.
- If this still did not improve symptoms, I would consider budesonide or surgery to bring out an ileostomy.
- If a patient had a rapid relapse or more than three episodes a year, I would leave the patient on maintenance therapy for 3 months (e.g., daily cipro-floxacin or VSL 3).

RECTAL CANCER

A 75-year-old man was seen by your ST6 in the 2-week wait colorectal clinic with a change of bowel habit. A tumour is found 6 cm from the anal verge. How will you manage this patient?

- Perform a PR and proctoscopy to assess tumour site (anterior/posterior) and length. Is it mobile or fixed, circumferential/obstructing? Take a biopsy for histology to confirm the diagnosis.
- Counsel the patient that I am suspicious he has a tumour, request standard preop investigations and assess his fitness for treatment (performance status, cardiovascular/respiratory history).
  - Blood tests—FBC, U+Es, LFTs, G+S
  - Colonoscopy (3% synchronous tumour)
  - Rectal cancer protocol MRI—assess T stage (depth of tumour penetration), N stage (lymph node involvement and circumferential resection margin)
  - CT chest/abdomen/pelvis
  - Transrectal USS (if considering local therapy)
- Discuss in MDT—is there an indication for neoadjuvant therapy or local excision versus a radical cancer resection?

Would a liver US be adequate for staging?

- USS sensitivity is only 55%.
- FDG-PET (90%), MRI (76%) and CT (72%) have a higher sensitivity, and CT is the initial staging test used.

When would you consider preop chemoradiation (CRT) in this gentleman? Why do we give it preop rather than postop?

- I would consider this if the tumour was T3 N0/1 or T4, there was a threatened margin (tumour or lymph node within 1 mm from the CRM) or multiple involved local nodes. I would also consider it if the tumour was anterior or the patient was male with a high BMI.
- The German rectal cancer group published a large RCT comparing preop versus postop CRT in stage 2 and 3 rectal cancer. Although there was no

difference in overall survival, there was a significant reduction both in local recurrence (6% versus 13%) and treatment toxicity in the preop group.

- It is also given preoperatively to downstage the tumour, increase tumour resectability and give a higher rate of sphincter preservation at surgery. A complete pathological response is achieved in 10%–25% of patients.

What is the in-hospital mortality for rectal cancer surgery?

- For elective surgery, it is 8% for the < 80 year-old and 16% for the > 80 year-old. The mortality increases with an anastomotic leak.

What is a total mesorectal excision?

- This is precise dissection in an areolar plane between visceral fascia (envelopes rectum and mesorectum) and parietal fascia (overlying pelvic structures).
- It was popularised by Professor Heald from Basingstoke.
- It leaves an intact mesorectum, negative CRM and distal margins.
- Local recurrence is 3% (5 years) and survival is 80%.
- It should be performed for all midrectal and low rectal cancers, including APER.

What is the difference between a high and low anterior resection, and when would you use a covering loop ileostomy?

- A high anterior resection is done for a tumour above the peritoneal reflection. A low anterior resection is done for a tumour below peritoneal reflection.
- An alternative distinction is high anterior (anastomosis >10 cm from anal verge), low anterior (anastomosis < 10 cm but > 6 cm from anal verge), ultralow anterior resection (anastomosis < 6 cm from anal verge).
- I would consider a covering ileostomy for all low anterior resection patients (especially in men and after radiation), ileo-anal pouch anastomosis, a technically difficult anastomosis, and for certain patient factors (immunosuppressed, smokers, diabetes, renal failure, moderate to severe cardiovascular disease).

What nerves do you encounter during an anterior resection? At what points might they be at risk of being damaged?

- Pelvic parasympathetic nerves (nervi erigentes) originate from the S2–S4 ventral nerve roots, join the hypogastric nerves (sympathetic) of the pelvic sidewall to form the inferior hypogastric plexus (pelvic autonomic nerve plexus).
  - There is risk of damage during lateral wall dissection and near the lateral ligament (nerves close to the middle haemorrhoidal artery).
  - Injury results in erectile dysfunction, impaired vaginal lubrication and voiding difficulty.

- POINT (parasympathetic)—erection
  - Pelvic sympathetic nerves originate from the T12–L3 ventral roots, forming preaortic superior hypogastric plexus. Distal to the aortic bifurcation, the superior hypogastric plexus forms hypogastric nerves.
  - There is a risk of damage during high ligation of IMA and during dissection on the sacral promontory and presacral region.
  - Injury results in increased bladder tone, decreased bladder capacity, voiding difficulty, impaired ejaculation, loss of vaginal lubrication and dyspareunia.
- SHOOT (sympathetic)—ejaculation
- Dissection near the seminal vesicles and prostate can damage the periprostatic plexus, leading to mixed parasympathetic/sympathetic injury.

SLOW TRANSIT CONSTIPATION

How would you manage a patient with a functional constipation referred by a GP? What are the causes?

- Functional constipation is due to slow colonic transit, problems with rectal evacuation or both.
- Secondary causes of slow-transit constipation are:
  - Neurogenic (MS, Parkinson's disease, spinal cord lesions, diabetic autonomic neuropathy)
  - Endocrine/metabolic (hypothyroidism, hypercalcaemia)
  - Anatomical (strictures, aganglionosis)
  - Drugs (anticholinergics, opiates, antihypertensives, antacids)

How will you assess the patient in clinic?

- Take a history to exclude red-flag symptoms, ascertain degree of constipation, history of prolapse or manual evacuation, previous laxatives that have been tried, and exclude secondary causes listed before.
- Examine the patient and feel for anal sphincter tone and sensation and a prolapse.
- Request FBC, U+Es, Ca and TFTs.

What investigations would you request?

- If any symptoms are of concern, exclude colonic pathology first (colonoscopy or CT colonography).
- A transit study should be conducted. Ten markers are ingested on 6 consecutive days and an abdominal x-ray is taken on the seventh day. Counting the number of markers and multiplying by 2.4 gives the colonic transit time in hours (Arhan's method). Delayed colonic transit is defined as a time > 48 hr or 20 residual markers.

What other conditions need to be excluded?

- Isolated slow transit constipation is now thought to be relatively uncommon (5% in recent data from Oxford).
- Other disorders which give rise to obstructive defaecation (e.g., anismus and internal rectal prolapse) need to be excluded. A significant proportion of patients previously diagnosed with STC actually have constipation secondary to outlet obstruction.

How would you manage a patient with isolated STC?

- Ensure adequate fibre intake (>20 g/day) combined with sufficient fluid intake (2+ L) and regular physical exercise. However, these lifestyle changes are rarely sufficient to improve symptoms.
- Osmotic laxatives are often prescribed. A small prospective, randomised, crossover RCT showed that lactulose resulted in significantly higher mean bowel frequency and improved stool consistency when compared to fibre. However, osmotic laxatives can cause diarrhoea, bloating and electrolyte disturbances.
- Polyethylene glycol is an exception, as it is not absorbed and contains no electrolytes, making it preferable in patients with renal/cardiac failure.
- Biofeedback which focuses on abdominal and pelvic coordination is also being offered in some specialist centres and has shown some benefit in selected patients.

Is there a role for sacral nerve stimulation in the management of patients with STC?

- Several small studies have shown improvement in symptoms of patients with medically refractory STC with the use of SNS. The ability to offer test stimulation with an external stimulator allows a trial period of 2–3 weeks in order to evaluate the effect of stimulation on symptoms. A >50% improvement in symptoms is often used as an indication for permanent stimulation.

REFERENCES

1. Quasar Collaborative Group, Richard Gray, Jennifer Barnwell, Christopher McConkey, Robert K Hills, Norman S Williams and David J Kerr. 2007. Adjuvant chemotherapy versus observation in patients with colorectal cancer: A randomised study. *Lancet* 370 (9604): 2020–2029.
2. Folkesson, Joakim, Helgi Birgisson, Lars Pahlman, Bjorn Cedermark, Bengt Glimelius and Ulf Gunnarsson. 2005. Swedish rectal cancer trial: Long lasting benefits from radiotherapy on survival and local recurrence rate. *Journal of Clinical Oncology: Official Journal of the American Society of Clinical Oncology* 23 (24): 5644–5650.
3. Peeters, Koen C M J, Corrie A M Marijnen, Iris D Nagtegaal, Elma Klein Kranenbarg, Hein Putter, Theo Wiggers, Harm Rutten, et al. 2007. The TME trial after a median follow-up of 6 years: Increased local control but no survival benefit in irradiated patients with resectable rectal carcinoma. *Annals of Surgery* 246 (5): 693–701.

4. Sebag-Montefiore, David, Richard J Stephens, Robert Steele, John Monson, Robert Grieve, Subhash Khanna, Phil Quirke, et al. 2009. Preoperative radiotherapy versus selective postoperative chemoradiotherapy in patients with rectal cancer (MRC CR07 and NCIC-CTG C016): A multicentre, randomised trial. *Lancet* 373 (9666): 811–820.
5. Sauer, R, R Fietkau, C Wittekind, C Rödel, P Martus, W Hohenberger, J Tschmelitsch, et al. 2003. Adjuvant vs. neoadjuvant radiochemotherapy for locally advanced rectal cancer: The German trial CAO/ARO/AIO-94. *Colorectal Disease: Official Journal of the Association of Coloproctology of Great Britain and Ireland* 5 (5): 406–415.
6. MERCURY Study Group. 2006. Diagnostic accuracy of preoperative magnetic resonance imaging in predicting curative resection of rectal cancer: Prospective observational study. *British Medical Journal* (clinical research ed.) 333 (7572): 779.
7. Clinical Outcomes of Surgical Therapy Study Group. 2004. A comparison of laparoscopically assisted and open colectomy for colon cancer. *New England Journal of Medicine* 350 (20): 2050–2059.
8. Lacy, Antonio M, Salvadora Delgado, Antoni Castells, Hubert A Prins, Vicente Arroyo, Ainitze Ibarzabal and Josep M Pique. 2008. The long-term results of a randomized clinical trial of laparoscopy-assisted versus open surgery for colon cancer. *Annals of Surgery* 248 (1): 1–7.
9. Jayne, David G, Pierre J Guillou, Helen Thorpe, Philip Quirke, Joanne Copeland, Adrian M H Smith, Richard M Heath and Julia M Brown, UK MRC CLASICC Trial Group. 2007. Randomized trial of laparoscopic-assisted resection of colorectal carcinoma: 3-Year results of the UK MRC CLASICC trial group. *Journal of Clinical Oncology: Official Journal of the American Society of Clinical Oncology* 25 (21): 3061–3068.
10. COLOR Study Group. 2000. COLOR: A randomized clinical trial comparing laparoscopic and open resection for colon cancer. *Digestive Surgery* 17 (6): 617–622.

7 Endocrine Surgery

Elizabeth Ball and Ashish Lal

CONTENTS

ADRENAL INCIDENTALOMA

A 63-year-old man having a CT colonography has had a 40 mm lesion detected on his right adrenal gland. A GP colleague of yours has asked for advice on this patient.

- It is important to determine the radiological (which can help with determining malignancy) and functional characteristics of this lesion.
- Of patients having an abdominal CT scan, 1% have an adrenal lesion identified.
- Initial assessment should focus on the patient.
- I would take a history, looking for the following symptoms:
  - Anxiety, palpitations, headaches, feeling of impending doom, dysmenorrhoea, hypertension, previous or current malignancy, family history of endocrine disease
- I would perform a general examination, looking for signs and symptoms of a pituitary–adrenal axis imbalance:
  - Obesity (includes facial and truncal), facial plethora, hirstutism, hypertension, proximal muscle weakness, striae
    - These symptoms occur in 50% or more of patients who are cushingoid.

What is the differential diagnosis of an adrenal incidentaloma?

- Functional:
  - Adrenal cortex—adenoma, nodular hyperplasia, carcinoma
  - Adrenal medulla—phaeochromocytoma, ganglioneuroma/blastoma
- Nonfunctional:
  - Adrenal masses—lipoma, cyst, haematoma, hamartoma, teratoma, amyloidosis, neurofibroma
  - Metastases—breast, lung, lymphoma
  - Leukaemia
  - Pseudoadrenal masses—lymph nodes, renal/pancreatic/splenic mass

What investigations would you request?

- Initial screening tests—U+Es, FBC and a CXR
- Serum or urinary catecholamines (10% of incidentalomas will be phaeochromocytomas)
- If hypertension—urinary and plasma cortisol, serum ACTH
- If inconclusive—dexamethasone suppression test
- Plasma sex steroids only if clinical signs of hyperandrogenism

All of the tests are normal. What would you do next?

- If there is a previous history of malignancy, request CT-guided FNA.
  - If cells resemble a primary tumour, this saves unnecessary diagnostic surgery.
  - This is not useful in patients without a history of cancer, as adrenal FNAs are difficult to interpret.
- Dynamic gadolinium-enhanced MRI may be helpful in combination with the CT scan.

How do you diagnose adrenal lesions on a CT scan?

- They are diagnosed by the Hounsfield units.
- The radiodensity of distilled water at standard temperature and pressure is 0.
- Other values include bone: 1000; muscle: 10–40; fat: −50–100; air: −1000.
- The CT should report the Hounsfield units of the lesion.
- If value is <10 µ, malignancy is unlikely.
- A benign lesion should have >60% contrast washout at 15 min in an IV-contrast enhanced CT.

The MRI and CT suggest this is a benign nonfunctioning tumour measuring 2.5 cm. How would you manage the patient?

- Adopt a watch and wait policy because it is <3 cm.
- Arrange for serial annual CT scanning.
- If the tumour grows, I would consider surgery.

Would your management plan change if the tumour were 5 cm?

- Yes—larger tumours have a significant risk of malignancy.
- I would recommend laparoscopic adrenalectomy.

APPENDICEAL CARCINOID

A 33-year-old male who underwent a laparoscopic appendicectomy 2 weeks ago has been referred to your endocrine clinic. The histology report confirms an 18 mm carcinoid tumour in the tip of the appendix. What is a carcinoid tumour?

- Carcinoid tumours are of neuroendocrine origin; the term now specifically applies to tumours of the midgut origin (jejuno-ileal and proximal colon).
- They predominantly secrete serotonin; stain with chromogranin A and synaptophysin immunostains.
- Appendix carcinoids are usually nonsecretory (commonly being picked up incidentally after an operation for acute appendicitis).

How are carcinoid tumours classified?

- Site of origin
  - Foregut—extra-GI tract, oesophagus and stomach
  - Midgut—small bowel
  - Hindgut—colon and rectum
- Degree of differentiation
  - Well-differentiated neuroendocrine—nonfunctioning, rarely invasive
  - Well-differentiated endocrine—functioning, often invasive
  - Poorly differentiated endocrine—nonfunctioning, invasive
  - Mixed exocrine–endocrine tumours

What is the differentiation classification based on?

- Histological appearance
- Mitotic index (number of mitoses per 2 mm^2 or 10 high-power fields)
- Ki67 proliferation index
  - Well-differentiated tumours—low mitosis and low proliferation index (generally <2%)
  - Poorly differentiated tumours—high mitosis and higher proliferation index (20%–40%)

What is the TNM classification of appendicial carcinoids?

- A TNM classification has been devised for well-differentiated (<2 mitosis per 10 high-power fields) carcinoids of the appendix:
  - T1a tumour: up to 1 cm
  - T1b tumour: 1–2 cm

- T2 tumour: 2–4 cm or extends to caecum
- T3 tumour: >4 cm or extends to ileum
- T4 tumour: breaches peritoneum and invades adjacent structures
- N1 node: positive
- M1: metastases present

Does this patient need further treatment?

- No, he has been fully treated. The indications for further surgery are:
  - Size > 2 cm (30%–60% metastasis rate)
  - Incomplete resection margins (suggest a caecal rather than appendicular primary)
  - High proliferation index
  - Positive lymph nodes
  - Angioinvasion
- These patients need a completion right-hemicolectomy
- Small tumours in the base of the appendix also require completion right hemicolectomy.
  - They may represent colonic (hind-gut) carcinoid tumour

How would you follow him up?

- No further follow-up is required.
- For those patients who needed a completion right hemicolectomy:
  - Request blood tests (5-HIAA, chromogranin A) at 3 months after resection.
  - Request CT scan/MRI/OctreoScan.

What is the 5-year survival rate for appendiceal carcinoid?

- Local disease: 84%
- Regional disease: 81%
- Distant metastases: 28%

How would your management plan change if the histology report confirmed a goblet-cell carcinoid tumour?

- This is a more malignant variant, also called an 'atypical' carcinoid.
- It does not express somatostatin receptors.
- Cannot be visualised by an octreotide scan
- There is a possibility of aggressive spread in the mesoappendix and intraperitoneally. This patient needs a completion extended ileocolic and mesenteric resection and may need chemotherapy.
- They have a less favourable survival (60% 10-year survival rate).
- For aggressive tumours, cytoreductive surgery can be offered (omentectomy, splenectomy and peritonectomy).

What is the carcinoid syndrome?

- This occurs when vasoactive substances produced by the tumour escape hepatic degradation.
- It is seen when GI carcinoids metastasise to the liver or in primary carcinoids in extraportal locations (e.g., bronchial carcinoids).
- It occurs in about 5% of carcinoids.
- Prominent symptoms include diarrhoea and flushing.
- Flushing affects the face and neck and typically lasts only a few minutes; it may be triggered by chocolate or alcohol.
- Other features include pellagra, telangectasiae and tricuspid regurgitation.

HYPERPARATHYROIDISM

A 50-year-old woman presents to her GP with fatigue, constipation and mild depression. Initial blood tests reveal a raised serum calcium and PTH. How would you manage this patient?

- The raised calcium and raised PTH suggest a diagnosis of primary hyperparathyroidism.
  - This commonly presents in women in their sixth decade, and fatigue is the most common presenting symptom.
- I would take a thorough history, looking for other symptoms of hypercalcaemia (stones, bones, groans, moans), history of renal disease/transplant, and a family history of endocrine disease (familial hyperparathyroidism, MEN 1 and 2a).
- I would examine her neck.
- I would request thyroid function tests, phosphate levels, urinary calcium (to exclude familial hypercalcaemic hypocalciuria) and an ECG.

What imaging would you request?

- I would request a neck USS and a Sestamibi scan.
- USS is operator dependent and only picks up glands > 5 mm in size.
  - Sensitivity is 71%–80%.
- The Sestamibi scan exploits differential uptake in hyperfunctioning and normal parathyroid and thyroid tissue.
  - It localises parathyroid adenomas in 80%–100% of cases.
  - Specificity is around 90%.

The USS and Sestamibi both show an abnormal left superior parathyroid gland. What operation would you perform?

- The operative decision is between bilateral neck exploration and minimally invasive parathyroidectomy (MIP).
- With concordant preoperative localisation, I would perform a MIP.

- A single adenoma is found in 87% of patients.
- There is less morbidity, quicker procedure, day-case procedure and better cosmesis.

What are the specific anatomical considerations of the minimally invasive operative approach?

- A 2–4 cm incision is made on anterior border of sternocleidomastoid.
- The plane is developed lateral (posterior) to the strap muscles and medial (anterior) to sternocleidomastoid.
- A key landmark is the carotid artery (often the recurrent laryngeal nerve [RLN] is not encountered in this operation).
- Many surgeons also advocate quick parathyroid hormone (QPTH) assay to exclude multigland disease.[1]

Give a brief description of parathyroid embryology.

- Superior parathyroids develop from the fourth branchial arch:
  - They are less variable in position.
  - They are almost always found somewhere between the angle of the mandible/carotid bifurcation and the intersection of the RLN and the inferior thyroid artery.
- Inferior parathyroids develop from the third branchial arch:
  - They are more variable in position.
  - Found behind inferior thyroid pole: 50%
  - Found in thyrothymic ligament: 25%
  - Found above the intersection between the RLN and inferior thyroid artery, in the thymus and the anterior mediastinum: 5%–10%

What would you do if you could not find the abnormal gland after a bilateral neck exploration?

- The gland is probably in the mediastinum.
- I would defer a median sternotomy until:
  - The diagnosis has been confirmed with imaging.
  - The adenoma is precisely localised.
- A left thoracoscopy or anterior mediastinotomy may be suitable; these are less invasive alternative approaches.

What imaging would you request to find the missing gland?

- There are three options, depending on facilities available and radiologist experience:
- CT scan with IV contrast:
  - Can produce artefacts after previous neck surgery
  - Need thin-cut slices
  - Sensitivity of 80% but 50% false positive rate

- T2-weighted MRI:
  - Excellent at localising ectopic glands
  - Cannot image glands < 5 mm in size
  - Difficulty localising superior glands (lie posterior to thyroid)
- SPECT—3D images which allow for better anatomical localisation, especially within the mediastinum

What are the postoperative biochemical changes after successful parathyroidectomy?

- PTH levels are almost undetectable 4 hr after surgery and then begin to return to normal.
- Plasma calcium returns to normal in 24–48 hr.
  - Significant postoperative hypocalcaemia is rare.
  - Preventive treatment for hypocalcaemia is not justified.
- Elevated serum PTH levels are observed in up to 30% of patients at 1 month postop despite normalisation of serum calcium levels.

MANAGEMENT OF SALIVARY GLAND STONES

A 55-year-old patient presents with a swelling in the submandibular triangle, associated with meals. What is the most likely diagnosis?

- Sialolithiasis:
  - Stone in distal/middle/proximal duct or impacted in the submandibular salivary gland
  - Primary or secondary
  - May be palpable in the floor of the mouth
  - Fifty times more common than parotid stones (due to more mucinous composition of secretion)
- Neoplasm—rare but must be excluded:
  - Pleomorphic adenoma (most common)
  - Warthins (smoking risk factor, 10% bilateral)
  - Cystic adenoid carcinoma (neurotropic spread a problem)
  - Mucoepidermoid carcinoma
  - Metastases (from head and neck/oropharangeal SCC)
- I would take a careful history and perform a full examination, including the oral cavity.

What imaging would you request, if any?

- Plain x-ray (Panorex view)—usually diagnostic
- Sialography/CT/MRI:
  - This is not routinely performed but can help diagnosis.
  - If neoplasm is suggested from history and examination or following FNA of the neck lump, then CT and MRI should be done for diagnosis and staging.

The x-ray confirms a stone in the submandibular salivary duct. What is your operative approach?

- This depends on the position on the duct and whether it is impacted.
- If the stone is palpable in the floor of the mouth (i.e., in the distal portion of the duct):
  - LA or GA, approach via oral cavity.
  - Grasp or put stay stitch proximal to the stone.
  - Make a longitudinal cut along duct to remove the stone.
  - Perform haemostasis, then leave the duct open.
- Duct excision (stone impacted in the gland/hilum/proximal duct):
  - Consent for nerve injury (marginal mandibular/lingual/hypoglossal) and a salivary fistula.
  - Incise 2 cm anterior to angle of the jaw and 4 cm inferior to this.
  - Extend from anterior border of SCM to anterior extent of the gland (posterior surface of anterior belly of digastric), just above the hyoid bone—avoid marginal mandibular nerve.
  - Dissect deep to subcutaneous tissue/platysma/deep cervical fascia and raise the flap dissecting onto the gland (from inferior to superior).
  - Divide the facial vein and artery.
  - The lingual nerve is avoided as the gland is pulled out of the wound (gets dragged down with traction).
  - Remove the stone and ligate the duct carefully (avoids fistula).

Are there any other techniques for removing stones?

- Minimally invasive techniques:
  - Irrigation, stenting and ductoplasty
  - Basket retrieval
  - Extracorporeal shock-wave lithotripsy

What are the clinical manifestations of nerve complications?

- Marginal mandibular nerve:
  - Paralysis of depressor anguli oris (not orbicularis ori)
  - Difficulty controlling saliva
  - Biting mucosal surfaces when chewing
- Hypoglossal nerve:
  - Deviation of tongue to affected side
  - Eventual fasciculation and wasting
- Lingual nerve:
  - Paraesthesia/loss of taste on affected side
  - Usually a partial injury; if problematic—divide the nerve

MANAGEMENT OF A THY 3 FNA

A 32-year-old woman presents to your clinic with a right-sided neck swelling. Her GP arranged a neck ultrasound which showed a 20 mm thyroid nodule. An FNA was performed, with a THY 3 result. She is visibly upset in clinic. How will you manage her?

- Take a history, looking for signs of hyperhyroidism, and check for a family history of thyroid disease or thyroid cancer, and pregnancy.
- Examine the neck and lymph nodes; look for thyroid eye signs and complete a general examination.
- Take blood for thyroid function tests, T3 and T4.
- Confirm whether an experienced radiologist performed the ultrasound. If not, repeat it.
- Assess the USS report.
  - Is this a solitary nodule?
  - Is there a cystic component?
  - Are there worrying features (e.g., enlarged lymph nodes)?

What does a THY 3 cytology report mean?

- This means that the FNA is suspicious for a follicular neoplasm (adenoma or carcinoma) (i.e., no atypical papillary cells or psammoma bodies have been identified).
- The malignant features of capsular invasion cannot be ascertained on FNA, and follicular carcinoma can only be diagnosed by formal tissue histology.

How will you treat the patient?

- I would explain that a THY 3 FNA means that there is a small chance that she may have a thyroid cancer (5%–15%) and that this cannot be accurately diagnosed without removing the nodule itself.
- I would recommend a thyroid lobectomy/isthmectomy.

If the final histology report confirms a follicular carcinoma, what further treatment will she need?

- She needs to be discussed at a thyroid MDT.
- If the tumour is small, capsular invasion is minimal and no angioinvasion is seen, a case can be made for no further surgery.
- If extracapsular extension and/or angioinvasion is present or a Hurthle cell variant is observed, completion thyroidectomy is advised.
- Hurthle cell tumours have poor uptake of radioactive iodine (RI), but do secrete thyroglobulin, which is why completion thyroidectomy is recommended.

MEDULLARY THYROID CANCER

A 28-year-old patient has been referred to your clinic with a neck lump and diarrhoea. How will you assess the patient?

- It is necessary to exclude medullary thyroid cancer.
- Take a history—how long lump has been present, associated symptoms (hoarse voice, difficulty breathing/swallowing), frequency of diarrhoea, family history of endocrine disease.
- Perform an examination—full neck exam including lymph nodes, general examination looking for evidence of Cushing's syndrome and metastatic disease.
- Diagnosis:
  - Neck USS and FNAC by experienced radiologist
  - Serum calcitonin and CEA
  - Exclude a phaeochromocytoma (24 hr urinalysis for catecholamine metabolites (vanillylmandelic acid [VMA], metanephrine)

What is medullary thyroid cancer?

- It originates from parafollicullar C-cells (neural ectoderm).
- It is often multifocal, more common in upper poles (C-cells).
- It can be sporadic (80%) or familial (20%) (autosomal dominant MEN 2A, MEN 2B).
  - Familial cases are always bilateral and multicentric.
- The tumour secretes calcitonin, as well as other hormones (CEA, serotonin and prostaglandins) and can cause carcinoid syndrome.
- Mutations in the RET proto-oncogene (chromosome 10) are classified into discrete subtypes, which confer varying degrees of risk.
- It spreads by lymphatics to regional nodes (45%–70% 10-year survival) and via the bloodstream to distant sites such as liver, lungs and bones (20% 10-year survival).

How would you prepare this patient for surgery?

- If cervical nodes are involved or calcitonin > 400 pg/ml, CT neck and chest, and/or MRI is needed to look for distant metastases.
- It is necessary to rule out phaeochromocytoma and hyperparathyroidism prior to surgery.
- Request USS of neck to rule out lymph node spread.

What is your operative approach?

- Total thyroidectomy (often multicentric and bilateral disease), central neck dissection, excision of Delphian node and thymus
- Frozen section of any suspicious internal jugular chain lymph node

- If positive, selective (at least level 2/3/4) structure-preserving neck dissection on that side

How will you follow this patient up?

- Serum CEA and calcitonin
  - No consensus on time frame
  - Probably best practice to do every 4 months for 2 years, every 6 months for 3 years, then annually
  - If raised, indicates recurrent or metastatic disease
    - Can be treated with tyrosine kinase inhibitors
- Annual check as appropriate if familial

This patient's newborn baby has a RET mutation consistent with MEN 2A. Would you offer surgery? If so, when?

- Current guidelines suggest prophylactic thyroidectomy should be offered between 4 and 7 years of age (no consensus on age).
- The age at which surgery is offered depends on level of risk according to the specific RET mutation.

PAPILLARY THYROID CANCER

A 38-year-old woman has been referred to you with a 30 mm papillary thyroid cancer with a confirmed THY5 FNA. How would you manage the patient in clinic?

- Review history—previous irradiation, family history of endocrine disease.
- Examine the patient—looking for symptoms and signs of local invasion or distant metastasis (e.g., hoarse voice, dysphagia).
- Arrange a neck USS—look for cervical adenopathy.
- Request serum TFTs, calcium levels and anti-Tg antibodies.
  - Anti-Tg antibodies are present in 25% of patients, which can make follow-up more difficult.
- Request a staging CXR.

What are the risk factors for developing papillary cancer?

- Environmental—living in iodine-rich areas
- Exposure to ionising radiation (e.g., Chernobyl) or direct irradiation of the neck
  - Radiation-induced thyroid tumours that are papillary: 85%
- Familial—rare

What are the pathological features of a papillary cancer?

- Macroscopically—hard whitish nodule, often multifocal, rare to have encapsulation

- Microscopically—Orphan Annie cells and psammoma bodies
  - Also follicular, encapsulated, diffuse sclerosing and tall cell variants
- Early lymphatic spread
- Late haematogenous spreading to lungs and bones

What are the key surgical steps involved?

- A total thyroidectomy, including clearance of pretracheal and paratracheal lymph nodes, should be done.
- Biopsy nodes in the lateral carotid chain for the frozen section.
  - If results are positive, perform modified neck dissection.
- Thymus ideally is not removed; avoid devascularising inferior parathyroids.
- Excise adjacent structures (e.g., trachea) if local invasion is present.
- The only indication for a lobectomy/isthectomy alone is if the tumour is <1 cm in low-risk disease.
- There is <3% incidence of permanent postoperative hypoparathyroidism.

How would you follow up the patient?

- In the immediate postoperative period, determine serum calcium and PTH.
- Discharge with T3 and arrange a radioiodine scan at 6 weeks.
  - Stop T3 2 weeks before the scan (allows an increase in TSH levels).
  - If there are residual thyroid remnants/mets, uptake at 24 hr < 1%.
  - Restart T3 and repeat radioiodine scan at 3 months.
  - If scan is negative, convert to T4 until TSH < 0.1 IU.
  - If the scan is positive, treat with radioiodine until the scan is clear.
- Thyroglobulin levels should be checked annually in clinic.
  - This indicates residual or recurrent disease on suppressive T4 dose.
- The frequency of USS is uncertain.
  - An annual USS for 2 years probably constitutes good practice.

The patient is concerned about needing radioiodine treatment and being radio-active around her children. How would you explain the treatment to her?

- The radioiodine is given as a capsule.
- In the immediate postadministration period, she should remain well hydrated and flush the toilet twice on voiding.
- On leaving the hospital, public transport may be taken for journeys < 3 hr.
- She can return to work the next day.
- Children need to be >1 m away for 9–15 days, depending on dosage.
- Only 15 min of close contact is allowed for the first 21–25 days after radioiodine.
- She can share a bed with her partner; however, a high-dose treatment requires separate beds for 4 days.
- All utensils used must be rinsed thoroughly.

- Clothing does not need to be separated unless there has been excessive sweating.
- If the patient is the sole caregiver for the child, arrangements for care may have to be made for up to 25 days. Some centres isolate the patient for 24 hr.

What is her prognosis?

- Prognosis of papillary thyroid cancer is generally good.
- There is more than 90% survival at 20 years.
- Using the MACIS calculator, this patient has a 99% survival chance at 20 years.
  - M: metastases (+3 if present)
  - A: age (add 3.1 if 0–39 years, or 0.08 × age if >39 years)
  - C: completeness of resection (+1 if incomplete)
  - I: invasiveness (+1 if locally invasive)
  - S: size (0.3 × tumour size in centimetres)
    - If size is <6, then there is a 99% 20-year survival.
    - If size is >8, there is a 24% 20-year survival.
- Other scoring systems in use are:
  - AGES scoring system (Mayo Clinic)—age, grade, extent and size
  - AMES (age, metastasis, extent and size)

PHAEOCHROMOCYTOMA IN PREGNANCY

A pregnant (20 weeks' gestation) 28-year-old lady presented to her obstetrician with hypertension, headaches, dizziness and tachycardia. After initial testing, they are strongly suspicious this may be a phaeochromocytoma. She has been referred to you for further management. What genetic syndromes are linked to phaeochromocytoma?

- MEN2a—medullary thyroid cancer, phaeochromocytoma, hyperparathyroidism
  - RET gene mutations (10q11.2)
  - Autosomal dominant inheritance
  - Biochemical abnormality by age 30: 90%; clinical manifestations by age 50: 40%; by age 60: 50%
- MEN2b—medullary thyroid cancer, phaeochromocytoma, mucosal neuromas, intestinal ganglioneuromatosis, marfanoid habitus, café-au-lait spots
  - RET gene mutations (10q11.2)
  - Autosomal dominant inheritance
- Neurofibromatosis—phaeochromocytoma occurs in 1% of NF Type 1
  - Autosomal dominant (17q11.2)
  - In order to diagnose:
    - Six or more café-au-lait macules
    - Axillary/inguinal freckling
    - Two or more neurofibromas or one plexiform neurofibroma
    - Two or more Lisch nodules

- – Optic glioma
- – Distinctive osseus lesion (e.g., sphenoid dysplasia)
- – First degree relative or known carrier of mutation
- Von Hippel–Lindau syndrome—CNS haemangioblastoma, renal cell carcinoma and phaeochromocytoma
  - Autosomal dominant inheritance (3p25-26)

What are the risks in treating a pregnant patient with a phaeochromocytoma?

- The tumour is potentially dangerous.
- There is a significant mortality risk for both the mother and the infant.

What is your management plan for her phaeochromocytoma?

- Include obstetrician, endocrinologist, paediatrician and anaesthetist.
- Need to treat the patient's symptoms, deliver the baby safely and operate to remove the tumour safely.
- Symptom control:
  - Alpha blockade to control hypertension (e.g., phenoxybenzamine or doxazosin)
    - Typically takes 2–4 weeks
  - Beta blocker such as atenolol if there is persisting tachycardia when hypertension is controlled
- Delivery of baby:
  - Caesarean section in third trimester with or without a synchronous open adrenalectomy
  - Vaginal delivery contraindicated
    - Maternal mortality up to 30%
- Surgical treatment of tumour
  - Open adrenaletomy at time of caesarean section
  - Laparoscopic adrenalectomy an alternative if gestation is <24 weeks
  - Early open or laparoscopic adrenalectomy once the uterus has healed and the patient is haemodynamically in her prepregnancy state.
  - The anaesthetist should be experienced in dealing with phaeochromocytoma and the profound intraoperative hypotension which may occur on removal of the tumour
  - Postoperative monitoring on ITU, including glycaemic control

THYROID GOITRE

A 70-year-old man has been sent to your clinic with an obviously enlarged thyroid gland. How will you assess him?

- I would take a history enquiring about the following symptoms:
  - Irritating cough, shortness of breath, stridor or hoarse voice
  - Pain—due to infarction or haemorrhage into a cyst

- Dysphagia
- Rapid growth—possible malignancy
- Previous head and neck irradiation at a young age
- Symptoms of hyper/hypothyroidism
- Family history of MEN (may be relevant if dominant nodule)

- I would assess the quality of his voice, listening for hoarseness and stridor, and ask about obstructive airway symptoms.
- I would examine the neck. Is there a dominant nodule (risk of malignancy is the same as with a solitary nodule), cervical lymphadenopathy, retrosternal extension? I would then check for tracheal deviation and percuss the manubrium to assess retrosternal extension and auscultate for a bruit.
- Finally, I would check for Pemberton's sign, to look for thoracic outlet obstruction:
  - The patient raises arms above his head, which blocks venous return, facial veins dilate and the face becomes red.

What further investigations would you request?

- This is probably a multinodular goitre. However, if it has rapidly increased in size, anaplastic carcinoma needs to be ruled out.
- I would request thyroid function tests (T4 and TSH) and arrange an initial USS ± FNA of any dominant nodule.
- If the goitre is retrosternal, and the patient wanted surgery, I would ask for a CT scan to assess the trachea and the degree of retrosternal extension and consider spirometry to assess the degree of airway compromise.

What are the causes of a multinodular goitre?

- Most MNGs are due to enlargement of a simple goitre, which develops due to TSH stimulation secondary to low levels of thyroid hormones.
  - Iodine deficiency causes an endemic simple goitre which appears in childhood and evolves into a colloid goitre at a later stage.
  - The increased demand for thyroid hormone in pregnancy and puberty causes enlargement of a goitre.
  - Dietary goitrous agents in brassica vegetables, lithium and carbimazole also induce goitres.
  - Rare hereditary congenital defects in thyroid metabolism also cause goitres.
- Sporadic MNG can occur, commonly affecting middle-aged women.
- Previous radiotherapy to the neck (e.g., lymphoma) can also cause goitres.

When would you offer surgery for a multinodular goitre?

- When there is a suspicion of malignancy
  - Rapid growth, FNA results

- Patients with pressure symptoms
  - Shortness of breath, dysphagia, stridor
- For cosmesis, in patients with a large neck swelling

What are the operative specific concerns?

- The patient should be made euthyroid prior to surgery.
- I would inform the anaesthetist beforehand and ask him or her to see the patient prior to surgery. Fibre-optic intubation may be required.
- If there is a large retrosternal element, then cardiothoracic assistance may be needed to split the sternum.
- Flexible laryngoscopy to assess the recurrent laryngeal nerve is not mandatory unless the patient describes voice changes or the clinician suspects hoarseness.
- A unilateral thyroid lobectomy can be performed if one-half of the gland is obviously compressing trachea.
  - This is acceptable with the understanding that all thyroid tissue on the compressed side would be removed and any future operation would be done on the previously unoperated side.

REFERENCE

1. Siperstein, Allan, Eren Berber, German F Barbosa, Michael Tsinberg, Andrew B Greene, Jamie Mitchell and Mira Milas. 2008. Predicting the success of limited exploration for primary hyperparathyroidism using ultrasound, sestamibi, and intraoperative parathyroid hormone: Analysis of 1158 cases. *Annals of Surgery* 248 (3): 420–428.

BIBLIOGRAPHY

Gopan, Thottathil, Erick Remer and Amir H Hamrahian. 2006. Evaluating and managing adrenal incidentalomas. *Cleveland Clinic Journal of Medicine* 73 (6): 561–568.

Guidelines for the surgical management of endocrine disease and training requirements for endocrine surgery (www.baets.org.uk).

Hay, I D, E J Bergstralh, J R Goellner, J R Ebersold and C S Grant. 1993. Predicting outcome in papillary thyroid carcinoma: Development of a reliable prognostic scoring system in a cohort of 1779 patients surgically treated at one institution during 1940 through 1989. *Surgery* 114 (6): 1050–1057 (discussion 1057–1058).

Moertel, C G, L H Weiland, D M Nagorney and M B Dockerty. Carcinoid tumor of the appendix: Treatment and prognosis. *New England Journal of Medicine* 317 (27): 1699–1701.

Oliva, Raymond, Peter Angelos, Edwin Kaplan and George Bakris. 2010. Pheochromocytoma in pregnancy: A case series and review. *Hypertension* 55 (3): 600–606.

8 HPB Surgery

Saurabh Jamdar, Jeffrey Lordan, Dermot O'Riordan and Manel Riera

CONTENTS

COLORECTAL LIVER METASTASES

You see a 67-year-old patient in clinic with newly diagnosed synchronous metastatic sigmoid cancer. He has a high BMI. He has four metastases in segments 6, 7 and 8 and a small metastasis in segment 2. He has not yet had a sigmoid resection. How would you manage this patient?

- There are three key points to discuss. Firstly, is the liver disease resectable? Secondly, is the patient fit enough for a liver resection? Thirdly, if the patient is fit for surgery, I will need to liaise with the colorectal surgeon regarding timing of surgery.
- Regarding the disease, I would make sure the patient has had a CT chest/abdomen/pelvis for accurate staging and arrange a liver protocol CT and MRI if necessary. I would request a baseline CEA for future monitoring and discuss the patient in the HPB MDT.
- I would establish the patient's performance status, and if the disease was potentially resectable, I would arrange CPEX testing and an anaesthetic assessment.

The patient has no other metastases. Are his multiple liver lesions a contraindication to surgery?

- Not anymore. Resectability is now based on whether an R0 resection is possible and is determined by the size of the future liver remnant.

- The American HPB Association guidelines state that metastases are resectable if they can be completely resected, two adjacent liver segments can be spared with adequate vascular inflow, outflow and biliary drainage and the future liver remnant is ≥ 20%. If > 70%–80% of the liver needs to be resected, there is an increased risk of hepatic insufficiency. I might consider portal vein embolization or a two-stage technique to increase the size of the remnant.
- The outcome is still favourable in patients with <1 cm resection margins.

The CT showed a small lung metastasis. Would you still consider a liver resection?

- Yes, this is not a contraindication to surgery.
- I would consider liver surgery in patients with the following extrahepatic diseases:
  - Resectable/ablatable lung mets
  - Resectable/ablatable isolated extrahepatic mets (e.g., spleen, adrenal)
  - Local invasion of liver metastases into diaphragm/adrenals that could be resected

What are your thoughts regarding the timing of the bowel and liver operations?

- The decision to resect the primary colorectal lesion or the liver metastases first is due to local policy, as there is no evidence that the order makes any long-term difference.
- I would be reluctant to do a combined procedure in this case as the liver resection would be extensive, and there would be an increased risk of morbidity and mortality.
- As the metastases are synchronous, I would consider treating the patient with neoadjuvant chemotherapy. The EPOC 1 and EPOC 2 studies have suggested that neoadjuvant chemotherapy and adjuvant chemotherapy (sandwich chemotherapy) may confer long-term benefit.
- In EPOC 1,[1] patients were treated with sandwich FOLFOX and had a 9% survival benefit compared with surgery alone. However, this did not quite achieve significance. The EPOC 2 study, where patients are treated with sandwich FOLFIRI and cetuximab in patients with K-RAS wild type colorectal cancer, is still running.

HEPATOCELLULAR CARCINOMA

A 65-year-old male, with history of nonalcoholic steatohepatitis (NASH), presents with weight loss, loss of appetite and vague discomfort over the right upper quadrant. On examination he is mildly jaundiced and has hepatomegaly. How would you investigate this patient?

- I would take a thorough history and examine the patient.
- I would request blood tests (FBC, U+Es, LFTs, amylase and α-fetoprotein) and an urgent ultrasound.

- If the USS was suspicious for malignancy, I would request a triple phase CT scan with IV contrast, to assess the lesion and to look for evidence of metastatic disease and assess whether surgery is appropriate.

The USS shows a 3 cm lesion in the liver that looks like a hepatocellular carcinoma. How would you confirm the diagnosis?

- Ultrasound can detect large HCCs with high sensitivity and specificity.
- A raised AFP will help confirm the diagnosis; however 2/3 HCCs 4 cm have AFP levels < 200 ng/ml, and up to 20% do not produce AFP.
- If the CT is also suggestive of an HCC, the patient does not need a biopsy. There is a 1%–3% risk of seeding tumour in the biopsy tract, and tissue is not needed to confirm the diagnosis.

What are the typical features of hepatocellular carcinoma on CT?

- Hypodense lesions >2 cm in size.
- Hyperdense lesion on the arterial phase, iso/hypodense lesion on the portal venous phase, washout on delayed phase.
- Smaller lesions between 1 and 2 cm on CT, with a normal AFP, may need biopsy as the diagnosis is uncertain.
- Lesions smaller than 1 cm are difficult to characterize and a surveillance policy is advised.

What are the risk factors for developing HCC?

- The main risk factor is liver cirrhosis; the risk is further increased in older male patients and those with diabetes.
- Chronic viral hepatitis (HBV, HCV) is a risk factor.
- Nonalcoholic fatty liver disease, hereditary haemochromotosis and primary biliary cirrhosis are also risk factors.

How do you screen and follow up patients at risk of developing HCC?

- Abdominal ultrasound and AFP measurements should be done every six months.
- The basis of surveillance is to pick up small lesions that are potentially curable, but there is no evidence to confirm that earlier detection leads to a survival advantage.
- I would consider this in the high-risk patients:
  - Hep B and Hep C cirrhosis
  - Cirrhosis due to haemochromatosis and PBC
  - Patients with alcohol-related cirrhosis, who are abstaining

What factors contribute to the prognosis?

- Tumour size (TNM, AJCC)
- Number of lesions (TNM, AJCC)

- Vascular invasion (TNM, AJCC)
- Portal thrombosis
- Degree of liver failure per the Child–Pugh or MELT models
- WHO performance status

What are the treatment options?

- Transplantation is the only treatment for cirrhotic patients that also treats the underlying disease; otherwise, recurrence is likely. However, donor shortages and the Milan criteria for transplantation mean that less than 10% of patients are suitable for transplantation.
- Resection can be performed for noncirrhotic patients.
- This should be considered in patients with a single, small lesion (<5 cm) or up to three lesions < 3 cm.
- Portal embolisation of the affected lobe will help the remnant liver regenerate.
- If surgery is not possible, percutaneous ethanol injection (PEI) and chemo-embolization have been shown to produce tumour necrosis in small lesions.

JAUNDICE AFTER HEMIHEPATECTOMY

You are asked to see a patient who underwent a right hemihepatectomy 5 days ago who has now become jaundiced. What are the possible causes?

- There are several potential causes for developing jaundice:
  - The patient could have hepatic insufficiency. The risks of developing insufficiency increase with preoperative steatohepatitis associated with excess alcohol use, neoadjuvant chemotherapy (the effects of which are cumulative), perioperative blood transfusions and postoperative sepsis.
  - Another cause of postoperative jaundice is a bile leak from the anastomosis, resulting in a 'biloma'.
  - The patient may have had an intraoperative injury to the contralateral hepatic duct, resulting in a bile leak or biliary obstruction.

How would you manage this patient?

- I would review the patient by assessing his or her ABCs and looking at the patient's observation, fluid balance and drug charts, the operative note and the current medical notes.
- I would take blood for FBC, U+Es, LFTs, clotting and group and save.
- I would prescribe a litre of IV Hartmann's solution and contact the outreach and ITU teams to consider transfer to a level 2 bed.
- Ultimately, however, the patient requires cross-sectional imaging, and I would arrange a liver-specific contrast-enhanced CT.

How would you manage a biliary injury in this scenario?

- A biliary injury causing a bile leak can be managed radiologically, endoscopically or surgically.
- Depending on the level of injury, my first choice would be a radiological approach via a percutaneous transhepatic cholangiogram (PTC).
- This would allow placement of a plastic or covered (removable) metal stent, which can be protected by either an external drain or an internal–external drain.
- The advantage of this is that a PTC can be repeated a few days later to ensure correct placement of the stent and can demonstrate anatomical flow of contrast and, therefore, bile.

MANAGEMENT OF A BILE LEAK FOLLOWING LAPAROSCOPIC CHOLECYSTECTOMY

You performed an elective laparoscopic cholescystectomy on a 56-year-old man. He developed abdominal pain in the afternoon and was kept in overnight. In the morning he is pyrexial and still in pain. How will you manage him?

- I would suspect that he has a bile leak until proven otherwise.
- I would resuscitate the patient (ABCs, oxygen, IV fluids, opiate analgesia) and take bloods for FBC, U+Es, CRP, amylase, LFTs, ABGs and blood cultures.
- I would arrange an urgent USS to look for a bile collection.
- I would treat the sepsis with broad-spectrum antibiotics including GN bacterial coverage (e.g., IV Tazocin).

The USS shows a fluid collection in the right subphrenic space, and you suspect a bile leak. How will you treat the patient?

- My priority is to control the sepsis and the ongoing bile leak.
- If the patient was peritonitic, I would book him for an urgent laparoscopy and washout and place abdominal drains.
- If he was not peritonitic, I would arrange radiological drainage, as undrained bile can be lethal.
  - The absence of bile in a drain does not exclude a bile leak, and I would need to correlate this with my index of clinical suspicion.
- I would then consider an MRCP to confirm the leak and help plan definitive management.

What are the principles of MRCP?

- Heavily weighted T2 pulse sequences ensure a very high signal from stationary liquids such as bile and pancreatic juice (in contrast to blood, which has no signal due to its high velocity).

- The column of bile stands out as a hyperintense signal against the background of hypointense liver tissue.
- Hence, most of the time a detailed image can be seen without the use of contrast.

The MRCP suggests a small CBD injury. You confirm this at ERCP. How will you manage the patient?

- I would insert a plastic pigtail biliary stent and repeat the ERCP at 6–8 weekly intervals, to replace the stent and assess the rate of healing.

How would your management change if the MRCP suggested complete transection of the CBD?

- If this was identified early, and there was minimal peritoneal contamination or sepsis, I would consider early surgical repair in an HPB unit.
- However, in this case, with significant sepsis, I would defer surgery for 4–6 weeks.
  - This allows for maturation of adhesions and tissues at the porta hepatis.
  - Rehab at home, with nutritional support, may be necessary.
- I would request a preop CT to ensure that the abdominal collections have resolved, exclude liver atrophy and assess vascular anatomy.
- At 4–6 weeks, I would perform a hepaticojejunostomy using a 70 cm Roux limb loop of jejunum.
- This minimises risk of enteric reflux and chronic damage to the biliary tree.

What are the postop complications following hepaticojejunostomy?

- Cholangitis is treated with IV broad-spectrum antibiotics
- For recurrent anastomotic strictures and hepatodocholelithiasis, stents can be placed percutaneously.
  - Construction of an access loop at initial operation allows percutaneous drainage and calculus extraction via the subcutaneous jejunal loop.
- Liver atrophy and cirrhosis can occur.
- The predictors of poor outcome are involvement of biliary confluence, repair by injuring surgeon and more than three attempts at repair.

PANCREATIC CARCINOMA

A 62-year-old previously fit man has been transferred to you from the on-call medical team, after presenting with painless obstructive jaundice. There is no evidence of sepsis, but an ultrasound has shown grossly dilated intra- and extra-hepatic ducts and no gallstones. How would you manage this patient?

- I would reassess the patient to check that he does not have cholangitis and is not septic.
- I would take a comprehensive history and examine the patient (feeling for a palpable gallbladder, Virchow's node, hepatomegaly), but I would be concerned about a malignant process that requires further imaging.

- I would repeat the blood tests and request tumour markers CA 19-9 and CEA.
- I would then organise a pancreatic protocol CT (triple phase) and a staging CT (thorax, abdomen and pelvis).

What are the typical presenting symptoms of pancreatic cancer?

- Unexplained obstructive jaundice (with or without pain)
  - Jaundice due to primary disease causing biliary obstruction or enlarged porta hepatitis nodes
- Unexplained weight loss
- Late-onset diabetes
- Endoscopy-negative epigastric and back pain

What are the risk factors for developing pancreatic cancer?

- Smoking and obesity
- Chronic pancreatitis (18-fold higher risk)
- Type 2 diabetes (relative risk 1.8)
- Gardner's syndrome, MEN I, Peutz–Jeghers syndrome, FAP

The CA19-9 is raised, and the CT shows a suspicious 1.2 cm lesion in the pancreatic head with no evidence of metastatic disease. The bilirubin is 250.

- This is likely to be a resectable pancreatic tumour and I would consider surgery (pylorus-preserving pancreaticoduodenectomy).
- Firstly, establish whether the tumour is resectable and whether the patient is fit enough for surgery.
- To complete the staging, I would arrange an EUS to obtain more information regarding local respectability and an FNA to determine the cytology.
- To assess the patient for surgical resectability, I would assess his performance status, and organise cardiopulmonary exercise testing. This determines the perioperative risk and helps counsel and consent the patient prior to surgery.

The patient is medically fit for surgery, and the EUS confirms resectability. His bilirubin is still 220. How will you treat his jaundice?

- The literature shows that there is no benefit to preoperative stenting for a bilirubin < 200–250. The morbidity of ERCP can be detrimental rather than beneficial. I would correct any coagulopathy with vitamin K.
- However, if the bilirubin > 250 or if the patient had cholangitis, I would consider a preoperative stent with a plastic or covered (removable) metal stent.

Your patient asks you about this new cyberknife that he read about on the Internet. How would you advise him?

- I would explain that although there are many modalities of treatment, including chemotherapy and radiotherapy, surgical resection offers the best chance of long-term survival in patients with resectable disease.[2]

- Cyberknife is a method of delivering focused radiotherapy. However, in pancreatic cancer, there is no evidence that radiotherapy is beneficial.
- The ESPAC-1[3] study is probably the most important study. This was a European multicentre prospective RCT that included 550 patients with resectable pancreatic cancer. There were four arms:

Treatment	5-Year survival
Surgery alone	10.7%
Surgery + chemoradiotherapy	7.3%
Surgery + chemotherapy	29%
Surgery + chemoradiotherapy + chemotherapy	13.2%

- The chemotherapy used was gemcitabine. Therefore, I would recommend surgery with adjuvant chemotherapy and not offer radiotherapy.

PANCREATIC SEROUS CYST ADENOCARCINOMA

You see a 24-year-old lady in your clinic who was referred to you with an incidental pancreatic cyst found on an USS performed to investigate biliary colic symptoms. How would you manage this patient?

- The differential is benign or malignant disease. Benign causes are a simple cyst or a pancreatic pseudocyst. Malignant causes include IPMN, MCN, neuroendocrine tumours and pancreatic adenocarcinoma.
- I would take a comprehensive history, asking about steatorrhoea, jaundice, weight loss, shivers, sweating, diarrhoea, family history, smoking and diabetes. I would also ask about alcohol intake and previous attacks of pain (which may represent episodes of pancreatitis) and then examine the patient.

The patient describes no sinister symptoms. What do you do next?

- The cyst requires investigation. I would organise a triple-phase (pancreatic protocol) CT and a gut hormone screen and I would consider an endoscopic ultrasound (EUS) with FNA.
- The FNA will help determine the nature of the cyst:

	Pseudocyst	Benign cyst	Malignant cyst
Epithelial cells	No	Yes	Yes
Raised CEA	No	No	Yes
Raised amylase	Yes	No	No
Mucin	No	No	Yes (IPMN, MCN)
Malignant cells	No	No	Yes

The CT and FNA confirm a malignant serous cyst adenocarcinoma. Your patient tells you she wants a laparoscopic Whipple procedure after reading about it on the Internet. What do you tell her?

- I would discuss all the available treatment options with her, including doing nothing, as part of routine consent for surgery.
- My preferred treatment would be a pylorus preserving pancreatico-duode-nectomy (PPPD).
- There is no evidence that a classic Kausch–Whipple resection or a total pancreatectomy confers oncological benefit over a PPPD.
- There were concerns that a PPPD may have an increased incidence of delayed gastric emptying compared with Kausch–Whipple, but the evidence is weak.
- Furthermore, a Kausch–Whipple involves resection of the distal stomach, which may increase symptomatic reflux of enteric contents into the stomach.
- With regard to the laparoscopic approach, although some centres around the world are practicing this, this is not widely practiced in the UK and there is no evidence currently that this benefits patients versus an open resection.

RECURRENT CBD STONES

A 62-year-old lady had a laparoscopic cholecystectomy 1 year ago. She has presented with obstructive jaundice. Following US and MRCP assessment, she is found to have a small mobile stone in the distal CBD that measures 1.1 cm, with mild intrahepatic dilatation. How will you remove the stone?

- ERCP is preferable to surgery in postcholecystectomy patients.
- Duct clearance is possible in 90%–95% of patients after a sphincterotomy.
- In selected patients with stones < 15 mm, some centres use papillary dilatation rather than sphincterotomy to reduce morbidity.
- Stones > 15 mm can be difficult to remove and may need stone fragmentation by lithotripsy.
- If CBD stone extraction is incomplete/impossible, a stent still provides biliary decompression and prevents stone impaction of distal CBD.
  - The stents can block but biliary drainage often continues around the stent.
  - They may need changing in unfit patients if jaundice develops.

What is the incidence of retained or recurrent CBD stones?

- 2–5%
- More common in patients with primary CBD stones, large CBD diameters (>15 mm) and periampullary diverticula

How do you consent a patient for an ERCP?

- I would explain the indications for the procedure—to remove the stone and decompress the biliary system—and the consequences of not doing the procedure (progressive jaundice and sepsis).

- I would describe the procedure—endoscopy under sedation, use of contrast, sphincterotomy and stent placement, which may be removed 6 to 12 months later.
- I would discuss the common side effects and complications, and the rare but potentially serious complications (failure of the procedure, bleeding, pancreatitis, cholangitis and duodenal perforation).

What are the complications following ERCP?

- Major complications occur in 10% of patients.
  - Acute pancreatitis occurs in 7%.
  - Haemorrhage occurs in 0.8%.
  - Cholangitis occurs in 0.8%.
  - Retroduodenal perforation occurs in 0.08%
  - There is procedural mortality of 0.1%.
  - Thirty-day mortality can reach 15% (reflects severity of underlying disease).
- Pain during the procedure is an important indicator of an increased risk of post-ERCP pancreatitis (27%).
- Other independent risk factors for post-ERCP pancreatitis are:
  - History of recurrent pancreatitis, previous ERCP-related pancreatitis, multiple cannulation attempts and pancreatic brush cytology

REFERENCES

1. Nordlinger, Bernard, Halfdan Sorbye, Bengt Glimelius, Graeme J Poston, Peter M Schlag, Philippe Rougier, Wolf O Bechstein, et al. 2008. Perioperative chemotherapy with FOLFOX4 and surgery versus surgery alone for resectable liver metastases from colorectal cancer (EORTC Intergroup Trial 40983): A randomised controlled trial. *Lancet* 371 (9617): 1007–1016.
2. Pancreatic Section, British Society of Gastroenterology, Pancreatic Society of Great Britain and Ireland, Association of Upper Gastrointestinal Surgeons of Great Britain and Ireland, Royal College of Pathologists, Special Interest Group for Gastro-Intestinal Radiology. 2005. Guidelines for the management of patients with pancreatic cancer periampullary and ampullary carcinomas. *Gut* 54 (Suppl 5): v1–v16.
3. Neoptolemos, J P, J A Dunn, D D Stocken, J Almond, K Link, H Beger, C Bassi, et al. 2001. Adjuvant chemoradiotherapy and chemotherapy in resectable pancreatic cancer: A randomised controlled trial. 2001. *Lancet* 358 (9293): 1576–1585.

BIBLIOGRAPHY

Connor, S and O J Garden. 2006. Bile duct injury in the era of laparoscopic cholecystectomy E. *British Journal of Surgery* 93 (2): 158–168.
Ryder, S D, British Society of Gastroenterology. 2003. Guidelines for the diagnosis and treatment of hepatocellular carcinoma (HCC) in adults. *Gut* 52 (Suppl 3): iii1–iii18.

9 Transplant Surgery

Zia Moinuddin, Rajesh Sivaprakasam and David van Dellen

CONTENTS

ACCESS FOR DIALYSIS

A 67-year-old man with end-stage renal failure with an eGFR of 16 ml/min is referred to the vascular access clinic for creation of access for haemodialysis. He remains predialysis and is otherwise in reasonably good health. How would you proceed with your assessment?

- Obtain a full history—ask for symptoms of heart failure. An arteriovenous fistula increases the preload. This can adversely affect patients with heart failure.
- Check right- or left-hand dominance. The nondominant arm is always the first choice for creation of an AV fistula where possible.
- Perform clinical examination—full venous, arterial and cardiovascular examination.
- Perform venous and arterial duplex scanning of upper limbs (either bedside or formal depending on personal preference and expertise).

The vein mapping shows good quality signals in the radial, brachial and ulnar arteries bilaterally. The cephalic vein is 1.9 mm at the wrist and forearm and 3.2 mm at the elbow bilaterally. The basilic vein is 2.4 mm at the elbow and arm. Where would you create the AV fistula in this patient, who is right-hand dominant?

- The general rules are as follows:
  - Choose the nondominant arm.
  - Use as distal a site as possible to preserve venous real estate.

- Use the cephalic vein where possible, as it is more superficial, and the upper limbs before the lower limbs for creation of arteriovenous fistulae.
- However, several studies have shown that 2.0 to 2.5 mm is the threshold for creation of a successful arteriovenous fistula, especially at the wrist.
- Radiocephalic fistulae created with veins less than 2.0 mm in calibre have a 16% 3-month primary patency as compared with 76% for those with more than 2.0 mm in diameter.
- Therefore, a left brachiocephalic fistula would be the ideal first choice in this patient.

What are the advantages and disadvantages of elbow fistulae as compared to wrist fistulae?

- Advantages:
  - There are higher flow rates and quicker maturation than with wrist fistulae.
  - The cephalic vein is easier to cannulate in the upper arm.
- Disadvantages:
  - There is less long-term patency.
  - There is a shorter vein length for needling once dialysis commences.
  - It can lead to more arm swelling.
  - There is a higher incidence of steal phenomenon when compared to wrist fistulae.
  - There is a higher incidence of cephalic arch stenosis.

A 70-year-old diabetic who had a left brachiocephalic fistula created 6-months ago is referred, complaining of a painful, cold left hand which worsens whilst he is on dialysis. How would you manage this patient?

- Take full history and complete arterial assessment.
- A duplex scan is needed to assess arteries to rule out any proximal or distal arterial disease and assess fistula flow.
- Physiological steal is common in fistulae. Symptoms can occur on dialysis, as venous return is lower, which leads to a reduction in cardiac output. This lowers the perfusion pressure in the fistula outflow artery and the collaterals supplying the hand.
- Persistent symptoms (rest pain and ulceration) occur in pathological steal when there is either proximal or distal arterial disease. This requires further imaging with angiograms and revascularisation of the hand.
- Revascularisation can be achieved through a variety of methods:
  - Ligation of fistula
  - Banding of fistula (if preservation required)
  - DRIL (distal revascularisation and interval ligation) procedure—not commonly performed

What are the risk factors for developing ischaemic steal syndrome?

- ESRF and diabetes mellitus both significantly increase the risk of peripheral arterial disease.
- Age > 60
- Women
- Multiple operations on the same limb
- Use of PTFE grafts

BRAIN-STEM DEATH

A 45-year-old hypertensive male presented to A+E with a 24 hr history of severe headache. GCS was 15 on arrival but the patient suddenly deteriorated to a score of 3. He was intubated, ventilated and transferred to the intensive care unit. The CT scan shows a large subarachnoid haemorrhage with pronounced midline shift. He is unresponsive to any stimuli. There is suspicion that he might be brain-stem dead (BSD). At what point can testing for BSD be performed?

- Before brain-stem testing is done, the following preconditions must be met:
    - The patient must be in apnoeic coma. He or she must be unresponsive and dependent on mandatory continuous ventilation.
    - The underlying cause must be irreversible structural brain damage due to a disorder that can possibly result in brain stem death.
    - All possibilities of potential drug intoxication (recreational and thera-peutic), temperature aberration (particularly hypothermia) and possible metabolic disturbances must be excluded.
    - Beware of other causes which may potentially mimic BSD (Guillan–Barre syndrome and pontine infarction).
- The timing of testing can be considered from when the preceding precondi-tions can be fulfilled.
- In an apnoeic coma occurring following radiologically confirmed intra-cerebral haemorrhage, subarachnoid haemorrhage or major neurosurgery, brainstem testing can be performed after 6 hr of ventilation.
- In cases of hypoxic brain injury, there should be a minimum of 24 hr of ventilation prior to consideration of undertaking testing.

The preconditions have been met and the decision is made to proceed with BSD testing. What tests are used to confirm the absence of brain-stem reflexes? How are they performed? Which cranial nerves do they test?

- BSD testing must be performed by two experienced clinicians, of whom at least one must be a consultant; neither can be a member of the prospective transplant team.
    - Conduct apnoea testing.
    - Preoxygenate for 10 min.
    - Check $P_aCO_2 > 5.3$ kPa.
    - Disconnect ventilator until $P_aCO_2 > 6.65$ kPa.

- Monitor for absence of any signs of respiratory efforts.
- Cranial nerve testing
- There should be no pupillary reflex—fixed pupils with no response to light directly shined into eyes.
  - Afferent—II (optic)
  - Efferent—III (oculomotor)
- There should be no corneal reflex—absence of blinking to direct stimulation of cornea (by cotton wool or other similar substance taking care to avoid potential corneal abrasions).
  - Afferent—V (ophthalmic branch of trigeminal nerve)
  - Efferent VII (facial)
- There should be no vestibulo-ocular reflex—absence of eye movements when the tympanic membrane is irrigated with 20–50 ml ice-cold water or saline. Eyes should normally move away from the stimulating side.
  - Afferent—VIII (vestibular)
  - Efferent VI (abducent)
- There are no cranial nerve motor responses to a painful stimulus over area of distribution (usually supraorbital pressure).
  - Afferent—V (trigeminal)
  - Efferent VII (facial)
- There is no gag or cough reflex—absence of response to deep bronchial suctioning.
  - Afferent—IX (glossopharyngeal)
  - Efferent—X (vagus)
- There is no oculocephalic reflex (not required by UK legislation, but recommended in absence of cervical spine injury)—also termed doll's eye test: When the eyes are held open and the head moved briskly side to side, no eye movement is detected. Movement of eyes in the opposite direction implies brain-stem activity.
  - Afferent—VIII (vestibular)
  - Efferent VI (abducens)
- All the tests must be repeated at least twice after an elapsed time that is a matter of clinical judgement. Time of death is recorded as the time that the second round of testing occurs.

A 1-month-old child with meningitis has not responded despite treatment for an intracranial haemorrhage for over a week. He is being considered as a potential donor. Can BSD testing be performed in this scenario?

- Brain-stem death cannot be declared in children < 2 months of age.
- In children > 2 months old, the adult guidelines apply.

CARDIAC RISKS IN TRANSPLANTATION

A 55-year-old man with end stage renal failure due to chronic pyelonephritis is being assessed for renal transplantation. His past medical history includes hypertension; he has tablet-controlled non-insulin-dependent diabetes mellitus

as well as being an ex-smoker. His blood sugars are well controlled with metformin and he is currently predialysis with an eGFR of 20 ml/min. How would you formally assess his cardiac risk for transplantation?

- Obtain a full history to identify evidence of symptomatic coronary artery disease (CAD), cerebrovascular or peripheral vascular disease.
- Conduct a cardiovascular examination—look for any evidence of aortic or iliac disease, which may preclude successful transplantation.
- He should have routine cardiological investigations including ECG, chest x-ray and echocardiogram.
- Although asymptomatic, because of his NIDDM and age, he is a high cardiovascular risk candidate and should therefore undergo further intensive imaging—either a dobutamine stress echo or myocardial perfusions scan.
- Cardiopulmonary exercise testing aids in potential risk stratification and is becoming more widely utilised, although it is not yet validated in a renal failure population.

The echocardiogram shows some LV hypertrophy, but otherwise there is good overall systolic function (ejection fraction estimated at >60%). However, abnormalities are demonstrated on the myocardial perfusion scan. How will you proceed?

- There is no consensus over the management of asymptomatic patients.
- Referral to a cardiologist for coronary angiography may be considered, although concerns exist as to the potential nephrotoxicity of contrast media used for the investigation.
- Although there is no evidence that routine revascularisation in the majority of patients is beneficial, some patients with prognostically important disease (three-vessel disease) do benefit from revascularisation.

How would you proceed if this patient had angina on moderate exertion?

- Patients with symptomatic ischaemic heart disease should all be referred to a cardiologist for coronary angiography.
- Revascularisation should be performed by either stenting or bypass for any significant disease.
- Following successful treatment, patients can be considered for transplantation.

A 25-year-old patient with end stage renal failure due to IgA nephropathy is being assessed for renal transplantation. Apart from being on haemodialysis he is in reasonably good health. How would your assessment of his cardiac risk differ from the previous diabetic patient with asymptomatic ischaemic heart disease?

- The relative risk of cardiovascular death is disproportionately high in young dialysis patients.

- Assessment of this patient would therefore proceed along the lines of assessment for any asymptomatic high-risk patient with end stage renal failure.
- He should have a routine ECG and echocardiogram despite his age. He would not have a routine myocardial perfusion scan or dobutamine stress echo and CPEX testing unless there was a definitive indication or a strong family history.
- The high-risk group includes:
  - Age > 50
  - Diabetes
  - Coronary revascularisation > 3 years ago
  - Evidence of cerebrovascular or peripheral vascular disease
  - Abnormal resting ECG or echocardiogram
  - Smoker

How does renal failure increase the risk of cardiovascular disease?

- Volume overload due to excess fluid and anaemia leads to left ventricular hypertrophy.
- Increased after-load on the heart also results in left ventricular hypertrophy due to the creation of high-output cardiac failure.
- Abnormal mineral metabolism and hyperparathyroidism lead to arterial medial calcification.
- Cardiac myocyte injury and myocardial fibrosis are due mainly to raised PTH, angiotensin II and uraemic toxins.
- There is oxidant stress and inflammation.
- Hyperhomocysteinaemia increases the risk of endothelial injury leading to atherosclerosis.

CHRONIC TRANSPLANT DYSFUNCTION

A 50-year-old man is seen in the transplant clinic with progressively rising creatinine. He underwent a cadaveric renal transplant 5 years ago and is currently on maintenance immunosuppression of tacrolimus (1 mg bd) and Myfortic (360 mg bd). His creatinine over the last year has gradually increased from a baseline of about 250 to around 350 μmol/l. He is otherwise systemically well and continues to pass normal amounts of urine with no evidence of outflow obstruction. How would you investigate and manage this patient?

- A gradual rise in creatinine over time is suggestive of chronic transplant dysfunction (CTD).
- I would review the history to look for any symptoms of peripheral oedema, claudication or underlying urological problems. In addition, I would confirm compliance with immunosuppression and nephrotoxic medications. I would also establish the number and severity of previous episodes of acute rejection.
- Examination would focus on clinical stigmata of hypertension, fluid overload or dehydration, and vascular disease.

- I would ask for the following tests:
  - Serum biochemistry (to establish trends of creatinine and glomerular filtration rate over time), calcium, albumin, glucose, and HbA1c if diabetic
  - Tacrolimus levels (both current and historical; reduced levels suggest poor compliance and increased levels suggest drug-induced nephrotoxicity)
  - FBC and coagulation
  - HLA antibody screen
  - Check virology PCR: CMV, EBV, BK/JC titres
  - Urine for urinalysis, protein:creatinine ratio, MSU and cytology
  - Ultrasound of transplant kidney with Doppler study of renal artery to look for transplant renal artery stenosis
  - I will also arrange for an elective transplant kidney biopsy if all preceding tests were normal

All the tests are completely normal. There have been no episodes of rejection at any point in the post-transplantation period. Renal biopsy demonstrates interstitial fibrosis and tubular atrophy (IFTA) with no evidence of ongoing cell- or antibody-mediated rejection (AMR). What would be your next step in the management of this patient?

- The most important risk factors contributing to the development of IFTA are pre-existing donor disease, acute rejection, subclinical ongoing rejection and prolonged calcineurin inhibitor exposure (tacrolimus or cyclosporin).
- In the absence of ongoing cell- or antibody-mediated rejection, the mainstay of treatment of IFTA is immunosuppression modification via reduction in CNI exposure.
- In addition to this, general measures applicable to all patients are targeted:
  - BP control—target of 130/80 (aim for 125/75 if diabetic or significant proteinuria)
  - ACE inhibitors or angiotensin receptor blockers if diabetes or proteinuria present
  - Prophylaxis against cardiovascular disease with aspirin and statins
  - Anaemia treated and bone biochemistry optimised

Do all patients require a biopsy?

No. In some patients, CTD can be assumed:

- Pre-existing donor disease
- Patients > 3 years post-transplant with:
  - Slowly progressing reduction in GFR
  - Normal urinalysis (therefore, recurrent GN or transplant glomerulopathy unlikely)
  - Normal urine cytology (BK virus nephropathy unlikely)
  - No detectable donor-reactive HLA antibody (chronic antibody-mediated rejection unlikely)

- In such patients CNI withdrawal is likely to be safe with confirmatory biopsy at a later date.

Would it be appropriate to consider tacrolimus withdrawal in the patient?

- The criteria for calcineurin inhibitor withdrawal are:
  - >12 months post-transplant
  - No episodes of acute rejection in preceding 3 months
  - Biopsy demonstrating absence of cell- or antibody-mediated rejection (in most cases)
  - No contraindications to mycophenolic acid or other antiproliferative therapy
- Based on these criteria, this patient would be suitable for consideration of tacrolimus withdrawal.

How would you withdraw tacrolimus in this patient?

- Establish therapeutic MMF (1 g bd) or MPA (720 mg bd) dose. Azathioprine is a reasonable alternative in MMF-/MPA-intolerant patients.
- Progressively reduce the calcinuerin inhibitor dose by 50% every 2–4 weeks until it is stopped.
- Patients should be reviewed before every dose reduction and every 2–3 weeks for 3 months.

What are the causes of chronic transplant dysfunction?

- CTD is the result of ongoing graft injury on the background of established graft damage. Factors affecting graft injury begin even before transplantation. They include:
  - Pre-existing donor disease
  - Injury at organ retrieval
  - Ischaemia-reperfusion injury

Post-transplant graft injury may be immune or nonimmune mediated:

- Immune-mediated graft injury
  - Acute cellular- or antibody-mediated rejection
  - Subclinical rejection
  - Chronic antibody-mediated rejection
  - Recurrent glomerulonephritis
- Non-immune-mediated graft injury
  - Obstruction (ureteric or bladder outflow)
  - Recurrent UTI with pyelonephritis
  - Renal vascular stenosis
  - Atheromatous vascular disease
  - Hypertension

- Calcineurin inhibitor toxicity
- BK virus nephropathy
- Diabetes mellitus

INFECTIONS FOLLOWING TRANSPLANTATION

A 40-year-old presents to the transplant clinic with a short history of fever, night sweats, arthralgia and anorexia. He is 5 months postcadaveric renal transplantation. His immunosuppressive regimen is mycophenolate mofetil and tacrolimus. Blood tests show slightly raised creatinine along with leucopenia and a mild transaminase rise. How will you manage this patient?

- I will review the history to identify signs and symptoms of common infections and then examine the patient.
- In addition to the U&Es, LFTs, FBC and CRP, request screening for viral infections (CMV, EBV, BK/JC) and also check drug (tacrolimus) levels.
- I would also check the donor and recipient CMV status at the time of transplantation and ascertain both the presence and duration of CMV prophylaxis treatment.
- Send blood and urine for culture and request a chest x-ray and USS of the transplant kidney.

The tacrolimus levels are 14 and CMV PCR is positive (log 3.2). How will you manage this patient?

- This patient has symptomatic CMV viraemia. Antiviral therapy with oral valganciclovir or IV ganciclovir is the mainstay of treatment.
- Treatment is usually for 2 weeks or until CMV PCR is negative. Tissue-invasive disease may require 4–6 weeks of therapy. Following treatment, I would continue with serial CMV monitoring for any disease reactivation.
- As his tacrolimus levels are high, I would reduce the tacrolimus dosage and monitor closely for any further relapses of infection. Overimmunosuppression often presents with intercurrent infection.

What do you know about CMV prophylaxis in transplant patients?

- The simplest strategy is to offer all high-risk patients prophylaxis:
  - All CMV-negative patients receiving organs from a CMV positive donor
  - Patients receiving T-cell depleting antibodies if either the donor or the recipient is CMV positive
- Valganciclovir is the most common antiviral in use for CMV prophylaxis:
  - Treatment is commenced within 10 days of transplantation.
  - The dose is based on the creatinine clearance.
  - Prophylaxis is currently recommended for 100 days in most cases.

What are the modes of CMV infection in transplant patients and when does it usually occur?

- Transplant patients develop CMV disease in several ways:
  - Transmission of virus with the donor organ:
    - Primary infection of nonimmune CMV recipients
    - Superinfection with a different CMV strain if seropositive
  - Reactivation of latent infection
- CMV infections (opportunistic and unconventional infections) typically occur between 1 and 6 months after transplantation, during the period of maximal immunosuppression. Infections within the first month are generally nosocomial and related to transplant surgery. After 6–12 months, infections are usually caused by conventional community pathogens.

How does CMV affect the transplant recipient?

- Direct effects:
  - CMV infection (asymptomatic viraemia) may occur.
  - CMV disease may occur:
    - Symptomatic viraemia
    - Tissue-invasive disease—gastrointestinal, pneumonitis, chorioretinitis or graft dysfunction
- Indirect effects:
  - Immunosuppression—CMV infection suppresses both T-cell- and B-cell-mediated immunity, leading to superimposed opportunistic infections.
  - Acute rejection—despite enhancing immunosuppression, CMV also increases HLA class I and II expression within the organ transplant, leading to increased acute rejection.
- Long-term effects:
  - CMV infection has been associated with the development of allograft vasculopathy and new onset diabetes after transplantation (NODAT).

LIVE KIDNEY DONATION

A 35-year-old woman with end stage renal failure, who has been active on the cadaveric renal transplant waiting list, presents to transplant clinic with her husband as a potential live donor. He is a medically fit and well 40-year-old man, apart from a history of hypertension. How would you proceed with your assessment of the donor?

- Obtain a full history focused particularly on:
  - Identification of possible risk factors for future development of renal disease
  - Exclusion of diseases potentially transmissible to recipient
  - Assessment of fitness of donor for surgery

- Hypertension is a risk factor for chronic kidney disease (CKD) and precludes organ donation if:
  - There is any evidence of end-organ damage—left ventricular hypertrophy or proteinuria.
  - The potential donor is on more than two antihypertensive agents.
- Measure the BMI: BMI > 35 is an absolute contraindication to donation. Ideally, BMI should be less than 30 to minimise potential risks to the donor.
- General examination should be focussed on previous surgery or other preclusions to successful donation.
- Urinalysis for blood, protein and pyuria should be done.
- Arrange initial investigations:
  - FBC, U&Es, LFT, Ca, coagulation
  - Fasting blood glucose
  - Virology—hepatitis B, C, HIV, CMV, EBV and syphilis serology
  - Urine protein/creatinine ratio and MSU
  - Chest x-ray and ECG
  - Echocardiogram to rule out left ventricular hypertrophy—especially important as he has hypertension
- If these investigations are satisfactory, I will then arrange:
  - Renal USS to look for the presence of two normal kidneys
  - Isotope renogram to check individual kidney function
  - CT angiogram to delineate renal anatomy

Urinalysis reveals microscopic haematuria, but all the other tests are normal. What would be your next course of action?

- All potential donors with microscopic haematuria should undergo a urological assessment and formal cystoscopy.
- If no cause is found and the assessment is otherwise normal, the potential donor should have a renal biopsy to rule out glomerulonephritis.

All investigations are satisfactory and you find the donor suitable to proceed pending review of the isotope scan and CT angiogram. The isotope scan reveals equal function in both kidneys. The CT angiogram reveals a single renal artery and vein on the right but two renal arteries and one vein on the left. How would you proceed?

- Results should be reviewed at a multidisciplinary meeting including the transplant coordinator, donor and recipient surgeons and radiologist.
- A left kidney with two arteries is usually still preferable to a right kidney with a single artery unless there is a significant difference in the divided function. This is due to the fact that the renal vein is longer facilitating ease of implantation.
- However, choice of kidney for donation remains for discussion between both retrieving and implanting surgeons, with various risks and benefits discussed with both patients if possible.

- Multiple arteries are usually reconstructed prior to implantation, to allow for a single arterial anastomosis.

RENAL GRAFT THROMBOSIS

A 63-year-old female underwent renal transplantation from an extended criteria donor. On the second postoperative day, she develops sudden-onset oliguria. How would you manage her?

- I would resuscitate her, exclude a blocked urinary catheter and take bloods to check the renal function and clotting.
- My main concern is that she has a graft thrombosis, which is a graft-threatening situation and needs urgent intervention.
- Patients typically present with increasing pain from the graft, oliguria or anuria and macroscopic haematuria.
- I would arrange an urgent Doppler scan of the kidney to look for a thrombus.

The USS showed a renal vein thrombosis. What are the risk factors for developing a thrombosis?

- Retrieval injury (e.g., traction-induced intimal tear)—more common in kidney-only retrievals and in donors after cardiac death
- Atherosclerosis of the donor and recipient vessels
- Evidence of external compression by haematoma/urinoma
- Episodes of hypotension in the peri and postoperative periods
- Hypercoagulable state

How will you treat her?

- Ensure that hyperkalaemia has been corrected and consider haemofiltration in theatre to reduce any operative delay.
- Consent the patient for an urgent exploration of the graft and take to theatre.
- Arrange for an appropriate graft preservative solution in theatre so that the graft can be perfused and assessed for the reimplantation.
- Warn the patient that she may need to have a graft nephrectomy.

The kidney appears dusky and a renal vein thrombosis is confirmed. After perfusion, there was also evidence of an arterial intimal tear. What is your approach?

- This is a difficult decision; contact a colleague to discuss the options for graft preservation.
- Unless the graft thrombosis is diagnosed early, thrombectomy will not salvage the graft, and graft nephrectomy is inevitable.

SIDE EFFECTS OF IMMUNOSUPPRESSION

A 40-year-old woman who underwent cadaveric renal transplantation 2 months ago is seen in the transplant clinic. She is taking tacrolimus (4 mg bd) and mycophenolic acid (720 mg bd) for immunosuppression. She is feeling well and has stable graft function. However, upon reviewing her bloods, you notice that her white cell count has been steadily drifting downwards and is currently at 2.8. How will you manage this patient?

- WCC will require close monitoring and therefore more frequent follow-up.
- If it continues to fall, mycophenolic acid (an antiproliferative) will need either dose reduction or withholding until the WCC improves, as one of the drug's side effects is marked bone marrow depression.
- Also, check if patient is taking valganciclovir, septrin or any other medication that can cause leucopaenia and stop them appropriately.
- A full virological screen will need to be undertaken as this can also result in unexplained refractory leucopaenias.
- If the WCC continues to fall despite all these measures, the patient will require granulocyte colony-stimulating factor (G-CSF) and prophylactic antibiotics.

A 46-year-old man is seen in the transplant clinic a month after a cadaveric renal transplant. His immunosuppressant regimen is tacrolimus (5 mg bd) and mycophenolic acid (720 mg bd). His main complaint is of diarrhoea of 2-week duration with him opening his bowels at least six times a day. His graft function remains stable and he is otherwise well. How will you manage this patient?

- Examine the patient, review inflammatory markers and send stool for microscopy and culture.
- The most likely cause of diarrhoea is drug induced.
- Both mycophenolic acid and tacrolimus can cause diarrhoea or bowel frequency, although antiproliferatives such as mycophenolic acid are more commonly responsible.
- In the absence of any infective or organic cause, the dose of antiproliferative can be split into smaller, more frequent doses (although this use is currently off licence). The other options include changing to another antiproliferative with equivalent actions, such as azathioprine or, alternatively, dose reduction (if sufficient immunosuppressive load from other drugs because of rejection risk).
- Monitor tacrolimus trough levels closely as they tend to go up in patients with diarrhoea.
- If the diarrhoea persists despite these measures and with potential infective causes excluded, further investigation to rule out other causes is warranted and should focus on imaging of the large and small bowel.

A 26-year-old man who underwent a cadaveric renal transplant 2 years ago is seen in the follow-up clinic. He complains of feeling tired, weight loss and lumps in his groin. He is of Asian origin and is currently on tacrolimus monotherapy. How will you manage this patient?

- The differential diagnosis is likely to be infective causes (particularly TB with the symptom and patient history) or potentially post-transplant lymphoproliferative disorder (PTLD).
- Take a full history and do a systematic examination, particularly focusing on respiratory examination for potential TB and an examination for potential lymphadenopathy or hepatosplenomegaly.
- Get a full set of screening tests, including graft function, and routine blood tests including LDH and virology (CMV, BK but particularly EBV serology)
- EBV infection is a common predisposing factor for PTLD development, especially in young transplant recipients.
- Request a chest x-ray.
- A lymph node biopsy can be used for histological diagnosis.

Biopsy shows a Burkitt's type lymphoma. EBV serology is positive. All other blood tests are normal, apart from a raised LDH. What are the next steps in the management of this patient?

- An oncological staging CT scan should be performed.
- Antiproliferative agents (azathioprine or MMF) should be stopped.
- Aim to reduce the calcineurin inhibitor dose by 50% over 2–4 weeks.
- Continue steroids or consider increasing the dose of steroids if acute rejection is a concern—the risk of graft loss needs to be countered by the oncological concerns of heavy immunosuppression.
- Consider replacing CNI with sirolimus (mammalian target of rapamycin (MTOR) inhibitor) as the immunosuppressant blocks growth-factor-driven proliferation of many cell types including malignant cells.
- Assess the patient's response by serial LDH measurements.
- Refer him to haematologists for oncological input.
- Chemotherapy might be required if these measures do not help or if acute rejection occurs with reduction in immunosuppression.
- The most common regime is CHOP (cyclophosphamide, doxorubicin, vincristine and prednisolone) ± rituximab.

What other malignancies are transplant patients particularly at increased risk of developing?

- Skin cancers—mainly nonmelanoma skin cancers (half of all post-transplant cancers) and especially basal cell carcinomas
- Melanomas and Kaposi sarcomas
- Squamous cell carcinoma of oral cavity, perineum, anus and penis

- Renal cell carcinoma, especially in patients with acquired cystic kidney disease
- Transitional cell carcinoma of the bladder, oesophageal, lung and colon cancer—a modest twofold increase with long-term immunosuppression
- Patients with pre-existing cancers—generally require a 5-year window period prior to being considered for transplantation, although lower risk cancers can be considered after 2 years of disease-free survival.

10 Upper GI Surgery

Naheed Farooq, Dermot O'Riordan,
Dimitri Pournaras, Manel Riera and Andy Tsang

CONTENTS

ACHALASIA

A 51-year-old female complains of dysphagia, retrosternal pain on swallowing and regurgitation of food. Discuss your management.

- Take a history—duration of symptoms, difficulty on swallowing fluids or solids, associated respiratory problems (due to regurgitation). These presenting symptoms suggest a possible diagnosis of achalasia.
- Clinical examination is generally normal.
- Arrange an urgent endoscopy to exclude pseudoachalasia due to a distal oesophageal tumour. In early achalasia, the typical findings of a dilated oesophagus containing undigested food and a tight gastric cardia may not be seen.
- If achalasia is suspected, the gold standard investigation is oesophageal manometry—hypertensive nonrelaxing lower oesophageal sphincter in response to wet swallows and loss of peristaltic activity in the oesophagus.

The endoscopy and manometry studies confirm achalasia. What are the treatment options?

- There are three treatment options—botulinum toxin injection, pneumatic dilatation and surgical cardiomyotomy. I would reserve Botox injections for patients unfit for other treatments, as they are the least effective.[1]

319

- Pneumatic balloon dilatation is effective in up to 90% of patients, but often needs repeating. There is evidence to support dilatation over surgery, provided the balloon size < 30 mm.[2]
  - The most serious complication of dilatation is perforation (up to 5%).
- Surgical cardiomyotomy is a definitive treatment.

Briefly describe how you would perform a surgical cardiomyotomy.

- Laparoscopic myotomy from the gastro-oesophageal junction, continued distally no further than 2 cm onto the stomach.
- It ensures that muscle fibres of the oesophagus, lower oesophageal sphincter region and cardia are adequately divided to expose the underlying mucosa.
- Simultaneously perform an antireflux procedure (partial anterior Dor fundoplication) because there is a high risk of gastro-oesophageal reflux after division of the lower oesophageal sphincter.
- Total fundoplication is often avoided because of the aperistaltic oesophagus, and increased risk of post-up dysphagia.

What determines the extent of your proximal oesophageal myotomy and why?

- As long as the thickened musculature of the lower oesophageal sphincter region is divided, the proximal extent is less important
- However, most surgeons will perform a proximal myotomy of about 6 cm.
- The myotomy should not extend high into the mediastinum—limited so as to limit the ability to suture repair a mucosal breach.
- Consider water-soluble contrast swallow (exclude mucosal breach).

BARIATRIC SURGERY

Why should surgery be offered for the treatment of morbid obesity?

- Obesity, with its associated comorbidities, is rapidly becoming a global epidemic. It is estimated that in England alone the cost to the NHS of treating obesity and its related disorders is £480 million and the impact on the NHS as a whole £4.3 billion.
- Obese subjects have a reduced life expectancy due to cancer-related deaths, coronary artery disease and diabetes with the obese person expected to die 11 years prematurely compared with a normal weight individual.
- Bariatric surgery has been shown to be the only effective treatment for weight loss and weight loss maintenance.
- In addition, it is now becoming recognised that bariatric surgery has profound metabolic benefits, in particular for patients with type 2 diabetes.[3] These effects may be more important than weight loss itself. This is reflected in the renaming of both the US and UK national bariatric surgical organisations to include the word 'metabolic'.

Which patients are eligible for bariatric surgery on the NHS?

- The NICE Guidance 2006[4] criteria:
  - Body mass index (BMI) > 40 or more with or without obesity-related disorders
  - BMI of 35–40 with obesity-related disorders (type 2 diabetes, obstructive sleep apnoea, hypertension and osteoarthritis)
  - Nonoperative measures at weight loss have failed and been attempted for at least 6 months.
- Patients who do not meet the criteria may be approved for CCA funding in exceptional cases on clinical grounds.
- CCAs may deny funding to suitable patients.

Which bariatric surgical procedures are available for the treatment of obesity?

- There are four operations available for the treatment of obesity:
  - Laparoscopic adjustable gastric band (LAGB)
  - Laparoscopic sleeve gastrectomy (LSG).
  - Laparoscopic Roux-en-Y gastric bypass (LRYGB)
  - Biliopancreatic diversion (BPD) and duodenal switch (DS)—now rarely performed

How does a gastric band work?

- The band is placed around the upper part of the stomach with the creation of a 20 ml volume pouch above it and the fundus sutured over the band to create an anterior tunnel to prevent slippage.
- The band is adjusted by fluid inflation or deflation via a port to restrict the passage of food into the distal stomach, thus creating the feeling of early satiety.
- The average loss of excess body weight at 2 years with an LAGB is 40%.

How does a sleeve gastrectomy work?

- The body and fundus of the stomach are excised vertically using a linear stapler to create a narrow gastric tube along the lesser curve with a capacity of approximately 150–200 ml.
- The average loss of excess body weight at 2 years with an LSG is 50%.

How does a Roux-en-Y bypass procedure work?

- This is the most effective surgical procedure with both weight loss and metabolic benefits.
- A small 20 ml gastric pouch is formed by division of the gastric body and fundus and a distal jejunal limb is anastomosed to the pouch.
- Approximately 100 cm of the distal jejunal limb is then bypassed before the proximal biliary jejunal limb is anastomosed to the distal jejunal limb.
- The average loss of excess body weight at 2 years with an LRYGB is 70%.

What are the advantages and disadvantages of each bariatric surgical procedure?

- Laparoscopic adjustable gastric band:
  - Advantages:
    - Safe (operative mortality < 0.1%), reversible, adjustable, and does not disrupt normal anatomy
    - Does not prevent further bariatric surgery
  - Disadvantages:
    - Complications (e.g., slippage/gastric prolapse that can lead to gastric ischaemia/infarction, band erosion [1%])
    - Regular follow-up needed in order to achieve good results
    - Interestingly, 10% of patients develop complications within 10 years and as many will request removal of their band due to these complications within the same time period.
- Laparoscopic sleeve gastrectomy:
  - Advantages:
    - Safe and very effective bariatric procedure with operative mortality of 0.2%
    - No adjustments required and therefore a single one-off procedure; technically simple to perform and no disruption to small bowel anatomy
    - Does not preclude further bariatric surgery
  - Disadvantages:
    - Staple line leakage, tube stenosis, and exacerbation of acid reflux
    - Potential weight regain
    - Irreversibility
- Laparoscopic Roux-en-Y gastric bypass:
  - Advantages:
    - Most effective weight loss treatment, single one-off procedure
    - Dramatic metabolic benefits leading to improved glycaemic control and remission of diabetes, improvement in hypertension and hypercholesterolaemia in a large proportion of patients
  - Disadvantages:
    - Operative mortality (0.5%), anastomotic leak, internal herniation, gastrojejunal stenosis, marginal ulceration, vitamin and mineral deficiency requiring lifelong supplementation of iron, vitamin B12, calcium, and multivitamins
    - Irreversible surgery

How would you decide what bariatric procedure is most suitable for an obese patient?

- There are no clear recommendations.
- Many factors must be considered, including patient choice and surgical expertise.

- The MDT is also responsible but the patient's choice is of paramount importance and all patients should be informed appropriately regarding the different types of procedures.
- Patients are encouraged to attend patient support groups allowing direct contact with patients who underwent different procedures. The surgeon performing the operation should be adequately trained for the individual procedure offered and the environment should be a centre in which weight loss surgery is performed in high volumes and at high frequency.
- Other factors that must be considered are the degree of obesity (each procedure has a different weight loss profile), associated comorbidities, risks of surgery, patient compliance and eating habits.
- There is a risk-to-benefit ratio for each operation. Choosing the lowest risk surgery may not benefit the patient in the long term, and the converse is also true. For example, an obese patient with a BMI of 70 with type 2 diabetes and obstructive sleep apnoea is unlikely to achieve the same benefits from an LAGB as an LRYGB, whereas a patient with a BMI of 35 but no metabolic disorders may benefit from a lower risk LAGB than the higher risk LRYGB.

Due to the high incidence of gallstones amongst the obese population, would you routinely perform a cholecystectomy at the same time as the bariatric operation?

- This is a controversial area, as about half of these patients will have symptomatic gallstones.
- ERCP after an LRYGB is notoriously difficult due to the altered anatomy. Conversely, laparoscopic cholecystectomy in morbidly obese patients can be technically challenging and there is no reason this cannot be performed at a later interval after laparoscopic bariatric surgery, particularly as adhesions are less likely to be troublesome.
- A complication of cholecystectomy in a patient who has also undergone simultaneous gastric bypass may be catastrophic due to the catabolic state these patients are in.
- Gastric banding includes the implantation of a foreign body and hence a cholecystectomy would increase the risk of infection. It should also be mentioned that additional ports may be needed for the cholecystectomy.
- Finally, a prophylactic cholecystectomy is not included in the current funding tariff for bariatric surgery and would therefore be a direct cost to the hospital itself. Although a prophylactic cholecystectomy is performed routinely in some parts of the United States, there is no recommendation for this in the UK.

BARRETT'S OESOPHAGUS

You perform an upper GI endoscopy on a 48-year-old man with symptoms of acid reflux and discover he has Barrett's oesophagus. What is Barrett's oesophagus (BE)?

- It is an endoscopically visible columnar epithelium within the oesophagus, with glandular metaplasia on histological examination.
- It is found more commonly in patients undergoing endoscopy for symptoms of gastro-oesophageal reflux and this is accepted as the leading cause of Barrett's metaplasia.
- The theory is that acid injures the squamous epithelium of the oesophagus and subsequent repair occurs, but the abnormal acid environment affects healing and columnar cells replace the native squamous epithelium.

How would you manage this patient?

- Barrett's oesophagus is a premalignant condition, with a 30- to 50-fold increased risk of developing oesophageal cancer; however, the actual incidence of cancer within BE remains low.
- Carcinogenesis follows a sequence from intestinal metaplasia to low- and high-grade dysplasia followed by invasive cancer.
- Systematic biopsies of the Barrett's segment are needed to assess for these changes (four quadrantic biopsies for every 2 cm length of BE).
- Surveillance involves endoscopic evaluation every 2 years—ideally, with high-resolution endoscopy and systematic biopsies.

This gentleman's biopsies demonstrated areas of high-grade dysplasia within the Barrett's oesophagus. How will you manage him?

- Repeat biopsies on PPI treatment to assess degree of dysplasia.
- I would then discuss the case with a specialist UGI MDT, and arrange EUS to ensure no invasive component.
- The standard of care used to be oesophagectomy.
- However, endoscopic mucosal resection is now considered appropriate management for areas of high-grade dysplasia within Barrett's oesophagus and for macroscopic oesophageal mucosal abnormalities.[5]
- EMR, in conjunction with ablative therapies (laser, electrocoagulation, cryotherapy or RFA depending on local expertise), for residual areas of dysplastic mucosa forms the basis of intensive follow-up.
- Acetic acid chromoendoscopy enhances the detection of occult neoplasia in BE.[6]

GASTRIC CANCER AND *HELICOBACTER PYLORI*

A 70-year-old lady is referred for an OGD to investigate epigastric discomfort and a microcytic anaemia. You find a malignant-appearing 3 cm ulcer in the gastric antrum. Biopsies confirm adenocarcinoma and *Helicobacter pylori*. What is the relevance of *H. pylori*?

- *Helicobacter pylori* organisms damage gastric mucosa by producing urease and ammonia, acetaldehyde, a vacuolating toxin and mucolytics. These attract inflammatory cells and produce free radicals, which cause acute and then chronic gastritis.

- Chronic superficial gastritis can progress to atrophic gastritis, intestinal metaplasia, dysplasia and eventually gastric cancer.
- *H. pylori* eradication reduces the inflammatory reaction and halts the development of intestinal metaplasia.
- There is no clear evidence, however, that *H. pylori* eradication prevents gastric cancer, but it does prevent progression of precancerous lesions.
- Paradoxically, it has been suggested that community-based programmes to eradicate *H. pylori* may actually be contributing to the rise in gastro-oesophageal junction cancers.
- It is thought that the hypochlorhydria associated with *H. pylori* and the ammonia produced by the bacteria from urea protect the lower oesophagus by changing the content of the refluxing acid content; this protective mechanism is lost by eradication of *H. pylori*.

What are the next steps in the management of this lady's malignant gastric ulcer?

- She needs staging (CT chest, abdomen and pelvis) to assess for metastatic disease.
- I will discuss the results in a UGI MDT.

Would you consider endoscopic treatment for this lady?

- I might, since the criteria have been extended by the Japanese Gastric Cancer Association from mucosal cancer, well differentiated nonulcerated small lesions (<2 cm) to any size (elevated), ulcerated (<3 cm) lesions including those of undifferentiated subtype.[7]
- However, mucosal disease is associated with a 0%–3% incidence of lymph node metastases and this rises to 20% for cancers extending to the submucosa.

This lady is fit for radical therapy. How would you proceed?

- She requires a diagnostic laparoscopy to assess for small-volume peritoneal disease and to assess the local spread of the tumour to ensure operability.
- In the UK, perioperative chemotherapy is the standard of care for patients with localised gastric or junctional adenocarcinoma.
- The MAGIC trial[8] randomised 503 patients with gastric, gastro-oesophageal junction or lower oesophageal adenocarcinoma to perioperative ECF (epirubicin, cisplatin and 5-FU), administered as three cycles before and after surgery, or to surgery alone.
  - In the group undergoing chemotherapy, there was evidence of tumour down-staging without an increase in postoperative complications.
  - Furthermore, this group had a statistically significant improvement in overall survival from 23% to 36%.

What type of operation would be appropriate for this lady?

- A distal gastrectomy with a modified D2 lymphadenectomy (i.e., pancreas and spleen preserving) would be appropriate.
- Limited gastric resections should only be used for palliation or the very elderly.
- The distal pancreas and spleen should only be removed if there is direct invasion of these organs and still a chance of curative R_0 resection in patients with proximal gastric cancers.

You are asked to see a 78-year-old lady on the medical ward admitted with vomiting and dehydration. A plain abdominal radiograph shows a grossly distended stomach. You suspect she may have gastric outlet obstruction (GOO). Discuss how you would manage her.

- Start IV fluid resuscitation and correct electrolyte abnormalities (hypochloraemic, hypokalaemic metabolic alkalosis).
- Take a history, looking for symptoms suggestive of malignancy or chronic peptic ulceration.
- Examine looking for signs of dehydration, a succussion splash, abdominal distension or mass.
- Place a large-bore nasogastric tube; lavage may be needed.
- Once resuscitated, arrange a CT scan with oral contrast to look for mechanical obstruction (intraluminal or extraluminal, benign or malignant).
- An OGD may be necessary to obtain biopsies to confirm malignancy, but only if the stomach has been adequately emptied via nasogastric aspiration.
- Therapeutic measures depend upon the cause of the obstruction. Localised malignant disease should be managed per MDT discussion.
- Options for palliation include endoscopic stents, gastroenterostomy (laparoscopic) and palliative distal gastrectomy.
- For benign causes, the options include balloon dilatation, endoscopic stents or gastroenterostomy (laparoscopic, Roux-en-Y).

GASTRO-OESOPHAGEAL REFLUX DISEASE

A 35-year-old male is referred to your clinic complaining of severe burning retrosternal pain typical of gastro-oesophageal reflux disease. He has been taking omeprazole (40 mg/day) for 6 months with minimal relief. How will you manage him?

- I would take a detailed history and examine the patient. Symptoms of regurgitation, stasis of food and dysphagia might suggest a hiatus hernia or oesophageal dysmotility.
- It is important to exclude dysmotility, as antireflux surgery may exacerbate this.
- I would arrange an OGD and 24 hr pH/manometry to obtain objective evidence of reflux before considering surgical management.

- However, up to 25% of patients with reflux may have a normal endoscopy and/or pH studies.
- My decision to offer antireflux surgery will take into account both clinical and investigative findings.
- There are two groups of patients form the main bulk of surgical candidates:
  - Patients with reflux who have had a partial or no response to medical treatment
  - Patients adequately controlled on medication but who do not wish to take tablets lifelong

What parameters form the basis of 24 hr pH studies? What are the normal values?

- There are six components that comprise a standard pH study (normal values in parentheses), and these are correlated with the patient's reflux episodes and symptoms:
  - Total reflux duration (<5%)
  - Upright reflux time (<8%)
  - Supine reflux time (<3%)
  - Number of reflux episodes (<50)
  - Number of episodes greater than 5 min in duration (<3)
  - Longest reflux episode
- The most useful parameters are the total reflux time and symptom correlation. A patient may have clinically significant reflux disease despite having normal total oesophageal duration of pH < 4 if the symptom correlation is almost 100%. Conversely, a patient with no correlation of symptoms with reflux episodes, despite having values above the normal range, may not have clinically significant reflux disease.

What is the DeMeester scoring system?

- The DeMeester score measures lower oesophageal acidity and correlates it with symptom duration. It is based on six parameters involving patient position, number and length of reflux.
- A normal score is <14.

What would you discuss when consenting a patient for an antireflux procedure?

- The outcome is successful in >90% of patients.
- Surgery is the only treatment that actually stops reflux.
- There is markedly reduced morbidity with laparoscopic procedure compared with open surgery.
- There are risks of postoperative dysphagia (usually temporary, resolves within 2–3 weeks), early satiety, bloating, increased flatulence, inability to vomit or belch, and risk of recurrence of symptoms.

What is the controversy surrounding total versus partial fundoplication?

- No evidence supports one technique over the other.
- Many surgeons perform a partial anterior or posterior fundoplication because of the risk of postoperative dysphagia, wind-related problems or concerns about exacerbating an existing dysmotility disorder.
- Evidence suggests there are fewer wind-related problems following a partial posterior compared with a total fundoplication, but whether dysphagia is less common is still not clear.[9]
- Similarly, evidence suggests there are less dysphagia and fewer wind-related problems following an anterior fundoplication, but possibly at the expense of a higher reflux recurrence rate.[10]

Does division of the short gastric vessels to create a floppy valve during a Nissen fundoplication reduce the incidence of postoperative dysphagia?

- Some surgeons believe that failure to divide the short gastric vessels leads to an increased incidence of early dysphagia.
- Published data, however, do not show any difference in dysphagia with or without short gastric division, but there is some evidence to suggest a higher incidence of wind-related problems following division of the short gastric vessels.[11]

GASTROINTESTINAL STROMAL TUMOURS

A 54-year-old male presents with a previous history of haematemesis and, on endoscopy, is found to have a large submucosal tumour. What is the most likely diagnosis?

- The most common tumour in this setting is a gastric GIST.
- Typically, biopsies do not help confirm the diagnosis as the biopsies are mucosal and the tumour is submucosal.
- GISTs arise from mesenchymal elements and form soft tissue sarcomas. They comprise about 1%–2% of all gastrointestinal tract tumours, with approximately 900 new cases each year in the UK.
- The common sites of origin are the stomach and small bowel, followed by oesophagus, mesentery and large bowel.

How would you investigate this patient?

- A CT scan allows the site of origin to be determined as well as the presence of distant metastases. A full-staging CT chest, abdomen and pelvis is usually performed for large tumours. This also aids surgical planning.
- An endoscopic ultrasound (EUS) typical finds a hypogenic mass. Small homogenous tumours <3 cm with a regular outline are most likely to behave in a benign manner. EUS-guided fine needle aspiration cytology is usually diagnostic.

- The most useful application for PET CT scanning is to determine the response of unresectable or metastatic GISTs to imatinib (Glivec).

What factors determine the potential malignancy of GISTs?

- Tumour size—small tumours (<2 cm) are very low risk; those > 10 cm are high risk.
- Mitotic count (per 50 high-power fields)—<5 is low risk; >10 is high risk.

What are the treatment options?

- Small asymptomatic incidental GISTs may be observed as long as there is no change in size on serial scanning.
- Large symptomatic GISTs should be resected, but only if complete resection can be achieved with negative resection margins (R0 resection). It is vitally important that the tumour not be ruptured during surgery as this and/or a positive resection margin leads to a dramatic reduction in survival.[12] Palliative surgery may have a role in selected patients for the alleviation of symptoms.
- Unresectable or metastatic GISTs can be treated with Imatinib (Glivec).

What is the mechanism of action of imatinib?

- GIST cells express the tyrosine kinase receptor KIT (CD117).
- Imatinib is a tyrosine kinase receptor inhibitor that inhibits the tyrosine kinases of KIT on GIST cells, leading to the inactivation of cell proliferation and the promotion of apoptosis. These kinases are not present in normal cells.
- Huge response rates of over 80% were seen after the introduction of imatinib, and more than 50% of patients with unresectable or metastatic GISTs will survive more than 5 years.

OESOPHAGEAL CANCER

A 62-year-old man with a long-standing history of gastro-oesophageal reflux presents with symptoms of intermittent dysphagia. How would you manage him?

- I strongly suspect that he has oesophageal cancer.
- I would take a history regarding the dysphagia (progressive vs. rapid onset, solids or liquids) and any associated weight loss. Smoking history is relevant. Respiratory symptoms may suggest aspiration of undigested food or a sign of more advanced disease (direct invasion of tracheobronchial tree by a tumour).
- I would examine the patient looking for signs of more advanced disease (supraclavicular/cervical lympadenopathy), hepatomegaly or abdominal nodal or omental masses.

- I would arrange an urgent OGD with biopsies (at least six biopsy samples for any suspected gastro-oesophageal malignancy).

The OGD demonstrates a malignant appearing tumour infiltrating the gastro-oesophageal junction from above. Biopsies confirm adenocarcinoma. How would you classify GOJ tumours?

- The Siewert classification:
  - Type I—adenocarcinoma of the distal oesophagus, which usually arises from an area with specialised intestinal metaplasia of the oesophagus (i.e., Barrett's oesophagus) and may infiltrate the GOJ from above.
  - Type II—true carcinoma of the cardia arising immediately at the GOJ.
  - Type III—subcardial gastric carcinoma that infiltrates the GOJ and distal oesophagus from below.

What staging investigations are appropriate for this man?

- Arrange a CT scan of chest, abdomen and pelvis with IV (if no contraindications) and oral contrast or water assess for metastatic disease and extent of local invasion for more advanced tumours.
- Use EUS for more accurate T staging of the primary tumour and to assess regional lymph node involvement, as FNA samples maybe obtained.
  - For T1 tumours, EMR is a more sensitive method of differentiating mucosal from submucosal penetration.
- PET-CT is also utilised to assess regional and distant nodal disease more accurately.
- Laparoscopy for direct visualisation of low-volume peritoneal and hepatic metastasis tends to be reserved for type II and III tumours and less for type I tumours, given the pattern of disease spread.

What are the next steps in his management?

- I will discuss his case in the UGI MDT.
- In the absence of metastatic disease, if he were medically fit, I would offer him an oesophagectomy after neoadjuvant chemotherapy.[13]
- The MRC OEO2 trial randomised 822 patients to surgery alone or two 3-weekly cycles of cisplatin + 5-FU prior to surgery. The group receiving chemotherapy was shown to have better disease-free and overall survival at 2 and 5 years (43% vs. 34%; 17% vs. 23% at 5 years).[14]
- The role of preoperative chemoradiotherapy in the management of oesophageal cancer is also evolving, but not yet fully accepted in the UK. The CROSS trial[15] compared chemoradiotherapy followed by surgery with surgery alone in patients with oesophageal and oesophagogastric-junction cancers. Overall survival was significantly better in the chemoradiotherapy group (49.4 months vs. 24.0 months), with acceptable adverse event rates.

What surgical approach could you use to resect this tumour?
Say which approach your would use, and whether YOU would use an open or a laparoscopic approach.

- There are three surgical approaches:
  - A one-stage oesophagectomy via a left thoraco-abdominal approach provides maximal exposure of the GOJ, allowing good opportunity to clear the maximal circumferential paraoesophageal tissue.
  - A two-stage oesophagectomy involves mobilisation of the stomach and the creation of a gastric conduit followed by a right thoracic approach to the oesophagus to resect the tumour and anastomose the conduit to the proximal oesophagus in the chest.
  - A three-stage oesophagectomy involves a prone thoracic phase for mobilisation of the oesophagus and tumour, followed by a laparoscopic abdominal phase to create a gastric conduit and a left neck incision to anastomose the stomach to the cervical oesophagus after removing the specimen through an extended abdominal port site.

POSTOP COMPLICATIONS AFTER BARIATRIC SURGERY

A 33-year-old female, with a BMI of 52, background of obstructive sleep apnoea, type II DM, hypercholesterolaemia and previous DVTs undergoes a laparoscopic Roux-En-Y gastric bypass. Your registrar rings you in the early morning because the patient has vague epigastric pain and feels nauseated. On examination, she has a pulse of 130 and is in pain. The abdomen is soft. What would you tell your registrar and what is your differential?

- Ensure the patient has received appropriate fluid resuscitation and analgesia.
- A patient in the early postoperative period following gastric bypass surgery who is in pain and tachycardic following surgery is presumed to have an anastomotic leak unless proven otherwise.

What would be the investigation of choice?

- If immediately available, a CT with water-soluble contrast (barium should not be used) is likely to diagnose a leak. For some bariatric patients, CT scanning may not be an option because of their weight and abdominal circumference.
- A laparoscopy should be contemplated to confirm or exclude a leak.

If a leak is found, how would you manage the patient?

- Drainage and nutrition are the treatment goals.
- A leak can be primarily sutured or sutured over a T-tube forming a controlled fistula if primary closure is not possible. Finally, I would perform a thorough washout with warm saline.

- Postoperatively, the patient should be managed on HDU.
- Nutritional support with parenteral nutrition of feeding jejunostomy may be needed.
- Analgesia should be optimised and vigorous chest physiotherapy offered.

What postoperative chest complications are common amongst these patients?

- Immediate complications include atelectasis and pneumonia (first 72 hr) as well as PE.
- All these patients are high risk and should receive thromboprophylaxis.

A 41-year-old female received a laparoscopic adjustable gastric band 12 months ago. Her current BMI is 29 with a preoperative BMI of 42. She had her band adjusted last week. Since then she has been getting progressive dysphagia and has not been able to swallow her own saliva in the last 10 hr. Your registrar rings late at night for advice. What would you tell your registrar and what is the main thing running through your mind?

- This patient needs an urgent deflation of her band, which should not wait overnight. This should be done ideally with a noncoring needle such as a Huber needle, but if one is not immediately available, a standard needle can be used instead. Full aspiration should lead to immediate resolution of symptoms. If not, band slippage should be suspected and further investigation is urgently needed.
- The management of a slippage is immediate band deflation followed by a barium swallow. If symptoms persist following the deflation, then urgent laparoscopy and band removal are needed as there is a risk of gastric ischaemia. This can be done by a general surgeon.

UGI TRIALS

- ST03[16]
    - MRC RCT compares different perioperative chemotherapy regimens in potentially curable gastric cancer (ECF, ECX-epirubicin, cisplatin, cepecitabine). Health-related quality of life (HQRL) issues are also addressed in this trial.
- Dutch D1D2 trial[17]
    - This 15-year follow-up demonstrated that D2 lymphadenectomy is associated with lower locoregional recurrence and gastric cancer-related death compared with D1 resection. The higher morbidity seen with D2 resection was associated with pancreaticosplenectomy. A safer spleen preserving D2 resection technique is the recommended surgical approach for patients with resectable and curable gastric cancer.
- USA intergroup 0116 trial[18]
    - On the basis of this trial, postoperative chemoradiation after gastrectomy is the standard of care in the United States. This is not accepted general practice in the UK.

- MRC OEO5 trial (ongoing)
  - This is evaluating the optimal preoperative chemotherapy regimens for patients with operable oesophageal adenocarcinoma and also includes a comprehensive assessment of HQRL.

REFERENCES

1. Leyden, J E, A C Moss and P MacMathuna. 2006. Endoscopic pneumatic dilation versus botulinum toxin injection in the management of primary achalasia. *Cochrane Database Systems Review* (4): CD005046.
2. Boeckxstaens, Guy E, Vito Annese, Stanislas Bruley des Varannes, Stanislas Chaussade, Mario Costantini, Antonello Cuttitta, J Ignasi Elizalde, et al. 2011. Pneumatic dilation versus laparoscopic Heller's myotomy for idiopathic achalasia. *New England Journal of Medicine* 364 (19): 1807–1816.
3. Sjöström, Lars, Kristina Narbro, C David Sjöström, Kristjan Karason, Bo Larsson, Hans Wedel, Ted Lystig, et al. 2007. Effects of bariatric surgery on mortality in Swedish obese subjects. *New England Journal of Medicine* 357 (8): 741–752.
4. National Institute for Clinical Excellence. 2006. Obesity: Guidance on prevention, identification, assessment and management of overweight and obesity in adults and children. NICE Clinical Guideline 43.
5. Pech, O, A Behrens, A May, L Nachbar, L Gossner, T Rabenstein, H Manner, et al. 2008. Long-term results and risk factor analysis for recurrence after curative endoscopic therapy in 349 patients with high-grade intraepithelial neoplasia and mucosal adenocarcinoma in Barrett's oesophagus. *Gut* 57 (9): 1200–1206.
6. Pohl, Juergen, Oliver Pech, Andrea May, Hendrik Manner, Annette Fissler-Eckhoff and Christian Ell. 2010. Incidence of macroscopically occult neoplasias in Barrett's esophagus: Are random biopsies dispensable in the era of advanced endoscopic imaging? *American Journal of Gastroenterology* 105 (11): 2350–2356.
7. Sugano, Kentaro. 2008. Gastric cancer: Pathogenesis, screening, and treatment. *Gastrointestinal Endoscopy Clinics of North America* 18 (3): 513–22–ix.
8. Cunningham, David, William H Allum, Sally P Stenning, Jeremy N Thompson, Cornelis J H van de Velde, Marianne Nicolson, J Howard Scarffe, et al. 2006. Perioperative chemotherapy versus surgery alone for resectable gastroesophageal cancer. *New England Journal of Medicine* 355 (1): 11–20.
9. Lundell, L. 2002. Laparoscopic fundoplication is the treatment of choice for gastrooesophageal reflux disease. Protagonist. *Gut* 51 (4): 468–471.
10. Baigrie, R J, S N R Cullis, A J Ndhluni and A Cariem. 2005. Randomized double-blind trial of laparoscopic Nissen fundoplication versus anterior partial fundoplication. *British Journal of Surgery* 92 (7): 819–823.
11. O'Boyle, Colm J, David I Watson, Glyn G Jamieson, Jennifer C Myers, Philip A Game and Peter G Devitt. 2002. Division of short gastric vessels at laparoscopic Nissen fundoplication: A prospective double-blind randomized trial with 5-year follow-up. *Annals of Surgery* 235 (2): 165–170.
12. Langer, C, B Gunawan, P Schüler, W Huber, L Füzesi and H Becker. 2003. Prognostic factors influencing surgical management and outcome of gastrointestinal stromal tumours. *British Journal of Surgery* 90 (3): 332–339.
13. Allum, William H, Jane M Blazeby, S Michael Griffin, David Cunningham, Janusz A Jankowski and Rachel Wong, Association of Upper Gastrointestinal Surgeons of Great Britain and Ireland, the British Society of Gastroenterology and the British Association of Surgical Oncology. 2011. Guidelines for the management of oesophageal and gastric cancer. *Gut* 60 (11): 1449–1472.

14. Allum, William H, Sally P Stenning, John Bancewicz, Peter I Clark and Ruth E Langley. 2009. Long-term results of a randomized trial of surgery with or without preoperative chemotherapy in esophageal cancer. *Journal of Clinical Oncology: Official Journal of the American Society of Clinical Oncology* 27 (30): 5062–5067.

15. van Hagen, P, M C C M Hulshof, J J B van Lanschot, E W Steyerberg, M I van Berge Henegouwen, B P L Wijnhoven, D J Richel, et al. 2012. Preoperative chemoradiotherapy for esophageal or junctional cancer. *New England Journal of Medicine* 366 (22): 2074–2084.

16. Yun, Jina, Jeeyun Lee, Se Hoon Park, Joon Oh Park, Young Suk Park, Ho Yeong Lim and Won Ki Kang. 1990. A randomised phase II study of combination chemotherapy with epirubicin, cisplatin and capecitabine (ECX) or cisplatin and capecitabine (CX) in advanced gastric cancer. *European Journal of Cancer* 46 (5): 885–891.

17. Songun, Ilfet, Hein Putter, Elma Meershoek-Klein Kranenbarg, Mitsuru Sasako and Cornelis J H van de Velde. 2010. Surgical treatment of gastric cancer: 15-Year follow-up results of the randomised nationwide Dutch D1D2 trial. *Lancet Oncology* 11 (5): 439–449.

18. Smalley, Stephen R, Jacqueline K Benedetti, Daniel G Haller, Scott A Hundahl, Norman C Estes, Jaffer A Ajani, Leonard L Gunderson, et al. 2012. Updated analysis of SWOG-directed intergroup study 0116: A phase III trial of adjuvant radiochemotherapy versus observation after curative gastric cancer resection. *Journal of Clinical Oncology: Official Journal of the American Society of Clinical Oncology* 30 (19): 2327–2333.

BIBLIOGRAPHY

Guidelines for the diagnosis and management of Barrett's columnar-lined oesophagus. British Society of Gastroenterology 2005 (http://www.bsg.org.uk/pdf_word_docs/Barretts_Oes.pdf).

11 Vascular Surgery

Tjun Tang, Janice Tsui,
Stewart Walsh and Michael Wu

CONTENTS

ACUTE ILIOFEMORAL VEIN THROMBOSIS

A 59-year-old woman presents with a 2-day history of a painful, swollen, discoloured left leg. There is no evidence of venous gangrene, compartment syndrome or arterial compromise. A venous duplex scan shows an extensive left iliofemoral deep vein thrombosis. What immediate management and investigations would you instigate?

- Elevation of the limb
- Blood tests including FBC, coagulation screen and fibrinogen, U+Es, LFTs
- Systemic anticoagulation
- CT pulmonary angiogram if indicated (in patients with a suspicion of pulmonary embolus)
- Consideration of catheter-directed thrombolysis (CDT)
- Investigations for underlying cause (thrombophilia, malignancy)

What is the aim of CDT?

- To reduce the morbidities associated with post-thrombotic syndrome (PTS)

What are the contraindications to CDT?

- Absolute:
  - Established cerebrovascular event (including transient ischaemic attacks within the last 2 months)
  - Active bleeding diathesis
  - Recent gastrointestinal or retroperitoneal bleeding (within the last 10 days)
  - Neurosurgery within the last 3 months
  - Intracranial trauma within the last 3 months
- Relative major:
  - Cardiopulmonary resuscitation within the last 10 days
  - Major nonvascular surgery or trauma within the last 10 days
  - Uncontrolled hypertension
  - Puncture of noncompressible vessel
  - Intracranial tumour
  - Recent eye surgery
- Minor:
  - Hepatic failure, particularly with coagulopathy
  - Severe renal failure
  - Bacterial endocarditis
  - Pregnancy and within 7 days postpartum
  - Diabetic haemorrhagic retinopathy
  - Significant thrombocytopenia or pre-existing coagulopathy

What is the role of IVC filters during CDT?

- There is no clear evidence that IVC filters improve outcomes or significantly reduce the occurrence of fatal pulmonary embolism.

What is the role of venous stents in patients with iliofemoral DVTs?

- Good results have been reported for iliac vein stents for May–Thurner syndrome (obstruction secondary to compression of the left common iliac vein by the right common iliac artery) following CDT.
- Stents placed for external compression have less favourable outcomes.
- There is insufficient evidence for femoral vein stents.

What systemic complication requires immediate management in patients with phlegmasia cerulean dolens?

- Due to massive fluid sequestration in the limb, patients may go into circulatory shock.
- Immediate fluid replacement is required.

ACUTELY ISCHAEMIC LEG

A 51-year-old man presents to A+E complaining of sudden-onset right leg pain and weakness whilst out walking his dog. How do you assess him?

- Take a history—cardiovascular disease (e.g., recent MI, AF), peripheral vascular disease (claudication, previous vascular limb surgery), family history of limb ischaemia, smoking and clotting problems.
- Examine the patient—check for sinus rhythm, exclude an abdominal aortic aneurysm, feel all peripheral pulses, using a hand-held Doppler probe if necessary, assess motor and sensory function of the affected leg.
- Take blood for FBCs, U+Es, clotting and a full coagulation screen prior to commencing anticoagulation.

He is in sinus rhythm. He has a palpable right femoral pulse but no distal pulses in the right leg. Left leg pulses were normal. He has reduced sensation and normal movements. There is no significant past medical or family history. What is your diagnosis and how would you proceed?

- This patient has an acutely ischaemic right leg, which appears viable (motor function intact).
- Differential diagnoses include an embolism secondary to cardiac arrhythmia; mural thrombosis; vegetations, cardiac tumours or proximal aneurysms; popliteal aneurysm thrombosis and arterial dissection.
- I would treat the patient with IV heparinisation to restrict thrombus propagation and further emboli. Give supplementary oxygen and fluid rehydration.
- I would book him for an urgent embolectomy with potential fasciotomies.
- The embolectomy may require a popliteal approach.

How would you carry out the fasciotomies?

- Four compartment fasciotomies should be performed via full length skin and fascial incisions.
- The anterior incision is placed about two finger-breadths lateral to the anterior border of the tibia (avoiding the peroneal nerve) to access the anterior and lateral compartments.
- The posterior incision is placed about two finger-breadths posterior to the medial condyle of the femur and medial malleolus (avoiding the long saphenous vein) to access the superficial and deep posterior compartments.

What further investigations would you carry out?

- Preoperatively, arrange for blood tests including full coagulation screen prior to commencing anticoagulation. If these have not been done, they will need to be taken after he has finished anticoagulation therapy.
- Intraoperatively, any material retrieved at embolectomy should be sent for histology ± microbiology.
- Postoperatively, request an ECHO, aortic ultrasound, lower limb duplex as guided by clinical findings and preliminary investigations.

When would you consider thrombolysis for an acutely ischaemic limb?

- Catheter-directed intra-arterial thrombolysis could be considered in patients with acute limb ischaemia where the limb is not immediately threatened (i.e., no sensory loss or paralysis, no significant calf tenderness) and the patient has no contraindications to thrombolysis.
- It may be of particular use in patients with occluded prosthetic grafts.

How would your management differ for an 88-year-old frail lady who presents with a 6 hr history of a cold, mottled left leg in atrial fibrillation?

- Elderly patients with underlying cardiac pathology presenting with acute limb ischaemia have high morbidity and mortality rates.
- These patients require cautious rehydration and anticoagulation, and any procedure may need to be carried out under local anaesthesia.
- With advanced ischaemia, the tissue damage may be irreversible and the systemic risks of reperfusion unacceptable.
- These patients should be considered for primary amputation or palliation.

ASYMPTOMATIC CAROTID STENOSIS

Describe the natural history of asymptomatic carotid stenosis.

- The risk of transient ischaemic attack (TIA) and stroke are proportional to the severity of the internal carotid stenosis. At 1 year, the risk of TIA or stroke in 0%–29% stenosis is 2.1% versus 5.7% for 30%–74% stenosis and 19.5% with 75%–99% stenosis.
- Over a 5-year follow-up period, stenoses < 75% have a TIA or stroke rate of 12.6% versus 60% in >75% stenosis.
- Calcified, echogenic plaques on ultrasound are less likely to be associated with TIA or stroke compared to soft echolucent plaque.
- Progressive narrowing of the plaque is also associated with an increased risk of TIA or stroke. In 1 year of follow-up, patients progressing from <80% to >80% stenosis carried a 46% risk of TIA, stroke or carotid occlusion compared to 1.5% in those with stable plaque.

What randomised controlled trial data are available to assess treatment of asymptomatic carotid stenoses?

- The Veterans Administration cooperative trial (VA),[1] the asymptomatic carotid atherosclerosis study (ACAS)[2] and the asymptomatic carotid surgery trial (ACST)[3] assessed best medical treatment (BMT) versus carotid endarterectomy (CEA) plus BMT of asymptomatic carotid stenoses. BMT comprised control of atherosclerotic risk factors and the use of aspirin.
- The VA trial[1] randomised over 400 men with 50%–99% carotid stenosis to aspirin alone versus aspirin plus CEA.

- The surgical group had a lower, but nonsignificant rate of ipsilateral stroke (4.7% vs. 9.4%) and no difference in 30-day stroke or death rate.
- ACAS[2] randomised over 1,600 adults with 60%–99% carotid stenosis to aspirin alone versus aspirin plus CEA.
  - The surgical group had a significantly lower rate of ipsilateral/perioperative stroke or death (5% vs. 11%). The rate of major stroke or death was lower in the surgical group but not significant.
- ACST[3] randomised over 3,000 patients with 60%–99% stenosis to either immediate CEA plus BMT or BMT with deferred CEA until the stenosis became symptomatic. In the immediate CEA group, only 50% received surgery within a month and 88% within a year. The stroke end point combined both ipsilateral and contralateral strokes to the treated carotid artery.
  - The 30-day stroke rate following CEA was 3.1%. The overall risk of stroke and death was nearly halved in the immediate CEA group (6.4% vs. 11.8%). The benefit of stroke prevention was demonstrable in both the ipsilateral and contralateral sides to the CEA, and significant in those less than 75 years of age
  - However, it should be noted that the net benefit of immediate CEA was not accrued till 2 years after surgery (worse event-free survival compared to deferred CEA).
- Both the ACAS and ASCT showed that the benefit of stroke prevention was the same in those with 70% carotid stenosis compared to those with 80% or 90% stenosis.
- A meta-analysis of ACAS and ACST data looking at the 5-year risk of any stroke or death found no benefit for women (OR 0.96) but a significant benefit for men (OR 0.49).
- Another important caveat is the evolution of BMT from the time of these trials to the modern day. The routine use of statins, newer antiplatelet agents such as clopidogrel and more aggressive management of hypertension, cigarette smoking and diabetes further narrow the benefit in the treatment of asymptomatic carotid disease.

A health screening scan has detected an 80% right internal carotid artery stenosis in an otherwise well 72-year-old woman who attends your clinic. Discuss your management.

- Initial history and examination should confirm whether this carotid stenosis is indeed asymptomatic. Although the trials differ in their definitions, absence of neurologic symptoms in the past 6 months would suffice.
- I would consider the use of antiplatelets, statin therapy and controlling hypertension, and smoking cessation, if relevant. The antiplatelet and statins assist in primary prevention of TIA/stroke and also contribute to a reduction in cardiovascular events.

She is already having best medical therapy and wants to know whether she needs surgery, as her GP mentioned that she might need it.

- There is no conclusive evidence that performing CEA in women with asymptomatic carotid stenosis prevents a stroke.
- If best medical therapy is instituted, then unless there is evidence to suggest progression of the carotid stenosis on serial ultrasonography, CEA would not be recommended.

CHRONIC MESENTERIC ISCHAEMIA

How would a patient with chronic mesenteric ischaemia present?

- The characteristic patient is a middle-aged woman who is cachectic, with a long smoking history, and presents with abdominal pain and weight loss (because of a fear of food).
- The pain is dull or colicky in nature, in the epigastric region with radiation to the back. Onset is 15–30 min after eating, in association with postprandial hyperaemia, and lasts for 1–3 hr.
- Physical examination, other than the preceding typical appearance, yields few clinical signs. Signs of vascular disease in other territories (e.g., carotid, peripheral) or the presence of abdominal bruits may be present, but are nonspecific.

What investigations would you request in a 45-year-old female with symptoms of CMI?

- Abdominal ultrasound should be requested (to exclude the presence of gallstones).
- Arrange for a CT of the abdomen to look for intra-abdominal masses or malignancy.
- Specific confirmatory investigations for CMI include:
  - Mesenteric duplex ultrasound
  - Catheter-based digital subtraction angiography (DSA)
  - CT angiography (CTA) or magnetic resonance angiography (MRA)
- Mesenteric duplex ultrasound has >80% sensitivity, specificity and PPV compared to DSA. A negative ultrasound essentially excludes CMI.
- DSA is the 'gold standard' test. Given the orientation of the coeliac axis and SMA to the aorta, a lateral aortogram is essential in the assessment of these vessels.
- CTA and MRA will identify significant coeliac and SMA stenoses, visceral collaterals, exclude other intra-abdominal pathologies and help plan treatment strategies.

How would you treat mesenteric occlusive disease?

- The two options are open surgery and endovascular surgery.
- Endovascular treatment (angioplasty and stenting of the coeliac axis and SMA) is associated with reduced morbidity and mortality compared to

surgical treatment, but has reduced long-term patency and increased rein-
tervention rates for recurrent stenosis/thrombosis.
- Surgical treatment options are:
  - Antegrade bypass from the supracoeliac aorta
  - Retrograde bypass from the infrarenal aorta or common iliac artery;
    tunnelling of the graft is problematic with potential for kinking
  - Endarterectomy
  - Reimplantation of affected vessels

**If you were considering an open bypass procedure, what type of conduit would
you use?**

- I would use a prosthetic conduit unless I had concerns regarding contamination (bowel ischaemia or infarction); I would then use an autogenous conduit.
- There is no evidence to show that one is superior to the other.

What is median arcuate ligament syndrome, and how do you treat it?

- The median arcuate ligament of the diaphragm compresses the origin of
  the coeliac axis. This can lead to reduced flow, chronic abdominal pain and
  mesenteric ischaemia.
- Unless the SMA is also diseased, it should provide sufficient collateral flow
  to obviate symptoms.
- Endovascular stenting is unlikely to relieve symptoms due to the extrinsic
  compression.
- Open or laparoscopic division of the ligament is the definitive treatment.

**During the workup for this 45-year-old female, she developed severe, constant
abdominal pain, with a raised white cell count and lactate. How will you manage her?**

- I am concerned that she now has ischaemic bowel. I will resuscitate her with
  oxygen, IV fluids and opiate analgesia and prepare her for urgent surgery.
- If time or patient condition allows, a CTA would allow assessment of the
  visceral circulation and also the extent of bowel compromise.
- I would perform a midline laparotomy, assess the bowel and attempt revascularisation before resecting the bowel, if necessary. A second-look laparotomy could be planned as an alternative to stoma formation if bowel
  viability was still borderline after revascularisation.
- A retrograde bypass with an autogenous conduit is a safer approach in an
  unwell patient and potentially soiled field.

DIABETIC FOOT

**A 55-year-old man with poorly controlled type 2 diabetes presents to your clinic
with a hot, swollen foot. How will you manage him?**

- Take a history—duration of symptoms, history of trauma, previous foot complications, known neuropathy/peripheral arterial disease, systemic symptoms (fever, rigors).
- Examine him—predominantly to differentiate between Charcot's neuro-arthropathy and foot sepsis (other differential diagnoses include soft tissue injury, fracture and other inflammatory conditions), assess for underlying neuropathy and peripheral arterial disease and identify systemic complications.
- Admit for further management involving the multidisciplinary foot team.
- Seek acute medical team/diabetic team input if he is systemically unwell.
- Swab areas of necrosis/gangrene, take bloods for FBC, U+Es, cultures, start broad-spectrum antibiotics and liaise with microbiology.
- Obtain a podiatrist's opinion to ensure immediate offloading of the foot.
- Arrange for urgent imaging to exclude an underlying collection if clinically unclear (XR of the foot, proceeding to MRI).
- Urgent surgical treatment of foot sepsis is needed.

The patient had a collection over the dorsum of his forefoot that has been drained and is now systemically well. What is your ongoing management plan?

- Continue broad-spectrum antibiotics until antibiotic sensitivities are available, and offload the foot.
- Conduct regular wound review and debridement as necessary.
- Review and optimise diabetes control and offer patient education about foot care.
- Request MRI and arterial duplex.

The wound becomes necrotic at the edges. The duplex shows a stenosis of the midsuperficial femoral artery (SFA) and heavily calcified infrageniculate vessels with likely multilevel disease. How would you proceed?

- Arrange an angiogram and angioplasty to treat the SFA stenosis, attempt to treat infrageniculate disease and assess runoffs
- There are some data showing improved patency rates of treatment of short, focal, infrageniculate lesions by drug-coated or drug-eluting stents.
- If the infrageniculate stent failed, I would consider a distal SFA—distal/pedal bypass following successful angioplasty of the SFA stenosis.

Following revascularisation, the wound improves. MRI shows no further collections, but osteomyelitis in the second and third metatarsals. What is your discharge plan for this patient?

- Continued long-course appropriate antibiotics and offloading
- Follow-up in the multidisciplinary foot clinic to monitor the wound, for antibiotic therapy and to ensure continued best medical therapy

- Surveillance for bypass graft if appropriate (no evidence for long-term surveillance after endovascular revascularisation)

What are the indications for primary amputation in this patient?

- Extensive soft tissue destruction with a nonviable foot
- Extensive infection
- No vascular reconstruction possible and ascending soft tissue necrosis

How would your revascularisation plan change if angiography showed mild disease above the knee, but heavily calcified and multiple stenoses in all three crural vessels. The anterior tibial runs to the foot.

There are three options: endovascular, surgical and a hybrid procedure:

- Endovascular:
  - Arrange for angiography ± angioplasty of the above knee disease to optimise inflow.
  - Treat the anterior tibial artery using 0.014 in. guide wires and small-diameter angioplasty balloons.
  - Treatment of long lesions may require tapered diameter balloons to minimise the duration and number of balloon inflations required.
  - Dilation of other crural vessels can be attempted to maximise the outflow available and to assist wound healing.
- Open surgical:
  - Determine inflow site—if significant SFA disease is present, then CFA and long bypass may need to be utilised. If SFA is relatively disease free, the popliteal artery can be used.
  - Determine the distal bypass site—either anterior tibial artery used in the midcalf via lateral approach or the dorsalis pedis artery at the ankle.
  - Determine conduit—length of ipsilateral vein available (LSV or SSV), size discrepancy of inflow and outflow sites and whether to use reversed, nonreversed or in situ bypass.
  - The results of prosthetic conduit in critical limb ischaemia and single vessel runoff are poor compared to autogenous conduit.
- Hybrid:
  - Use endovascular techniques to optimise SFA and popliteal flow.
  - Use below-knee popliteal artery as inflow site to minimise bypass length.
  - The outflow site is determined via previous angiogram to midcalf anterior tibial or dorsalis pedis at the ankle.

HYPERHIDROSIS

A 23-year-old woman is referred by her GP with palmar and axillary hyperhidrosis. How would you assess her in the clinic?

- I would take a history and perform an examination to distinguish between primary and secondary hyperhidrosis and to establish the severity of the symptoms and the disability caused. I would ask about:
  - Generalised versus localised sweating
  - Sites affected (whether bilateral and symmetrical)
  - Age of onset of symptoms
  - Frequency, duration and timing of symptoms, and triggers
  - Effect on social life and occupation
  - Family history
  - Symptoms and signs of diseases associated with secondary hyperhidrosis
- Primary hyperhidrosis is usually associated with the following:
  - Age of onset ≤ 25 years of age
  - At least weekly episodes
  - Bilateral and symmetrical symptoms
  - Affects primarily the palms, axillae, soles, face and scalp
  - Absent at night
  - Positive family history

What conditions are associated with excessive sweating?

- Diabetes mellitus
- Hypothyroidism
- Hyperpituitarism
- Phaeochromocytoma
- Neurological conditions (e.g., Parkinson's disease)
- Reflex sympathetic dystrophy/chronic pain syndrome
- Malignancy
- Tuberculosis (usually night sweats) and other infections
- Drugs (e.g., propanolol, tricyclic antidepressants, serotonin reuptake inhibitors)
- Menopause

Are there any tests that can be used to confirm the diagnosis?

- In the starch–iodine test, an iodine solution is applied to the affected area and starch is then sprinkled on it. The starch–iodine combination turns black over areas of excess sweating.

The patient appears to have primary hyperhidrosis, which is significantly affecting her work as a public relations officer. What treatment options would you discuss with her?

- Medical:
  - Topical agents (e.g., aluminium chloride; side effects include skin irritation, stains on clothes])
  - Systemic anticholinergics (side effects include dry mouth and eyes, blurred vision, urinary retention, constipation)

- Ionotophoresis—may be useful for palmar and plantar hyperhidrosis
- Botulinum toxin injections (requires repeated treatments)
- Surgical:
  - Thoracoscopic sympathectomy—at second and third thoracic ganglia (T2 and T3) for palmar hyperhidrosis, at T4 for axillary hyperhidrosis
  - Surgical excision/subcutaneous liposuction to remove/destroy sweat glands for axillary hyperhidrosis

What complications of thoracoscopic sympathectomy would you discuss with her?

- Compensatory sweating (up to 90% of patients)
- Gustatory sweating
- Pneumothorax
- Horner's syndrome
- Intercostal neuralgia
- Recurrence
- I would also mention a small mortality risk, since this is surgery for a benign condition

INFRAINGUINAL OCCLUSIVE DISEASE

How would you initially investigate a 70-year-old man referred to you from the medical team with rest pain and dry gangrene of his left great hallux?

- Opiate analgesia
- Baseline blood tests—FBC, U+Es, CRP, clotting
- Plain x-ray of the left foot
- Duplex ultrasound of left lower limb arteries

Duplex ultrasound demonstrates a long (25 cm) occlusion of his left SFA with runoff via posterior tibial and peroneal arteries. Discuss revascularisation options.

- Endovascular:
  - Angioplasty ± stenting of the SFA occlusion
    - Antegrade (from left CFA, crossing SFA occlusion via subintimal space and breaking back into the lumen of the popliteal)
    - Retrograde via the SAFARI (subintimal arterial flossing with antegrade–retrograde intervention) technique, whereby the posterior tibial artery is also punctured and a wire is introduced retrograde to meet a catheter introduced via the antegrade direction—passed through-and-through the catheter to allow passage of angioplasty balloons or stents along this
  - Open surgery—femoropopliteal or distal bypass, preferably with vein conduit

During angiography, it was not possible to cross the SFA occlusion successfully. Vein mapping reveals no usable vein in either of his lower limbs. What are your surgical options now?

- Look for venous conduit of the upper limbs—splicing of cephalic and basilic vein segments may be needed.
- If there is insufficient vein for the previous action, it is possible to choose to perform a composite graft (prosthetic proximal section with vein distal section and anastomosis joining the two) or
- Perform prosthetic bypass graft to the target vessel with a segment of vein harvested to form either a Miller cuff or St Mary's boot at the distal anastomosis.
- Perform remote endarterectomy of the SFA—(proximal CFA) and distal (BK popliteal) exposure and connect the two sites using remote endarterectomy (Moll) wire.

The femorodistal bypass performed was complicated by a groin wound lymphocoele and secondary infection by MRSA. Pus is now discharging from the groin wound. What are your surgical options now?

- Is the infected area superficial (i.e., pus is separated from the bypass graft via a fascial layer) or has the graft itself been compromised? If the former, drainage of the pus, debridement, appropriate antibiotic therapy and wound care may be sufficient.
- If the graft itself has become infected, then it is likely that the CFA anastomosis will eventually give way, leading to catastrophic bleeding.
- Is the patient fit enough or the limb affected still salvageable for another attempt at revascularisation? If so, the redo procedure will inevitably involve extra-anatomic bypass such as via the obturator canal or laterally around the groin.
- Furthermore, depending on whether the initial target vessel was the posterior tibial or peroneal artery, it may not be possible to revascularise the same vessel or use the same approach to the vessel
- If the decision is made to perform limb amputation (probably at above knee level), then the groin wound infection will also need to be debrided.
- Excision of the bypass graft, debridement of the infected material and, potentially, ligation of the superficial, profunda and/or common femoral arteries may need to be performed. A sartorius flap may need to be raised to cover the soft tissue defect.

INFRARENAL ABDOMINAL AORTIC ANEURYSM

A 73-year-old male smoker with COPD and hormonally controlled prostate cancer attends your clinic. He has a 6 cm infrarenal abdominal aortic aneurysm. What is your management plan?

- He has an annual risk of rupture between 10% and 20%.
- I would strongly counsel him on the benefits of smoking cessation, not only to reduce the risk of rupture but also for its cardiovascular benefits.
- Medical management of the aneurysm needs to be optimised with antihypertensive agents and a statin.
- I would request baseline blood tests, ECG and a CXR. If renal function is normal, I will arrange for a CT angiogram to assess suitability of the aneurysm for endovascular repair.
- I would then request pulmonary function tests and, if necessary a referral to a respiratory physician and anaesthetist to assess fitness for surgery.
- I would ask for a urology opinion to check that the prostate cancer is adequately treated and there are no concerns regarding metastatic spread and reduced life expectancy.
- I would discuss his results at a vascular MDT to determine whether he is anatomically suitable for an endovascular repair and fit enough for an open repair if the former is not possible.

What are the risk factors for developing an AAA?

- These include increasing age (men over 50, women over 60).
- Smoking and family history are independent risk factors.
- Diabetes and female gender reduce the risk.
- In the Western world, it is 3%–10% prevalent.

What is the natural history of an infrarenal AAA?

- Of ruptured AAAs, 50% do not reach hospital, and of those that reach hospital, 30% are not fit/suitable for surgery.
- The operative mortality rate is around 50% for emergency open aneurysm repair.
- The UK small aneurysm trial (UKSAT)[4] reported that the rupture risk greatly increases at 5 cm (4.0–4.9 cm rupture risk, 1.5% p.a.; 5.0–5.9 cm rupture risk, 6.5% p.a.). This rupture rate increases to 40% p.a. if it is >8 cm.
- AAA expansion of >1 cm in 1 year is also associated with a higher risk of rupture, and women have a higher rupture risk than men for a given AAA size.
- The threshold for elective surgical treatment is 5.5 cm in men and 5 cm in women.

What is the operative risk of open repair versus endovascular repair?

- For elective open repair, operative mortality in the United States is 5%, and in the UKSAT it was 5.6%.
- For elective endovascular aneurysm repair, the operative mortality in the United States is 1.3% and in the EVAR-1[5] trial was 1.6%.

- The morbidity of endovascular repair is also significantly less than that of open repair, partly due to a much shorter hospital length of stay.
- Quality of life measures at the 12-month mark and beyond are similar when comparing the open and endovascular groups.
- Multiple scoring systems are available to assess the operative risk for aneurysm surgery. Most include raised creatinine, congestive heart failure, ECG evidence of cardiac ischaemia, pulmonary dysfunction, history of cerebrovascular disease, advanced age and female gender.
- Higher volume centres and surgeons performing regular aneurysm surgery have reduced operative mortality and morbidity.

What randomised control trial data are available in assessing the role of endovascular repair of infrarenal abdominal aortic aneurysms?

- EVAR-1[5] and the Dutch randomised endovascular aneurysm management (DREAM)[6] are two RCTs that examined the outcomes of open versus endovascular repair of infrarenal abdominal aortic aneurysms > 5.5 cm.
- EVAR-1 looked at over 1,000 patients between 1999 and 2003, with a 30-day mortality of 1.7% in the endovascular repair group and 4.7% in the open repair group.
  - At 4-year follow-up, all-cause mortality was the same between groups, but there was a reduction in aneurysm-related death in the endovascular repair group (4% vs. 7%).
  - At this time point, 20% of endovascular repair groups needed reinterventions compared to 6% in the open repair group.
  - Follow-up at 10 years showed equivalent all-cause and aneurysm-related mortality in both groups.
- EVAR-2[7] is an RCT that examined whether endovascular repair is beneficial in those who are unfit for open repair of their aneurysm. It was run concurrently with EVAR-1. Over 300 patients were randomised to endovascular repair or no intervention. The mean forced expiratory volume at 1 s was 1.7 l.
  - The 30-day mortality of the endovascular repair group was 9%.
  - At 1 year, all-cause mortality was 42%, with an aneurysm-related mortality of 12%.
  - At 4 years, all-cause mortality was 64%.
  - There was no demonstrable benefit in all-cause or aneurysm-related mortality in the endovascular repair group.
- Endovascular repair of ruptured infrarenal abdominal aortic aneurysms has been widely reported and adopted around the world. Current evidence consists of experiences at different centres rather than a completed RCT. The immediate management of the patient with rupture: open versus endovascular repair (IMPROVE) trial is currently underway in the United Kingdom to compare the mortality and morbidity of open versus endovascular repair with a clinical diagnosis of ruptured abdominal aortic aneurysms.

INTERMITTENT CLAUDICATION

A 55-year-old man complains of calf pain on walking 400–500 yards. How would you assess him further?

- Take a history and examine him to confirm the cause, the severity and the disability it is causing, and to identify his cardiovascular risks and any previous vascular interventions.

He appears to have calf claudication that is inconvenient when he goes on holiday, but does not significantly affect his usual day-to-day activities. He has hypertension and smokes 15 cigarettes a day. He is not diabetic and has no history of hypercholesterolaemia, ischaemic heart disease or cerebrovascular disease and is unaware of any family history. How would you manage him further?

- Patients with intermittent claudication have significantly increased risks of cardiovascular events. Therefore, controlling his cardiovascular risks is the main priority.
- He should stop smoking (refer to smoking cessation team), ensure his blood pressure is well controlled (ACE inhibitor) and be started on antiplatelet and statin therapy.
- He should also be enrolled in a supervised exercise programme to improve his walking distance.

What are statins?

- Statins are cholesterol-lowering drugs which act by competitively inhibiting the enzyme HMG-CoA reductase, the rate-limiting enzyme in cholesterol biosynthesis in the liver.

What adverse reactions are associated with statins?

- Deranged liver function
- Myalgia
- Myositis, myopathy and rhabdomyolysis (increased risk if used in combination with a fibrate)
- Increased risk of diabetes (possibly with higher doses)

What pharmacological agents are used in the management of intermittent claudication?

- Naftidrofuryl oxalate—oral peripheral vasodilator (selective 5-hydroxytrptamine 2 receptor inhibitor)
- Cilostazol—oral phosphodiesterase III inhibitor
- Pentoxifylline—oral peripheral vasodilator

- Inositol nicotinate—oral peripheral vasodilator (slows release of nicotinic acid)
- Only naftidrofuryl oxalate recommendation in the treatment of intermittent claudication by NICE (Guidance TA223)

KEY TRIALS AND GUIDELINES IN VASCULAR SURGERY

- Aneurysms
  - The UK endovascular aneurysm repair (EVAR) trials[8] showed a clear operative mortality benefit of EVAR over open repair in patients fit for both procedures. However, no long-term survival advantage was found. For patients unfit for open repair, EVAR reduces long-term AAA-related mortality but not all-cause mortality.
- Carotids
  - The study of Murad et al.[9] included 13 RCTs involving both symptomatic (80%) and asymptomatic patients. It concluded that carotid artery stenting is associated with an increased risk of any stroke and decreased risk of myocardial infarct compared to CEA.
  - ACST-1[10] assessed the long-term effects of CEA for asymptomatic carotid stenoses. CEA was found to reduce 10-year stroke risks in patients younger than 75 years of age.
  - The ACST-2 trial to compare CEA with carotid artery stenting in the prevention of stroke in patients with asymptomatic carotid stenosis is now open and aims to recruit over 5,000 patients.
- Peripheral bypass
  - A trial[11] randomised patients with critical limb ischaemia to bypass surgery-first or balloon angioplasty-first revascularisation strategies. No significant differences in amputation-free survival or overall survival were found between the two groups overall. However, for patients who survived for at least 2 years, the bypass surgery-first strategy was associated with significant increase in subsequent overall survival.
- Varicose vein management
  - Craig et al.[12] concluded that radiofrequency ablation (RFA) and endo-venous laser therapy (EVLT) are at least as effective as surgery in the treatment of long saphenous varicose veins.
  - One study[13] included 28 RCTs. RFA and EVLT were found to be associated with lower wound complications, less pain and faster return to normal activities.

THORACIC AORTIC DISSECTION

How do you classify thoracic aortic dissection?
There are four classification systems:

- Acute (present for 14 days or less) and chronic (present for more than 14 days)

- The Debakey classification, based on anatomy:
  - Type 1—ascending aorta, across the arch and into descending thoracic aorta
  - Type 2—ascending aorta only
  - Type 3—descending aorta ± retrograde across the arch; tear usually distal to left subclavian artery
- The Stanford classification, based on the prognosis of the affected areas:
  - Type A—ascending aorta ± arch involvement
  - Type B—descending thoracic aorta distal to left subclavian artery
    - Both the Debakey and Stanford classifications have subtypes a and b, with the former confined to above the diaphragm and the latter involving the visceral/abdominal aorta.
- The Task Force on Aortic Dissection of the European Society of Cardiology has specifically defined the different variants of thoracic aortic dissection disease into a spectrum known as acute aortic syndrome:
  - Class 1—classical aortic dissection, with the presence of an intimal flap between the true and false lumen
  - Class 2—intramural haematoma with haemorrhage into the media
  - Class 3—eccentric bulge at tear site, but no haematoma
  - Class 4—penetrating aortic ulcer, usually subadventitial, may or may not have haematoma
  - Class 5—iatrogenic or traumatic aortic dissection

What investigations would you request in a patient with a suspected acute dissection?

- The purpose of imaging is to classify and define the anatomical involvement of dissection and to look for potential complications such as aneurysmal degeneration and malperfusion of end organs.
- A progress study during the acute stages can help to define if the dissection is uncomplicated or complicated.
- CT or MR angiography is the usual initial investigation.
- The angiogram needs to extend from the neck to the femoral bifurcations.
  - This allows assessment of the arch configuration, great vessel involvement, the thoracic and abdominal aorta and lower limb perfusion and potential access issues for endovascular repair.
  - It also allows assessment of visceral perfusion, haemothorax or pleural effusions suggestive of complications.
  - Acute growth of the dissected segment or a false lumen greater than three-fourths of the total lumen diammeter tends to result in aneurysmal degeneration and increased risk of rupture.
- Digital subtraction angiography is reserved to answer specific questions prior to open or endovascular repair.
- Adjuncts include echocardiography (pericardial effusions or aortic valve regurgitation) and ultrasound of the carotid or upper extremity vessels to assess the vertebral perfusion in the planning for repair.

What management strategies are employed in acute dissection?

- Initial management is medical stabilisation of the dissection.
- The patient is admitted to ICU/HDU with arterial line monitoring of blood pressure and heart rate.
- Blood pressure is lowered to a mean arterial pressure of 70 mmHg.
- There is reduction in wall stress (dP/dt) of the dissection with beta-blockade down to a heart rate of 60–70 beats per minute. This may also assist in blood pressure monitoring.
- Monitoring for potential complications such as coronary, cerebral, visceral or lower extremity malperfusion.
- The beta-blockers used include IV metoprolol and esmolol infusions. Esmolol is shorter acting and can be more tightly titrated to the patient's blood pressure and heart rate.
- Specific blood pressure lowering agents (e.g., vasodilators [IV GTN and sodium nitroprusside infusions]) may be required if beta-blockade is insufficient.
- Repeat CT/MR angiography in 5–7 days to look for acute expansion of the dissected segment, thrombosis of the false lumen and complicating factors such as malperfusion or pleural effusions. Depending on the comorbidities of the patient, the presence of these will lead to consideration of repair of the dissection with open or endovascular techniques.
- The goals of operative repair are:
  - Closure of the entry tear of the dissection to depressurise the false lumen and induce thrombosis
  - Preservation ± revascularisation of end organs affected to prevent or reverse any malperfusion

What are the sequelae as the dissection progresses into the chronic stage?

- The false lumen is usually larger than the true lumen, due to the preferential flow of blood through this lower pressure channel.
- If the false lumen does not thrombose, then over time this becomes a weak point of the vessel and can eventually dilate to become aneurysmal.
- In the INSTEAD trial,[14] 20% of cases treated conservatively progressed to aneurysmal dilation to greater than 60 mm that required endovascular or open repair.
- This emphasises the importance of ongoing surveillance in patients who are not offered initial surgical repair.

REFERENCES

1. Freis, E D. 1974. The Veterans Administration cooperative study on antihypertensive agents. Implications for stroke prevention. *Stroke: A Journal of Cerebral Circulation* 5 (1): 76–77.

2. Executive Committee for the Asymptomatic Carotid Atherosclerosis Study. 1995. Endarterectomy for asymptomatic carotid artery stenosis. *Journal of the American Medical Association* 273 (18): 1421–1428.

3. Mohammed, Naufal and Sonia S Anand. 2004. Prevention of disabling and fatal strokes by successful carotid endarterectomy in patients without recent neurological symptoms: Randomized controlled trial. MRC asymptomatic carotid surgery trial (ACST) collaborative group. *Lancet* 363:1491–1502.

4. Powell, J T, R M Greenhalgh, C V Ruckley and F G Fowkes. 1996. The UK small aneurysm trial. *Annals of the New York Academy of Sciences* 800:249–251.

5. Greenhalgh, Roger M, Louise C Brown, Janet T Powell, Simon G Thompson, David Epstein and Mark J Sculpher, United Kingdom EVAR trial investigators. 2010. Endovascular versus open repair of abdominal aortic aneurysm. *New England Journal of Medicine* 362 (20): 1863–1871.

6. Prinssen, Monique, Eric L G Verhoeven, Jaap Buth, Philippe W M Cuypers, Marc R H M van Sambeek, Ron Balm, Erik Buskens, Diederick E Grobbee and Jan D Blankensteijn, Dutch randomized endovascular aneurysm management (DREAM) trial group. 2004. A randomized trial comparing conventional and endovascular repair of abdominal aortic aneurysms. *New England Journal of Medicine* 351 (16): 1607–1618.

7. EVAR trial participants. 2005. Endovascular aneurysm repair and outcome in patients unfit for open repair of abdominal aortic aneurysm (EVAR trial 2): Randomised controlled trial. *Lancet* 365 (9478): 2187–2192.

8. Brown, L C, J T Powell, S G Thompson, D M Epstein, M J Sculpher and R M Greenhalgh. 2012. The UK endovascular aneurysm repair (EVAR) trials: Randomised trials of EVAR versus standard therapy. *Health Technology Assessment* (Winchester, England) 16 (9): 1–218.

9. Murad, Mohammad Hassan, Anas Shahrour, Nilay D Shah, Victor M Montori and John J Ricotta. 2011. A systematic review and meta-analysis of randomized trials of carotid endarterectomy vs. stenting. *Journal of Vascular Surgery* 53 (3): 792–797.

10. Halliday, Alison, Michael Harrison, Elizabeth Hayter, Xiangling Kong, Averil Mansfield, Joanna Marro, Hongchao Pan, et al. 2010. 10-Year stroke prevention after successful carotid endarterectomy for asymptomatic stenosis (ACST-1): A multicentre randomised trial. *Lancet* 376 (9746): 1074–1084.

11. Bradbury, Andrew W, Donald J Adam, Jocelyn Bell, John F Forbes, F Gerry R Fowkes, Ian Gillespie, Charles Vaughan Ruckley and Gillian M Raab, BASIL trial participants. 2010. Bypass versus angioplasty in severe ischaemia of the leg (BASIL) trial: An intention-to-treat analysis of amputation-free and overall survival in patients randomized to a bypass surgery-first or a balloon angioplasty-first revascularization strategy. *Journal of Vascular Surgery* 51 (5): 5S–17S.

12. Nesbitt, Craig, Ron Kg Eifell, Peter Coyne, Hassan Badri, Vish Bhattacharya and Gerard Stansby. 2011. Endovenous ablation (radiofrequency and laser) and foam sclerotherapy versus conventional surgery for great saphenous vein varices. *Cochrane Database Systems Review* 10:CD005624.

13. Siribumrungwong, B, P Noorit, C Wilasrusmee, J Attia and A Thakkinstian. 2012. A systematic review and meta-analysis of randomised controlled trials comparing endovenous ablation and surgical intervention in patients with varicose vein. *European Journal of Vascular and Endovascular Surgery: Official Journal of the European Society for Vascular Surgery* 44 (2): 214–223.

14. Nienaber, Christoph A, Hervé Rousseau, Holger Eggebrecht, Stephan Kische, Rossella Fattori, Tim C Rehders, Günther Kundt, et al. 2009. Randomized comparison of strategies for type B aortic dissection: The investigation of stent grafts in aortic dissection (INSTEAD) trial. *Circulation* 120 (25): 2519–2528.

BIBLIOGRAPHY

Enden, Tone, Ylva Haig, Nils-Einar Kløw, Carl-Erik Slagsvold, Leiv Sandvik, Waleed Ghanima, Geir Hafsahl, et al. 2012. Long-term outcome after additional catheter-directed thrombolysis versus standard treatment for acute iliofemoral deep vein thrombosis (the CaVenT Study): A randomised controlled trial. *Lancet* 379 (9810): 31–38.

NICE Guideline CG119. Inpatient management of diabetic foot problems.

Setacci, Carlo and Jean-Baptiste Ricco, European Society for Vascular Surgery. 2011. Guidelines for critical limb ischaemia and diabetic foot—Introduction. *European Journal of Vascular and Endovascular Surgery: Official Journal of the European Society for Vascular Surgery* 42 (Suppl 2): S1–S3.

Bibliography

ACADEMIC VIVA

Gosall, N, and G Gosall. 2009. *The doctor's guide to critical appraisal,* 2nd rev. ed. PasTest.
Greenhalgh, Trisha. 2010. *How to read a paper.*
The basics of evidence-based medicine, 4th ed. Hoboken, NJ: Wiley-Blackwell.

CLINICAL VIVA

Black, John, William Thomas, Kevin Burnand and Norman Browse. 2005. *Browse's introduction to the symptoms & signs of surgical disease,* 4th ed. London: Hodder Arnold.
Lumley, J S P., ed. 2014. *Hamilton Bailey's physical signs: Demonstrations of physical signs in clinical surgery,* 19th ed. Boca Raton, FL: CRC Press.

CRITICAL CARE VIVA

Anderson, Ian D. 2010. *Care of the critically ill surgical patient,* 3rd ed. London: Hodder Arnold.
Brooks, Adam, Keith Girling, Bernard Riley and Brian Rowlands. 2005. *Critical care for postgraduate trainees.* London: Hodder Arnold.
Kanani, Mazyar. 2002. *Surgical critical care vivas.* Cambridge, UK: Cambridge University Press.
————. 2004. *Applied surgical physiology vivas.* Cambridge, UK: Cambridge University Press.

EMERGENCY VIVA

American College of Surgeons. 2008. *ATLS student course manual,* 8th ed. Chicago, IL.
Boffard, Kenneth D, ed. 2003. *Manual of definitive surgical trauma care,* 2nd ed. Boca Raton, FL: CRC Press.
Schein, Mosche, Paul Rogers and Ahmad Assalia. 2010. *Schein's common sense emergency abdominal surgery: An unconventional book for trainees and thinking surgeons,* 3rd ed. New York: Springer.

GENERAL VIVA

Chaudry, M Asif, and Marc C Winslet. 2009. *Surgical oncology* (Oxford specialist handbooks in surgery). Oxford, UK: OUP Oxford.
Cuschieri, Alfred, Pierce A Grace, Ara Darzi, Neil R Borley and David I Rowley. 2003. *Clinical surgery,* 2nd ed. Hoboken, NJ: Wiley-Blackwell.
Jibawi, Abdullah. 2009. *Current surgical guidelines.* Oxford, UK: Oxford University Press.
Paterson-Brown, Simon. 2009. *Core topics in general & emergency surgery: A companion to specialist surgical practice,* 4th ed. London: Saunders Ltd.

SUBSPECIALTY VIVAS

BREAST DISEASES

Dixon, J Michael. 2012. *ABC of breast diseases (ABC series),* 4th ed. Hoboken, NJ: Wiley-Blackwell.

BREAST SURGERY

Dixon, J Michael. 2009. *A companion to specialist surgical practice,* 4th ed. London: Saunders Ltd.

COLORECTAL SURGERY

Phillips, Robin K S. 2009. *A companion to specialist surgical practice,* 4th ed. London: Saunders Ltd.

ENDOCRINE SURGERY

Lennard, Thomas W J. 2009. *A companion to specialist surgical practice,* 4th ed. London: Saunders Ltd.

HEPATOBILIARY AND PANCREATIC SURGERY

Garden, O James. 2009. *A companion to specialist surgical practice,* 4th ed. London: Saunders Ltd.

OESOPHAGOGASTRIC SURGERY

Griffin, S Michael, and Simon A Raimes. 2009. *A companion to specialist surgical practice,* 4th ed. London: Saunders Ltd.

RENAL TRANSPLANTATION

Torpey, Nicholas, Nadeem E Moghal, Evelyn Watson and David Talbot. 2010. *Oxford specialist handbooks.* Oxford, UK: OUP Oxford.

TRANSPLANTATION

Forsythe, John L R. 2009. *A companion to specialist surgical practice,* 4th ed. London: Saunders Ltd.

VASCULAR AND ENDOVASCULAR SURGERY

Beard, Jonathan D and Peter A Gaines 2009. *A companion to specialist surgical practice,* 4th ed. London: Saunders Ltd.

USEFUL WEBSITES

http://www.asgbi.org.uk
http://www.associationofbreastsurgery.org.uk
http://www.bcshguidelines.com/4_HAEMATOLOGY_GUIDELINES.html
http://www.bsg.org.uk/clinical/general/guidelines.html
http://www.frcsrevision.co.uk
http://www.intercollegiate.org.uk
https://www.iscp.ac.uk/surgical/syllabus.aspx

http://www.nice.org.uk
http://www.sign.ac.uk
http://www.surgicalnotes.co.uk
http://www.thecochranelibrary.com

FRCS REVISION COURSES

http://www.surgicalcourses.org.uk
http://www.liv.ac.uk/surgery/courses/FRCS_Course/index.htm
http://www.wxmec.org.uk/courses/HSC.html
http://www.derbyhospitals.nhs.uk/education-research/royal-derby-training-centre/training/
    frcs-going-for-gold/
http://www.courses.doctorsacademy.org.uk
http://www.asit.org/events/conferences/2013/pre-courses/FRCS
http://www.chm.rcsed.ac.uk/site/3142/frcs_course.aspx
http://www.cancerni.net/events/frcsexitexamrevisioncourseingeneralsurgery

Index